A Rational Approach to Clinical Infectious Diseases

A Rational Approach to Clinical Infectious Diseases

A Manual for House Officers and Other Non-infectious Diseases Clinicians

Editor:
ZELALEM TEMESGEN, MD, FIDSA

Professor of Medicine
Director, Mayo Clinic Center for Tuberculosis, a World health Organization
Collaborating center in Digital health and Precision Medicine for Tuberculosis
Director, HIV Program
Division of Infectious Diseases
Mayo Clinic
Rochester, MN
USA
Editor-in-chief, Journal of Clinical tuberculosis and other mycobacterial diseases

Associate Editors:
LARRY M. BADDOUR, MD, FIDSA, FAHA

Professor Emeritus of Medicine
Division of Infectious Diseases, Departments of Medicine and Cardiovascular Disease
Mayo Clinic College of Medicine and Science
Rochester, MN
USA

STACEY RIZZA, MD, FIDSA

Professor of Medicine
Executive Medical Director of Practice, Mayo Clinic International
Associate Dean, Mayo Clinic School of Health Sciences
Division, Infectious Diseases, Mayo Clinic
Rochester, MN
USA

ELSEVIER

Elsevier
1600 John F. Kennedy Blvd.
Ste 1800
Philadelphia, PA 19103-2899

A RATIONAL APPROACH TO CLINICAL INFECTIOUS DISEASES: A MANUAL
FOR HOUSE OFFICERS AND OTHER NON-INFECTIOUS DISEASES CLINICIANS   ISBN: 978-0-323-69578-7

Notice

Practitioners and researchers must always rely on their own experience and knowledge in evaluating
and using any information, methods, compounds or experiments described herein. Because of
rapid advances in the medical sciences, in particular, independent verification of diagnoses and drug
dosages should be made. To the fullest extent of the law, no responsibility is assumed by Elsevier,
authors, editors or contributors for any injury and/or damage to persons or property as a matter of
products liability, negligence or otherwise, or from any use or operation of any methods, products,
instructions, or ideas contained in the material herein.

Library of Congress Control Number: 2020947889

Senior Content Strategist: Charlotta Kryhl
Director, Content Development: Ellen M. Wurm-Cutter
Content Development Manager: Meghan B. Andress
Publishing Services Manager: Deepthi Unni
Senior Project Manager: Manchu Mohan
Design Direction: Bridget Hoette

Printed in India

Last digit is the print number: 9 8 7 6 5 4 3 2 1

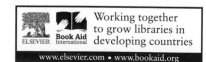

Working together
to grow libraries in
developing countries

www.elsevier.com • www.bookaid.org

Omar M. Abu Saleh, MBBS
Division of Infectious Diseases
Mayo Clinic
Rochester, MN
USA

Micah Beachy, DO, FACP, SFHM
Chief Quality Officer
Nebraska Medicine
Omaha, NE
USA
Associate Professor
Section of Hospital Medicine, University of
    Nebraska Medical Center
Omaha, NE
USA

Adarsh Bhimraj, MD
Head, Section of Neurologic Infections
Infectious Diseases
Cleveland Clinic Foundation
Cleveland, OH
USA

Erin M. Bonura, MD, MCR
Associate Professor of Medicine
Division of Infectious Diseases
Oregon Health & Science University
Portland, OR
USA

Kelly Cawcutt, MD, MS, FACP
Associate Director of Infection Control and
    Hospital Epidemiology
Nebraska Medicine
Omaha, NE
USA
Assistant Professor of Medicine
Divisions of Infectious Diseases &
    Pulmonary and Critical Care Medicine
University of Nebraska Medical Center
Omaha, NE
USA

Patricia Cornejo-Juárez, MD, MSc
Head
Department of Infectious Diseases
Instituto Nacional de Cancerologia
Mexico City, Mexico

Daniel C. DeSimone, MD
Division of Infectious Diseases
Mayo Clinic
Rochester, MN
USA

Dimitri M. Drekonja, MD, MS
Chief
Infectious Disease Section
Minneapolis VA Health Care System
Associate Professor of Medicine
University of Minnesota
Minneapolis, MN
USA

Srilatha Edupuganti, MD, MPH
Associate Professor of Medicine
Emory University School of Medicine
Division of Infectious Diseases
Atlanta, GA
USA

Silvano Esposito
Department of Infectious Diseases
University of Salerno
Italy

Inge C. Gyssens, MD, PhD
Department of Internal Medicine and
    Radboud Center for Infectious
    Diseases
Radboud University Medical Center
Nijmegen, The Netherlands
Faculty of Medicine
Research Group of Immunology and
    Biochemistry
Hasselt University
Hasselt, Belgium

Mary Jo Kasten, MD
Associate Professor of Medicine
Mayo Clinic Alix School of Medicine
Rochester, MN
USA

John C. O'Horo, MD, MPH
Associate Professor of Medicine
Division of Infectious Diseases
Joint Appointment
Division of Pulmonary and Critical Care
  Medicine
Mayo Clinic
Rochester, MN
USA

Robert Orenstein, DO
Professor
Mayo Clinic College of Medicine and
  Science
Division of Infectious Diseases
Mayo Clinic Arizona
Phoenix, AZ
USA

Pasquale Pagliano, MD, PhD
Assistant Professor of Medicine
Department of Infectious Diseases
University of Salerno
Italy

Raj Palraj, MBBS
Consultant, Division of Infectious Diseases
Assistant Professor of Medicine
Mayo College of Medicine
Rochester, MN
USA

Talha Riaz, MD
Division of Infectious Diseases
Mayo Clinic
Rochester, MN
USA

Elizabeth Salazar Rojas, MD
Consultant Dermatologist
Dermatology-Oncology Clinic Research
  Division Universidad Nacional Autónoma
  de México
Mexico City, Mexico

Audrey N. Schuetz, MD
Director, Initial Processing
Co-Director, Bacteriology
Department of Laboratory Medicine and
  Pathology
Mayo Clinic
Rochester, MN
USA

Brian Schwartz, MD
Professor of Medicine
Division of Infectious Diseases
University of California San Francisco
San Francisco, CA
USA

Arlene C. Seña, MD, MPH
Medicine
University of North Carolina at Chapel Hill
Chapel Hill, NC
USA
Medical and Laboratory Director
Durham County Department of Public
  Health
Durham, NC
USA

Aditya Shah, MD
Division of Infectious Diseases
Mayo Clinic
Rochester, MN
USA

James M. Sosman, MD
Division of Infectious Disease
Department of Medicine
University of Wisconsin School of Medicine
  and Public Health
Madison, WI
USA

Anna Maria Spera, MD, PhD
Department of Infectious Diseases
University of Salerno
Italy

Aaron J. Tande, MD
Division of Infectious Diseases
Mayo Clinic
Rochester, MN
USA

Zelalem Temesgen, MD, FIDSA
Professor of Medicine
Director, Mayo Clinic Center for Tuberculosis,
  a World health Organization Collaborating
  center in Digital health and Precision
  Medicine for Tuberculosis
Director, HIV Program
Division of Infectious Diseases
Mayo Clinic
Rochester, MN
USA
Editor-in-chief, Journal of Clinical
  tuberculosis and other mycobacterial
  diseases

Jaap ten Oever, MD, PhD
Department of Internal Medicine and
  Radboud Center for Infectious Diseases
Radboud University Medical Center
Nijmegen, The Netherlands

Elitza S. Theel, PhD
Director, Infectious Diseases Serology
  Laboratory
Department of Laboratory Medicine and
  Pathology
Mayo Clinic
Rochester, MN
USA

Jessica S. Tischendorf, MD, MS
Division of Infectious Disease
Department of Medicine
University of Wisconsin School of Medicine
  and Public Health
Madison, WI
USA

Diana Vilar-Compte, MD, MSc
Professor
Hospital Epidemiology
Department of Infectious Diseases
Instituto Nacional de Cancerologia
Mexico City, Mexico

Richard R. Watkins, MD, MS, FACP, FIDSA, FISAC
Professor of Medicine
Northeast Ohio Medical University
Rootstown, OH
USA
Division of Infectious Diseases
Cleveland Clinic Akron General
Akron, OH
USA

Infectious diseases are a tremendous burden and a significant cause of morbidity and mortality globally, both in resource-rich and resource-limited countries. Advances in our understanding of these diseases, the organisms that cause them, and the host response to them, coupled with advances in diagnostics and therapeutics, have resulted in improved outcomes. However, unnecessary and inappropriate diagnostic testing and antimicrobial prescription have resulted in the emergence of antimicrobial resistance as a major public health threat and imposed a large financial burden on an already enormously overburdened health care system in many areas of the world. In the United States, infections due to antimicrobial-resistant organisms affect nearly 3 million people and result in the deaths of more than 35,000 people annually. Globally, high rates of resistance to antimicrobials frequently used to treat common bacterial infections have been observed. Overuse and misuse of antimicrobials are the main drivers for the development of resistance. Antimicrobials are among the most commonly prescribed drugs used in human medicine, yet many problems have been associated with this large volume of antibiotic use, including prescription for illnesses that do not require antibiotics; incorrect selection, dosing, and/or duration of antibiotic therapy; and adverse drug events.

There is no field of medicine that is not affected by infections, and all medical practitioners will have to manage patients with infectious diseases, which will require the institution of appropriate diagnostic and therapeutic interventions. We offer this book as a resource to clinicians who have not had formal training in infectious diseases, with the hope and intent that it will instill a rational approach to the diagnosis and treatment of infections that they will encounter, resulting in a decrease in both antimicrobial resistance and adverse drug events that ultimately result in improved patient outcomes.

Larry M. Baddour, MD, FIDSA, FAHA
Stacey Rizza, MD, FIDSA
Zelalem Temesgen, MD, FIDSA

CONTENTS

A Rational Approach to
Clinical Infectious Diseases

CHAPTER 1

General Approach to Infectious Diseases Evaluation

Omar M. Abu Saleh ■ Zelalem Temesgen

CHAPTER OUTLINE

Infections are disorders or diseases caused by microorganisms such as bacteria, viruses, fungi, or parasites. Infections manifest themselves by a myriad of signs and symptoms in a variety of combinations. It is not possible to discuss in a meaningful way the various permutations and combinations of signs and symptoms associated with infectious diseases. However, some signs and symptoms are, rightly or wrongly, widely regarded as cardinal manifestations of infection and are discussed here.

Fever

Fever is defined as an elevation of normal body temperature. Definitions of normal temperature have evolved over the years through studies that have attempted to incorporate potential confounding factors such as time of day, age, gender, and body site of temperature measurement in their evaluations. Based on data from these studies, fever is defined as an oral temperature of $\geq37.2°C$ (99.0°F) in the morning or an oral temperature of $\geq37.8°C$ (100°F) at any time during the day.

Fever is a component of a complex physiologic reaction often, but not exclusively, in response to invasion by microorganisms or their products. Body temperature is regulated by a complex process that involves a variety of body structures, including the immune system, heat and cold receptors in the skin and organs, and the spinal cord and the brain. Thus fever may be caused by a variety of other noninfectious conditions (Table 1.1). Alternatively, fever may not be present though the patient clearly has an infection (e.g., typhoid fever, tularemia, brucellosis, and dengue).

TAKE-HOME POINTS BOX 1.1

Take-Home Points:
1. Infections commonly present with fever.
2. Infections can present without fever.
3. There are many noninfectious causes of fever.

TABLE 1.1 ■ Noninfectious Causes of Fever

Disease Conditions	Examples
Malignancies	Lymphoproliferative disorders
	Renal cell cancer
	Hepatocellular cancer
Autoimmune/connective tissue diseases	Vasculitis
	Temporal arteritis
	Systemic lupus erythematosus
	Sarcoidosis
	Still disease
Thromboembolic disease	Deep venous thrombosis
	Pulmonary emboli
	Acute stroke
Drugs	Antibiotics
	Antineoplastics
	Allopurinol
	Contrast dye
	Interferon
Others	Inflammatory bowel disease
	Gout
	Rheumatic fever

LEUKOCYTOSIS

The stem cells in the bone marrow that form the various blood cells—hematopoietic stem cells—produce erythroblasts, megakaryoblasts, lymphoblasts, and myeloblasts. Erythroblasts further differentiate into red blood cells, megakaryoblasts into platelets, and lymphoblasts into lymphocytes. Myeloblasts differentiate into monocytes and granulocytes, and granulocytes are further categorized into neutrophils, basophils, and eosinophils. The term *white blood cell (WBC)* denotes the cells derived from lymphoblasts and myeloblasts. Upon maturation, most (80% to 90%) of the WBCs remain in the bone marrow, a few (2% to 3%) circulate freely in the peripheral blood, and the remainder are stored in the spleen or deposited along the walls of the blood vessels.

Leukocytosis—an increase in the total number of WBCs due to any cause—is a reaction to a wide range of events that result in the release of various cytokines, which in turn mediate the release of leukocytes and their precursors from the marrow, spleen, and vessel walls. A rise in the absolute number of neutrophils is most commonly responsible for the overall leukocytosis, but increases in the numbers of the other components of WBCs—lymphocytes, monocytes, eosinophils, or basophils—may also play a role.

Infections are common causes of leukocytosis. However, leukocytosis can also be the result of a variety of other stimuli and conditions, including malignancies, inflammatory conditions, drugs, stress, and trauma (Table 1.2).

Occasionally, the magnitude of leukocytosis exceeds 50,000 cells/mm^3, requiring distinguishing it from leukemia. This is called a *leukemoid reaction* and is commonly caused by severe infections.

At times, leukopenia (a decrease in total WBCs) and not leukocytosis may be the presenting feature of certain infections. These infections include influenza, infectious mononucleosis, HIV, rickettsiosis, ehrlichiosis, typhoid fever, tuberculosis (TB), brucellosis, tularemia, leishmaniasis, and malaria. Sepsis, or any overwhelming infection, can also present with leukopenia.

TABLE 1.2 ■ Noninfectious Causes of Leukocytosis

Disease Conditions	Examples
Malignancies	Lymphoproliferative disorders Renal cell cancer Sarcoma
Autoimmune/connective tissue diseases	Vasculitis Rheumatoid arthritis Systemic lupus erythematosus
Physiologic	Strenuous exercise Emotional disorders Pregnancy
Drugs	Corticosteroids Epinephrine Endotoxin Lithium Ranitidine Serotonin Histamine Heparin Acetylcholine
Others	Inflammatory bowel disease Rheumatic fever Acute hemorrhage

---

TAKE-HOME POINTS BOX 1.2

Take-Home Points:
1. Infections commonly present with leukocytosis.
2. Infections can also present with leukopenia.
3. There are many noninfectious causes of leukocytosis.

Inflammatory Markers

Inflammatory markers are certain proteins that are released into the bloodstream as part of the body's response to an inflammatory insult or injury such as infections and systemic rheumatologic/autoimmune disorders. The inflammatory markers most commonly used in clinical practice are C-reactive protein (CRP) and erythrocyte sedimentation rate (ESR). The ESR measures the rate of fall of red blood cells to the bottom of a test tube in 1 hour. When blood contains higher amounts of certain inflammatory proteins such as fibrinogen and immunoglobulins, the red blood cells fall more rapidly. Thus the rate of erythrocyte sedimentation is increased. Any condition, including noninflammatory conditions such as age, anemia, obesity, and pregnancy, can cause increases in ESR. CRP is produced by the liver in response to inflammatory cytokines, with the rate of production proportional to the magnitude of the inflammation. In general, clinicians use CRP and ESR to identify a generalized inflammatory state—including infections—to monitor disease activity, or to monitor response to treatment. Infections that have been classically associated with elevations of CRP and/or ESR include cellulitis, necrotizing skin and soft tissue infections, osteoarticular infections, endocarditis, and TB. The utility of these inflammatory markers in infections is as a nonspecific tool for identifying these conditions and to monitor their response to therapy as an adjunct to overall clinical assessment and other, more specific diagnostic tests.

TAKE-HOME POINTS BOX 1.3

Take-Home Points:
1. Inflammatory markers can aid in identifying certain infections.
2. Inflammatory markers can aid in monitoring response of certain infections to treatment.
3. Inflammatory markers are nonspecific and are elevated as a result of a variety of inflammatory and noninflammatory conditions.
4. When used in diagnosing and/or managing infections, inflammatory markers play a subordinate role to overall clinical assessment and other, more specific diagnostic tests.

MIMICKERS OF INFECTION

A variety of local or systemic conditions, including malignancies, autoimmune diseases, inflammatory conditions, and drug effects, may mimic an infectious process (Table 1.3). Familiarity with these conditions is important for appropriate diagnosis and management and avoidance of unnecessary antimicrobial treatment.

TABLE 1.3 ■ Mimickers of Infection

Condition	Presentation	Cause
Calcified tendinitis	Acute pain involving the tendon sheath Most commonly affects rotator cuff tendons	Calcium deposits in or around a tendon
Venous stasis dermatitis	Bilateral presentation Absence of pain, warmth, or systemic signs of infection	Incompetent venous valves leading to leaking and pooling of blood in the extracellular compartment
Lymphedema	Nonpitting edema with erythema and induration in the absence of systemic signs	Accumulation of interstitial fluid due to disruption in normal lymphatic flow
Gout	Acute onset of monoarticular pain, swelling, warmth, and redness Classically affects the first metatarsophalangeal joint	Inflammation caused by monosodium urate crystals
Pyoderma gangrenosum	Papule, pustule, or vesicle resulting from trauma that progresses to form a nonhealing cutaneous ulcer	Neutrophil-predominant infiltration of skin
Erythema nodosum	Tender, erythematous nodules on bilateral shins	Delayed-type hypersensitivity reaction resulting from exposure to various pathogens
Pyogenic granuloma	Presents as a small red papule that grows over weeks to months involving skin or mucous membranes	Neovascular response to an angiogenic stimulus; can be due to trauma or drug induced
Contact dermatitis	Erythema, pain, burning, stinging vesicle formation Occurs within minutes to hours of exposure to offending agent Mostly well demarcated at the site of exposure History of exposure to physical or chemical irritants	Hypersensitivity reaction to physical or chemical irritants
Drug-induced pneumonitis	Cough, fever, bilateral interstitial infiltrates, hypoxia	Alkylating agents, analgesics, antibiotics (e.g., daptomycin), chemotherapeutic agents, etc.
Relapsing polychondritis	Redness, erythema, and swelling involving cartilaginous structures (e.g., auricular involvement, scleritis, episcleritis, nasal cartilage inflammation)	Immune-mediated condition, may be associated with vasculitis, connective tissue disorders, or myelodysplasia in one-third of patients

Syndrome	Infectious Etiology	Noninfectious Mimic
Cellulitis	Beta-hemolytic streptococci, most commonly group A (*Streptococcus pyogenes* in children and non–group A streptococci in adults) *Staphylococcus aureus* **Less common:** *Haemophilus influenzae, Clostridium* species *Streptococcus pneumoniae* **Related to specific exposures:** *Pasteurella multocida* *Aeromonas hydrophila* *Vibrio vulnificus* *Pseudomonas aeruginosa, Erysipelothrix rhusiopathiae*	Venous stasis Contact dermatitis Relapsing polychondritis Eosinophilic cellulitis Diabetic myonecrosis
Recurrent UTI	Chronic bacterial prostatitis, perinephric abscess, infected renal stone, urinary tract obstruction, genitourinary structural abnormalities	Interstitial cystitis Kidney stone Loin pain hematuria syndrome
Nonresolving pneumonia	Mycobacterial, fungal, bronchiectasis	Malignancy, interstitial lung disease, hypersensitivity pneumonitis
Chronic meningitis	*Mycobacterium tuberculosis* Bacterial (*Brucella, Nocardia, Tropheryma whipplei, Leptospira, Borrelia burgdorferi,* etc.) Viral (HSV, HIV, CMV, HTLV, Enterovirus), fungal (*Cryptococcus, Blastomyces, Coccidioides, Histoplasma, Sporothrix,* etc.) Parasitic (*Toxoplasma,* Acanthamoeba, Angiostrongylus, etc.)	Connective tissue disease, malignancy, paraneoplastic, medication induced, genetic
Acute meningitis	Bacterial (*Streptococcus pneumoniae, Haemophilus influenzae, Neisseria meningitidis, Listeria monocytogenes*) Viral (HSV, VZV)	Medication induced, connective tissue disease
Infected ulcers	Bacterial Mycobacterial Parasitic (*Leishmania*) Fungal	Pyoderma gangrenosum Necrosis lipoidica
Septic arthritis	*Staphylococcus aureus* Streptococci Gram-negative bacilli	Crystal-induced arthropathy Hemarthrosis Pigmented villous nodular synovitis
Multifocal osteomyelitis	Hematogenous dissemination due to endovascular infection	SAPHO
Infective endocarditis	*Staphylococcus aureus,* Viridans group streptococci, Enterococci, Coagulase-negative Staphylococci, *Streptococcus bovis,* Nutritionally variant streptococci, *Abiotrophia and Granulicatella* species, HACEK, Fungi	Anti-phospholipid antibody syndrome Libman-Sacks endocarditis Marantic endocarditis Degenerative valve changes
Chronic diarrhea	Parasitic (*Cryptosporidium, Cyclospora, Entamoeba histolytica, Giardia, Microsporidia,* etc.) Viral (*Norovirus, Rotavirus,* etc.) Bacterial (*Clostridioides difficile*)	Inflammatory bowel disease Celiac disease Cystic fibrosis Pancreatic insufficiency Malabsorption Hyperthyroidism Irritable bowel syndrome Medications (laxative, etc.)
Fever of unknown origin	Mycobacterial infections Osteomyelitis Infective endocarditis Occult abscesses	Malignancy (leukemia, lymphoma, renal cell carcinoma, hepatocellular carcinoma, atrial myxomas) Connective tissue disease Miscellaneous

CMV, Cytomegalovirus; *HACEK, Haemophilus* species, *Aggregatibacter* species, *Cardiobacterium hominis, Eikenella corrodens,* and *Kingella* species; *HSV, Herpes simplex* virus; *HTLV-1,* human T lymphotropic virus 1; *SAPHO,* synovitis, acne, pustulosis, hyperostosis, and osteitis; *UTI,* urinary tract infection; *VZV, Varicella zoster* virus.

CLINICAL EVALUATION FOR INFECTIOUS DISEASES

Obtaining a complete history and performing a thorough physical examination is the cornerstone of good clinical practice. This is even more so in infectious diseases, where understanding the interplay among the causative microorganisms, the environment, and the host is essential for identifying the infection and instituting the appropriate treatment.

Obtaining a complete medical history will aid in identifying the infection by elucidating signs and symptoms; localizing its effect; determining triggers, if present; understanding the sequence of events, and thus the natural history of the infection; ascertaining a pattern, if there is one; and discovering a clue to the identity of the infection through a better understanding of the patient's life and work environment. The history of present illness should ascertain the presence of localizing signs and symptoms and their duration and pattern, as well as the presence of nonspecific symptoms such as fever, weight loss, anorexia, fatigue, night sweats, arthralgias, and headaches. This information should further be supplemented by information about occupation; geographic residence; travel history (recent and lifetime); sick contacts; exposure history (e.g., dust, waterways, animals, insects, chemicals); comorbidities, including possible immunosuppression; previous infectious illnesses and associated microbial susceptibility profiles; family history of infections; leisure activities; medication history; history of substance use; dietary habits; and sexual history.

A thorough physical examination, in particular in cases of unexplained fever or other indicators of infection, is invaluable in determining the focus of infection and suggesting a likely etiology. Some components of a physical examination may not always be fully appreciated and get performed at all or may be performed in a perfunctory manner. However, they may play a critical role in identifying sources of infection. Examples include:

Oral cavity—The mouth is often overlooked or perfunctorily examined, but examination of the mouth may provide clues to the source and etiology of various disorders. Examination of the teeth may reveal an abscess. The presence of tooth decay and/or associated periodontitis may suggest, in the right circumstances, consideration of cervicofacial infections. Coating of the tongue or palate may be due to *Candida* infection. A swollen and inflamed tonsil with uvular deviation and systemic toxicity should raise concern for a tonsillar or peritonsillar abscess. Oral ulcerations may be due to a wide range of conditions, with infections figuring prominently in the differential diagnosis. Potential infectious causes of oral ulcerations include herpes simplex virus, Coxsackie virus, syphilis, HIV, and invasive fungal infections (e.g., mucormycosis, aspergillosis, histoplasmosis, blastomycosis).

Lymph nodes—Localized or generalized enlargement of lymph nodes may provide a clue to an infectious disease or other processes such as malignancy. Thus physical examination should include evaluation of peripheral lymph nodes (size, consistency, tenderness, mobility) in the areas where they are accessible (e.g., cervical, axillary, inguinal).

Skin—Evaluation of the skin in a patient presenting with clear symptoms of a cellulitis of an extremity is intuitive. However, less attention is paid to skin changes over cardiac devices, intravenous lines, surgical incisions, surgical drains, and pressure ulcers, which are important potential foci of infection.

Prosthesis—The presence of a medical device (e.g., cardiac devices, joint prosthesis, indwelling catheters, surgical drains, vascular grafts) may not have been ascertained from the history and may not be apparent during a cursory physical examination. Thus, an important potential focus of infection would be missed if a thorough history and physical examination are not done.

The most valuable tool and the first step is thorough clinical evaluation with a detailed history and physical examination, supplemented by basic laboratory evaluation when indicated.

At the end of the clinical evaluation a clinician should be able to have a clear understanding of the host unique features, specific details and the evolution of the signs and symptoms, and the setting or exposures in which the signs and symptoms originated and evolved. At this point, a clinician should be able to formulate a syndromic diagnosis specific to the host in that setting; this often predicts the microbiologic diagnosis and guides further diagnostic and therapeutic interventions (see Table 1.1).

The collective clues from the host, syndrome, and relevant exposure frame the next management steps. Some examples are provided here:

- In a patient with a history of travel and suspected parasitic infection, eosinophilia may provide supportive information.
- Similarly in a teenager with sore throat and generalized malaise and fever, atypical lymphocytosis may suggest Epstein–Barr virus (EBV) infection. Abnormal liver enzymes, although nonspecific, are not part of all infectious syndromes and may help narrow down the differential diagnosis. In addition, liver and renal function may be essential before making dosage recommendations for antimicrobials.
- Inflammatory markers, as described earlier, are nonspecific and may be abnormal with a number of noninfectious disorders. However, they may be especially helpful when history and physical exam indicate compatible infectious disease diagnoses, such as osteomyelitis and prosthetic joint infections.
- Acute onset of productive cough, pleuritic chest pain, and fever form a clinical pattern suggestive of pneumonia. The differential diagnosis of pneumonia will depend on the clinical and epidemiologic scenario:
  - In an immunocompetent host with otherwise nonspecific exposures, it is often labeled *community-acquired pneumonia* for which there is a predictable microbiology and treatment.
  - The thinking about the same patient will be different in the following scenarios:
    - If he had recent travel to a TB-endemic area
    - If he failed to respond to a beta-lactam
    - If he had concomitant gastrointestinal (GI) symptoms and abnormal liver enzymes
    - If this was his fourth febrile respiratory illness in the last 6 months
    - If he was a rheumatoid arthritis patient who received a tumor necrosis factor (TNF) alpha inhibitor
    - If he developed this syndrome after a long flight or had a history of malignancy

The details in each of the scenarios require additive analytical thinking to modify the syndromic and microbiologic differential, which will lead to a different diagnostic and therapeutic strategy. In the first patient an evaluation for TB would be appropriate. If the patient failed to respond to beta-lactam monotherapy, then that would be inadequate for CAP treatment since beta-lactams do not provide coverage for organisms (ie, Mycoplasma pneumoniae, Legionella species, and Chlamydia pneumoniae) that cause "atypical pneumonia". Therefore, a macrolide or doxycycline would be needed.

Additional information that may be helpful includes the following:

- Presence of systemic inflammatory response, especially fever
- Timeline: prodromal illness, duration (acute, chronic, recurrent), season
- Clinical course and evolution (progressive, persistent-stable, self-resolved)
- Response to empiric therapy when applicable
- Supplementary clues from physical examination, synchronous symptoms, laboratory tests, and imaging

Diagnostic Evaluation in Infectious Diseases

The decision regarding diagnostic evaluation is often driven by the pretest probability for an infection, the severity of the illness, the unique host, and the syndrome and exposure clues. The purpose of the diagnostic evaluation is elaborated in the next few sections.

FURTHER DEFINE THE SYNDROME

1. **Confirm the clinical suspicion of a syndromic diagnosis** (obtaining chest imaging to confirm the suspicion of pneumonia or lung abscess).
2. **Evaluate for disease-specific complications** or dissemination outside the primary site of infection. An example would be obtaining a transesophageal echocardiogram in patient with *Staphylococcus aureus* bloodstream infection.
3. **Rule out an alternative diagnosis** (like malignancy or pulmonary embolism or deep venous thrombosis [DVT] when appropriate).
4. **Identify high-yield targets for invasive evaluation**; for example, in patients with fever of unknown origin, obtaining cross-sectional imaging of the body or a positron emission tomography (PET) scan can not only identify the source of fever but also help identify high-yield targets for biopsy.

SECURING A MICROBIOLOGIC DIAGNOSIS

Generally speaking, microbiologic evaluation is not indicated in all cases of suspected infection. As a general rule, mild to moderate infections, which have predictable microbiology and which can be treated as an outpatient with a short course of antimicrobials or with observation, do not require microbiologic confirmation unless there is a public health impact. Examples of such infections include:
- Mild to moderate community-acquired pneumonia
- Uncomplicated cystitis in a young female
- Mild to moderate nonpurulent cellulitis
- Mild influenza-like illness during influenza season in a low-risk patient

In some cases, it may be best to just do clinical observation instead of performing further testing or treatment. For example, upper respiratory tract symptoms in an otherwise immunocompetent individual should be managed conservatively without any additional testing or antibiotic treatment unless there are clear signs of bacterial infection (e.g., purulent sinus drainage, persistent fever, etc.). Examples of infections where microbiologic diagnosis is crucial include:
- Infections in immunocompromised hosts
- Severe infections requiring hospitalization
- Infections that require an extended treatment (like osteomyelitis)
- Recurrent and relapsing infections
- Presumed infection that fails appropriate empiric therapy
- Infections with public health consequences (e.g., TB, sexually transmitted infections)

Many of the commonly encountered mild to moderate infections in immunocompetent hosts can be managed without the involvement of the infectious disease specialist. However, in more complex situations, involvement of the infectious disease consult service is known to affect survival, cost of care, length of stay, and antimicrobial stewardship.

Infectious diseases specialists should be involved in all cases of:
- Life-threatening infections, like *S. aureus* bacteremia, meningitis, endocarditis, and necrotizing fasciitis
- Infectious in immunocompromised hosts
- Presumed infectious syndromes that failed to respond to appropriate empiric therapy
- Infections with public health impact
- Recurrent and relapsing infections

THERAPEUTIC CONSIDERATIONS

The process of treating infectious diseases requires a comprehensive integration of all the information obtained during the clinical and diagnostic evaluation. A good rule to remember is that fever in immunocompetent patients is not an indication for antibiotics—a clinical suspicion for infection is. When making a therapeutic plan, the main questions to answer are:

1. **Should we start antibiotics immediately?** The likelihood of infection, severity of presentation, immune status of the patient, predictability of the involved microbiology, and the toxicity of the treatment involved are the main considerations for this question. For example, immediate empiric therapy for patients presenting in septic shock is lifesaving. However, for patients presenting with probable diskitis who otherwise are hemodynamically stable and have no neurologic deficits, a diagnostic evaluation should be the initial focus.

2. **Which antibiotic to start?** Multiple considerations come into play when trying to answer this question.

   A. **Spectrum:** The initial antimicrobial regimen is often empiric and based on the most likely involved pathogen. Nonpurulent cellulitis is often caused by beta-hemolytic streptococci for which a first-generation cephalosporin is an appropriate *empiric* therapy. Nosocomial pneumonia is less predictable; the potential involvement of multidrug-resistant Gram-negative pathogens or methicillin-resistant *S. aureus* mandates a complex empiric regimen pending microbiologic confirmation with sputum culture, after which an empiric therapy can be changed into *targeted* therapy.

   B. **Efficacy:** Choosing the most effective antimicrobial regimen is very important. For example, both vancomycin and cefazolin are effective against methicillin-sensitive *S. aureus*. However, cefazolin is superior and has a better safety profile; thus it should be used over vancomycin for infections caused by this pathogen.

   C. **Toxicity:** Whenever possible, the most effective, least toxic agent should be used. For example, antipseudomonal beta-lactams are favored over aminoglycosides.

   D. **Pharmacokinetics (PK):** A basic knowledge of key antimicrobial PK issues is very important. For example, when treating meningitis or prostatitis, it is important to utilize an antibiotic that is not only effective but also capable of reaching a clinically significant concentration at the target compartment.

   E. **Allergies:** Ten percent of hospitalized patients report an allergy to antimicrobial agents. Conversely, 95% of patients who report a penicillin allergy actually tolerate penicillin. It is very important to accurately obtain an allergy history and consult an allergy specialist for penicillin skin testing when appropriate before accepting the allergy label that would preclude a patient from receiving a first-line therapy.

   F. **Drug interactions:** Recognizing the potential risk of drug interactions early in the course of treatment can prevent toxicity and treatment failure.

   G. **Comorbidities:** Certain comorbidities might be a contraindication to a class or more of antibiotics. For example, patients with myasthenia gravis should not receive agents that may augment neuromuscular blockade, like aminoglycosides or fluoroquinolones. Patients with advanced chronic kidney disease should not receive nephrotoxic agents.

3. **Duration of antibiotics:** The Infectious Diseases Society of America provides management guidelines regarding the duration of treatment for the key clinical syndromes commonly encountered. It is important to understand that it may not be possible to predetermine treatment duration for some infections. For example, for abscesses in various parts of the body with ongoing attempts at source control, the duration of treatment should be defined by prospective clinical and radiographic follow-up rather than selection of an arbitrary number of weeks early in the course of treatment.

4. **Other therapeutic interventions include the following:**

   A. **Source control:** Identifying source of infection and providing adequate control is a key component of infection treatment—sometimes it is more important than antimicrobial therapy. A good example for that will be skin and soft tissue abscesses, intraabdominal infections, and line-related bloodstream infections. A delay in identifying and addressing the source often leads to treatment failure, relapse of the infection, and prolonged and repeated exposure to antimicrobial therapy. Source control intervention includes surgical debridement, percutaneous drainage, relief of any obstruction, removal of infected foreign bodies, etc.

B. **Identifying and addressing any reversible immune defects**

C. **Identifying patients at high risk of recurrence and providing preventive measures:** For example updating the pneumococcal influenza vaccination in a patient admitted with pneumonia, or considering secondary prophylaxis for a patient with recurrent lower extremity cellulitis in addition to aggressive lymphedema management and treatment of tinea pedis.

D. **Utilizing adjunctive therapies when there is a good evidence:** For example, utilization of corticosteroids in bacterial meningitis.

Syndrome	A syndrome is defined as a group of symptoms and signs that consistently occur together, or a condition characterized by a set of associated symptoms and signs. Formulating a syndrome, where possible, instead of merely listing signs and symptoms helps focus attention on the most likely infection scenarios and pathogens in the case under review so that downstream activities result in a rational selection of diagnostic tests and antimicrobial treatment.	
Host	Defining the host characteristics that may affect: -Unique vulnerability or risk for certain infection or infection complication -Comorbidities that may change management (allergies, baseline organ dysfunction)	
	Age	• Vulnerability to certain pathogens: *Listeria* risk in patients >65 years old • Impact on presentation: Euthermic infections and atypical presentation • Risk of complications: Risk of chronic hepatitis B is less in adults compared with neonates. *Clostridium difficile* infection most likely to relapse in elderly.
	Gender	• Risk for certain infection: UTI is more common in females compared with males. • Presentation: *Chlamydia* can be asymptomatic in females > males • Menopause and pregnancy: Risk of listeriosis in pregnant females
	Immune status	Immunocompromised patients secondary to primary or acquired immune deficiency and iatrogenic immunosuppression often present with infections: • Of unusual frequency • Infections caused by opportunistic pathogens • Unusual severity and atypical presentation
	Altered anatomy or physiology	• Risk of certain infection: Biliary strictures and risk for cholangitis, lymphedema, and risk of cellulitis • Colonization with certain pathogens in patients with bronchiectasis or CF
	Medical devices	Device-specific infections can be difficult to diagnose: • Presence of endovascular, orthopedic, or CNS hardware
	Comorbidities	• Disease-specific infection: Peritonitis in patients receiving peritoneal dialysis, spontaneous bacterial peritonitis in patients with cirrhosis • Vulnerability to certain pathogens: Liver cirrhosis and *Cryptococcus* infection • Impact on diagnostic decisions: Use of contrast in patients with kidney disease, accuracy of serology in patients with hypogammaglobulinemia • Impact on therapeutic decisions: Presence of advanced kidney disease in avoidance of nephrotoxins, drug interactions, history of seizure disorder, prolonged QT, etc. • Provide alternative diagnosis: Nonresolving cellulitis in a patient with probable inflammatory bowel disease can be erythema nodosum • Immunocompromising (cancer, transplant, autoimmune condition)

Exposures	Host-specific, syndrome-relevant exposures are the key to accurate diagnosis and targeted workup	
	Occupational	Risk for zoonosis, laboratory or health care–related infections, hypersensitivity reactions, and intoxication
	Endemic	Risk for endemic mycosis, vector-borne illness, TB, parasites varies by geography (present and previous addresses)
	Hobbies	Hunting, spelunking, gardening, farming
	Water exposure	Drinking water: GI illnesses, heavy metal toxicity Recreational water\beach activities: Skin and soft tissue infections, aerosol-related infections, hot tub–related syndromes
	Dietary habits	Undercooked food, unpasteurized milk or milk products, raw seafood
	Sexual history	Screening for high-risk behavior, number of partners, history of STI, etc.
	Substance abuse	Tobacco, alcohol, IV substance abuse, and other drugs of abuse; may put the patient at high risk for blood-borne pathogens, bacteremia, endocarditis; may affect treatment decisions
	Travel history	Detailed recent and remote travel history can be very informative
	Sick contacts	Can be the earliest clue of an outbreak or a specific pathogen
	Health care exposure	Likelihood of nosocomial pathogen is higher; subsequently empiric therapy may be different
	Seasonality	Whereas some viral illnesses (e.g., influenza, norovirus) have a well-recognized seasonal predilection, bacterial infections that cause skin and soft tissue infections have a seasonal (spring, summer) prevalence.

CF, Cystic fibrosis; *CNS,* central nervous system; *UTI,* urinary tract infection.

CHAPTER 2

Interacting with the Clinical Microbiology Laboratory

Elitza S. Theel ■ Audrey N. Schuetz

Introduction

The clinical microbiology laboratory offers an increasingly diverse menu of diagnostic assays, including maintenance of traditional methods first developed in the early 1900s, to implementing increasingly complex molecular assays and, most recently, implementing whole-genome and next-generation sequencing assays for pathogen detection, typing, and assessment of antimicrobial susceptibility. The laboratory is also becoming increasingly automated, from the adoption of automated enzyme immunoassay (EIA) processors, to nucleic acid extraction and amplification platforms, to the implementation of total laboratory automation systems. Regardless of the diagnostic method, the accuracy and relevance of results generated by the microbiology laboratory are dependent on multiple factors, including whether the right specimen was collected and transported to the laboratory appropriately, whether the correct test was ordered for that specimen type, and when the specimen was collected relative to patient presentation and antibiotic initiation, among others. This chapter aims to provide general commentary regarding important features of specimen collection, to present the advantages and limitations of common diagnostic assays, and to address a number of common questions and points of confusion among health care workers.

Specimen Collection: What, When, and From Where

SPECIMEN COLLECTION AND PREANALYTIC VARIABLES IN MICROBIOLOGY TESTING

Proper specimen collection and transport to the laboratory are critically important for appropriate patient management. Submission of poorly collected specimens may lead to failure to recover or detect significant pathogens. Results may be difficult to interpret when specimens are improperly collected due to recovery of colonizing, nonpathogenic organisms. If a laboratory performs testing on a specimen that experienced prolonged transport time or was submitted under improper transport conditions, false-negative or false-positive results are likely. Downstream consequences may include an inaccurate diagnosis and/or inappropriate treatment. Administration of unnecessary treatment or procedures may in turn result in increased length of hospital stay, drug side effects, and/or additional costs.

Rejection of specimens may be due to improper sample labeling, delay in transit to the laboratory, collection in an improper container, or improper specimen type. As testing menus vary among laboratories, so do the specimen collection devices and guidelines. Differences in laboratory collection guidelines are due in part to the differences in the types of assays performed. Test manufacturer's guidelines specify the type of specimen validated for that particular assay, and laboratories should adhere to these guidelines. Therefore clinicians should be familiar with the specimen collection guides of their laboratories. Such guides often outline collection instructions, transport conditions, volume of specimen required, and rejection criteria. General specimen collection and transport guides focused on microbiologic tests are also available.[1] Table 2.1 outlines examples of specimen collection and transport guidance based on various body sites.

TABLE 2.1 ■ **Examples of Specimen Collection and Transport Guidelines for Microbiologic Tests**

Specimen Type	Collection Guidelines	Transport Guidelines	Comments
Abscess, including wounds	Cleanse surface with sterile saline or alcohol. Do not submit swabs.	Utilize anaerobic transport system for anaerobic cultures.	Tissues or aspirates are superior to swabs. Contamination with surface material may occur with colonizing organisms unless the site is well cleaned.
Blood	Collection of serum, plasma, or whole blood may differ depending on testing requested. Disinfect culture bottle top and patient skin.	For blood culture bottles: as rapidly as possible; within 2 hours is optimal.	Collect more than one set, including aerobic and anaerobic bottles for routine blood cultures.
Body fluid	Cleanse surface with sterile saline or alcohol. Do not submit swabs.	Utilize anaerobic transport system for anaerobic cultures.	If inoculation of blood culture bottles with body fluid is performed by clinician, a separate sterile tube of fluid is required for direct Gram stain.
Catheter	Blood cultures may be drawn from blood catheters for assessment of line infections.	Sterile screw-cap container.	Do not submit urinary Foley catheters to the laboratory for culture.
Cerebrospinal fluid (CSF)	Disinfect area before collection.	Never refrigerate CSF.	Refrigeration prevents growth of some clinically significant organisms.

Continued

TABLE 2.1 ■ Examples of Specimen Collection and Transport Guidelines for Microbiologic Tests—cont'd

Specimen Type	Collection Guidelines	Transport Guidelines	Comments
Decubitus ulcer	Cleanse surface. Obtain biopsy of base of ulcer or bone. Do not submit swabs.	Sterile tube for tissue for aerobic bacterial culture; anaerobic transport for anaerobic culture.	Due to high probability of colonizing microorganisms, swabs of decubitus ulcers should be rejected.
Ear	Collect fluid via aspiration or flexible swab, if needed.	As rapidly as possible; within 2 hours is optimal.	For otitis externa, vigorous swabbing of external surface is often necessary.
Eye	Moisten conjunctival swabs with sterile saline before collection.	As rapidly as possible; within 2 hours is optimal.	Clinicians who inoculate media themselves should work closely with the laboratory to ensure appropriate media are used.
Feces	Many different collection devices are available for ova and parasite examination of stool.	Cary–Blair is commonly used as a transport medium for culture and other studies.	Loose, not solid, stool should be collected for *Clostridioides (Clostridium) difficile* testing. Rectal swabs are inferior collection specimens compared with feces.
Genital	Swabs may be used for certain locations, such as the urethra.	As rapidly as possible; within 2 hours is optimal.	Refer to local laboratory guidelines for collection and transport needs for *Chlamydia* spp. and *Neisseria gonorrhoeae* testing.
Respiratory	Expectorated sputum should be collected after deep cough to avoid oral flora. Nasopharyngeal or throat swabs may be collected.	Swabs should be kept moist during transport.	Anterior nose cultures are reserved for detection of *Staphylococcus* carriers or visible nasal lesions. Endotracheal aspiration specimens are frequently contaminated with colonizing organisms and are suboptimal specimens to assess for respiratory infection.
Skin	Scrapings may be obtained for virus detection. Skin, hair, or nail collections may be obtained for detection of fungi.	Smears should be rapidly transported to the laboratory.	Smears may be performed by the clinician and rapidly transported to the laboratory for studies. Oral mucosal lesions may be tested for virus or other pathogens.
Tissue	Sterile saline should be added to keep pieces of tissue moist.	Utilize anaerobic transport system for anaerobic cultures.	Submit as much tissue as possible. Avoid submitting swabs that have been rubbed over the tissue surface.
Urine	First-void urine is required for *Chlamydia* and *N. gonorrhoeae* molecular testing. Midstream urine should be collected for bacterial culture.	Boric acid is commonly used as transport medium for culture and other studies.	Utility of urine cultures from indwelling catheters is limited.

SPECIMENS AND COLLECTION DEVICES

Although convenient for collection, swabs are suboptimal collection devices for culture for a variety of reasons. Most importantly, limited patient material is captured on a swab. If multiple culture-based or molecular assays are ordered from a single swab, insufficient material is available to distribute among the tests. Recently, flocked swabs have replaced traditional spun cotton swabs at many institutions due to the superior recovery of organisms compared with traditional nonflocked swabs. Flocked swabs are made from nylon fibers that are sprayed onto a shaft, allowing for optimal specimen absorption and release. Microorganisms are less likely to be caught within the fibers of a flocked swab compared with spun swabs. Regardless of whether flocked or nonflocked swabs are used, comparatively limited material is captured on a swab. Additionally, some swab types are toxic to specific organisms and will inhibit their growth in culture. For instance, calcium alginate swabs inhibit growth of *Neisseria gonorrhoeae* and some viruses. Wooden-shafted swabs are toxic to viruses and some bacteria. Swabs should not be submitted for anaerobic bacterial culture. Some molecular assays are inhibited with the use of certain swabs. When swabs must be used to collect very small amounts of fluid in limited spaces (e.g., collection of fluid from the inner or middle ear), they should not be allowed to dry. Swabs for respiratory virus testing may be polyester, rayon, or Dacron material with either plastic or aluminum shafts.

Medical devices or prosthetic material may be removed to assess for infection. Such devices are either sonicated or vortexed to remove the biofilm material for culture or other tests. Tissue biopsies must be maintained in a moist environment with sterile gauze moistened with sterile saline and placed in a sterile screw-capped container. Biopsies should be transported to the laboratory as rapidly as possible. In general, larger pieces of tissues are desirable. When multiple tests are desired, a piece or pieces of tissue approximately 1 to 2 cm^3 in size (i.e., about the size of one to two green peas) are required. When skin or deep tissue biopsies are collected, cleansing of the skin should be performed to avoid contamination with colonizing skin flora. When osteomyelitis is suspected, the bone itself should be collected rather than the overlying skin or subcutaneous tissue, after adequate cleansing of the overlying tissue.

For suspected bloodstream infections, blood cultures are critical. At a minimum, two blood cultures sets per order should be drawn from two different sites for adults, with each set composed of at least two blood culture bottles: one for isolation of aerobic pathogens and one for isolation of anaerobic organisms. The preferred blood volume per bottle for adult patients is 10 mL, for a minimum of 40 mL of blood drawn per blood culture order. Many factors are involved with optimal performance of blood culture testing, starting with complete disinfection of the skin surface to minimize contamination with normal human skin flora (e.g., coagulase-negative staphylococci, *Corynebacterium* spp., *Bacillus* spp. [not *B. anthracis*], etc.). Generally, although a single blood culture bottle positive for one of these bacteria represents contamination, recovery of the same organism from multiple serially drawn blood cultures is more likely to represent clinically significant bacteremia. The majority of laboratories strive to maintain a contamination rate of <3%. The number of blood cultures sets drawn, the number and type (i.e., aerobic vs. anaerobic) of blood culture bottles per set, and the amount of blood drawn per bottle also affect the efficiency of pathogen recovery from septic patients.

It is also imperative that proper collection containers are used for blood obtained for serologic, molecular, or other studies. Serum, plasma, whole blood, or other blood components may be required, depending on the type of testing performed. In blood, plasma is the liquid component of the blood—minus the white and red blood cells—before the blood has been allowed to clot and thus contains clotting factors. Serum is the liquid component of the blood minus clotting factors and cells. The type of anticoagulant also affects testing.

SELECT IMPORTANT CONSIDERATIONS FOR SPECIMEN COLLECTION AND TRANSPORT

Bacteriology

Cerebrospinal fluid (CSF) collected for bacterial culture should never be refrigerated, because certain bacteria such as *Neisseria meningitidis* may not survive at low temperatures. Direct inoculation of synovial fluid and other body fluids into blood culture bottles has been shown to improve recovery of most organisms compared with direct plating of specimens in the laboratory onto solid agar media. This practice has also been applied to fluid other than joint fluids, such as peritoneal and pleural fluids. If body fluids are inoculated at the bedside by clinicians, a sterile tube of fluid should also be collected and submitted to the laboratory for a direct Gram stain.

Fresh urine collected without preservatives must be transported immediately to the laboratory within 30 minutes for culture; otherwise, urine may be stored in a sterile container at refrigerated temperatures for 24 hours before plating for culture. Urine may also be collected in boric acid preservative. Midstream (also known as *clean-catch*) urine is recommended for bacterial culture and requires cleansing of mucosal or skin surfaces before collection. First-voided urine (i.e., voiding the first 20 to 30 mL of urine into a collection container) is recommended for detection of the sexually transmitted pathogens *Chlamydia trachomatis*, *N. gonorrhoeae*, and *Trichomonas vaginalis*. Collection of urine from urinary catheters for culture is discouraged due to biofilm production and colonization of the catheters, unless the collection occurs by straight catheterization rather than via an indwelling catheter. Urinary Foley catheters themselves should never be submitted for culture.

Sinus contents for bacterial culture should be collected by aspiration rather than by swabbing due to contaminating normal flora.

For assessment of *Clostridioides (Clostridium) difficile*, loose stool should be collected from patients with diarrhea (i.e., three or more loose stools within a 24-hour period). Formed stool should not be collected for *C. difficile* due to the likelihood of detecting colonizing *C. difficile* organisms.

Swabs should not be submitted for anaerobic culture, as the majority of anaerobes will not survive on the swab. Rather, such specimens should be collected in approved anaerobic transport vials, which often have indicators that monitor the maintenance of an anaerobic environment.

Virology

Samples for virologic culture and other studies are typically collected in a liquid transport medium, which protects viruses from dying. Swabs are also commonly used for molecular viral studies from certain body sites, such as the nasopharynx. Nasopharyngeal swabs are optimal collection devices for molecular testing for influenza, respiratory syncytial virus, and other respiratory viruses. Throat swabs are inferior for viral detection compared with nasopharyngeal swabs. Although sputum is also suboptimal for viral culture, it may be an acceptable source for molecular viral testing. Viral studies on blood may be performed using various blood fractions (e.g., serum, plasma, or whole blood). Specimens for viral culture studies must not be stored at −20° C due to the freeze–thaw cycling of such freezers, which damages the organisms.

Mycology

Transport of specimens for fungal studies is best achieved at room temperature. However, if Mucorales (also referred to as *Zygomycetes*) infection is clinically suspected, rapid transport of the specimen to the laboratory is necessary for adequate recovery in culture due to the fastidious nature of such organisms. In addition, crushing of tissue with a grinder might damage the

Mucorales hyphae. Because most laboratories grind tissue to break apart the specimen for easier plating across various media, clinicians should notify laboratories when Mucorales infection is suspected. If notified, laboratories will often mince the tissue into small pieces with a sharp blade before plating, rather than grinding or crushing. CSF for fungal culture should be held at room temperature before plating.

Mycobacteriology

Specific collection tubes or bottles for mycobacterial blood cultures may be utilized in some laboratories. Gastric aspirates collected for mycobacteria should be transported immediately to the laboratory because acid-fast bacilli may not survive the high acidity environment of the stomach.

Parasitology

Blood smears for examination of parasites should be prepared optimally within 1 hour of collection for best morphology. Thick and thin smears allow for examination of the parasitemia percentage, as well as species-level identification of *Plasmodium*. Stool specimens for ova and parasite (O&P) examination may be performed on fresh stool or stool in appropriate preservatives. EIAs and molecular studies may also be performed on stool. Various enema preparations may interfere with stool O&P or other parasitologic stool assays; therefore specimen collection may need to be delayed for a period after enemas.

Diagnostic Methods in the Clinical Microbiology Laboratory

The clinical microbiology laboratory has become an incredibly diverse space with respect to the diagnostic and confirmatory testing methods that are offered and maintained for routine patient care. These methods range from traditional stain and culture-based techniques for bacterial, mycobacterial, fungal, viral, and parasitic pathogens to increasingly complex nucleic acid amplification tests (NAATs) (e.g., single-target assays vs. syndromic, multitarget panels), whole-genome sequencing (WGS) and next-generation sequencing (NGS) assays for direct-from-specimen pathogen detection, strain typing, and identification of antimicrobial resistance markers. It is important that clinicians be aware of how these methods generally work, including their advantages and limitations, so that results are appropriately interpreted. This section will provide brief overviews on select, commonly performed testing methodologies in clinical microbiology laboratories.

STAINS

Many different stains are used in the microbiology laboratory for the detection and visualization of microorganisms directly from patient specimens and/or after growth in culture; however, only those most commonly used will be reviewed here (Table 2.2). Stains can be classified as either "simple" contrast stains, differential stains, or fluorescent stains. Contrast stains contain charged dyes that are either attracted to or repelled from microorganisms. This includes lactophenol blue, which nonspecifically stains fungal cell walls, and the classic India ink stain for detection of *Cryptococcus neoformans/gattii* in CSF. In contrast, differential stains require more than one stain, have multiple steps (i.e., stain, decolorize, counterstain), and allow for a distinction between cellular morphology and organization. The most widely used differential stains include the Gram stain for bacteria, acid-fast stains for detection of *Mycobacterium* spp., and modified acid-fast stains for visualization of select members of the aerobic actinomycetes (e.g., *Nocardia* spp.) and certain intestinal parasites (e.g., *Cyclospora* spp., *Cryptosporidium* spp., *Cystoisospora*) (see Table 2.2). Briefly, Gram-positive cells (bacteria and yeast) stain bluish/purple due to intercalation of the crystal violet dye within the thick peptidoglycan layer of the cell wall and retain the stain after decolorization using a mild alcohol (Fig. 2.1). In contrast, although Gram-negative cells also have cell wall peptidoglycan, it is significantly less abundant and cannot retain the crystal violet after

TABLE 2.2 ■ Commonly Used Stains for Detection and Identification of Microorganisms Directly from Patient Specimens and/or Culture

	Primary Application	Key Laboratory Pearls
Contrasting Stains		
India ink	*Cryptococcus* spp.	• Used to detect *Cryptococcus* spp. in CSF; however, less sensitive than antigen testing, culture, or molecular diagnostics.
Lactophenol aniline blue	Fungi	• Lactophenol aniline blue is a nonspecific fungal cell wall stain. Used to visualize the microscopic features of fungi after growth in culture.
Differential Stains		
Gram stain (GS)	Bacteria, yeast	• Gram-positive bacteria and yeast stain blue/purple. • Gram-negative bacteria stain red/pink. • NOT useful for *Treponema, Borrelia, Mycoplasma, Ureaplasma,* and others. • *Mycobacterium* spp. generally do not stain by GS. • Aerobic actinomycetes (e.g., *Nocardia* spp.) appear Gram-positive and beaded.
Acid-fast (e.g., Ziehl–Neelsen, Kinyoun, modified Kinyoun stains)	*Mycobacterium*, aerobic actinomycetes, select parasites	• Acid-fast organisms (e.g., *Mycobacterium* spp.) appear red/pink. • Modified acid-fast stains are used for partially acid-fast organisms: *Nocardia* spp., *Cyclospora* spp., *Cryptosporidium* spp., *Cystoisospora* spp.
Trichrome, modified trichrome, iron–hematoxylin	Intestinal protozoan trophozoites/cysts, microsporidia	• Performed on fresh or fixed stool fixed to slides. • Cytoplasm of trophozoites is bluish-green, whereas cysts appear purplish with nuclei and inclusions appear red.
Giemsa and Wright–Giemsa	Parasites in blood	• *Plasmodium* spp., *Babesia* spp., *Trypanosoma* spp., microfilaria, etc.
Fluorescent Stains		
Acridine orange	Bacteria	• Used to confirm presence of bacteria in blood culture bottles that signal positive but are negative or questionable on GS.
Auramine–rhodamine	*Mycobacterium* spp.	• Equivalent to acid-fast staining, but easier to interpret in primary specimens.
Calcofluor white	Fungi, select parasites	• Calcofluor white nonspecifically binds to chitin in fungal cell wall. Used primarily to evaluate patient samples directly. • *Pneumocystis jirovecii, Acanthamoeba* spp., microsporidia will fluoresce.
Direct fluorescent antibodies	Varies	• Organism-specific antibodies labeled with a fluorescent dye may be utilized.

decolorization. Gram-negative cells appear reddish-pink due to retention of the safranin counterstain (see Fig. 2.1). Importantly, the Gram stain is not useful for detecting very thin or small bacteria (e.g., *Treponema* spp., *Borrelia* spp., etc.), bacteria without a cell wall (e.g., *Mycoplasma* spp., *Ureaplasma* spp.), and *Mycobacterium* spp. Acid-fast stains are required for members of the *Mycobacterium* genus due to the thick, hydrophobic layer of mycolic acid in the cell wall of these organisms. Multiple different

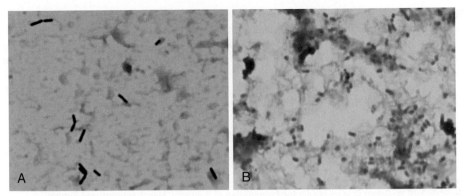

Fig. 2.1 Gram stain of (A) Gram-positive and (B) Gram-negative bacilli from blood culture bottle.

acid-fast staining procedures have been developed, primarily differing in the method used to penetrate the thick lipid layer, either by heating the slides using the Ziehl–Neelsen method or using a higher concentration of the primary carbolfuchsin stain, which has a lipid-soluble phenol group allowing the stain to penetrate the cell wall without heat (see Table 2.2). After the primary stain, slides are decolorized with an acid–alcohol and counterstained with methylene blue. Resistance to decolorization by the acid–alcohol after carbolfuchsin staining (i.e., "acid-fast") is required for an organism to be termed "acid-fast" and will appear pinkish-red. Some organisms are partially acid-fast (e.g., *Nocardia* spp., *Cryptosporidium* spp., *Cyclospora* spp., etc.), meaning that they do not stain evenly with carbolfuchsin using standard acid-fast staining methods. Modified acid-fast stains utilize milder decolorization acids for better visualization of such organisms (see Table 2.2). Because most laboratories do not routinely perform modified acid-fast stains on direct patient specimens, clinicians should notify the laboratory when nocardiosis is on the differential. Additional differential stains, their application, and "key laboratory pearls" are listed in Table 2.2.

Finally, fluorescent stains are considered among the most sensitive stains, as microorganisms will fluoresce against a largely black background, making them easier to detect (see Table 2.2). Commonly used fluorescent stains are the acridine orange stain, which intercalates with microorganism nucleic acid and can be used to confirm the presence of microorganisms in blood culture bottles that signal positive but for which the Gram stain result is questionable or difficult to interpret. The auramine–rhodamine stain is frequently used to detect *Mycobacterium* spp. in primary patient samples; both compounds are nonspecific fluorochromes that bind mycolic acid and resist decolorization. The calcofluor white stain is used to detect fungi in primary patient samples and is a nonspecific fluorochrome, binding β-1,3 and β-1,4 polysaccharides (e.g., cellulose, chitin) in the fungal cell wall.

Finally, it is important to indicate that direct examination of biopsy material, aspirates, or other body fluids for infectious agents by histopathology and cytology can provide invaluable diagnostic information. Many of the stains described earlier are routinely used by pathologists to detect and identify pathogens in tissue sections, in addition to other more targeted stains for visualization of specific structures (e.g., mucicarmine stain for staining of the capsule from *Cryptococcus* spp.). Clinical microbiology laboratory directors, both PhD and MD/DO trained, are an additional resource to review histopathology slides suspicious for infectious processes and should be contacted by health care providers and/or pathologists when confounding cases arise.

CULTURE

The cultivation of microorganisms from patient samples in liquid broth media or solid culture media has been the mainstay of clinical microbiology laboratories since their inception, and although molecular assays are increasingly deployed, culture remains the reference method for detection and identification of most bacterial, fungal, and mycobacterial pathogens. Over 100 different types of culture media have been developed, ranging from nonselective media (e.g., sheep blood agar), enabling the growth of most pathogens and primarily used to culture specimens from otherwise sterile sites, to selective media for isolation of targeted pathogen classes (e.g., Gram-negative bacteria on MacConkey agar) while suppressing the growth of other organisms, to differential media, which is selective media containing additional dyes, biochemical compounds, or antibiotics for recovery of specific pathogens (e.g., buffered charcoal–yeast extract [BCYE] agar for isolation of *Legionella* spp.) (Table 2.3). It is beyond this scope of this chapter to review all of the available culture media types; however, commonly used media in the clinical microbiology laboratory are listed in Table 2.3.

TABLE 2.3 ■ Select Culture Media for Propagation of Bacterial, Mycobacterial, and Fungal Pathogens

	Examples of Organism(s) Recovered	Key Laboratory Pearls
Bacterial Culture Media		
Blood agar	Gram-positive and Gram-negative bacteria	General media for isolation and detection of many bacterial pathogens; allows for visualization of hemolytic activity.
Chocolate blood agar	*Haemophilus* spp., *Neisseria* spp., and many fastidious (i.e., difficult to grow) organisms	Preferred for recovery of fastidious pathogens.
MacConkey agar	*Enterobacterales* and related enteric Gram-negative bacilli	Differential media with crystal violet and bile salts inhibiting growth of Gram-positive organisms.
Eosin methylene blue (EMB)		Differential media, with eosin and methylene blue inhibiting growth of Gram-positive organisms.
Hektoen enteric (HE) agar	*Salmonella* spp., *Shigella* spp.	Differential media to suppress growth of normal fecal flora.
Thiosulfate citrate bile salts (TCBS) sucrose agar	*Vibrio* spp.	Selective and differential media; growth of *Enterobacterales* in stool is suppressed.
CAMPY Cefoperazone vancomycin amphotericin (CVA) agar	*Campylobacter* spp.	Selective media; suppresses growth of fecal flora. Requires incubation in microaerophilic (85% N_2, 10% CO_2, 5% O_2 at 42° C) environment for recovery of *Campylobacter* spp.
Cefsulodin irgasan novobiocin (CIN) agar	*Yersinia enterocolitica*	Selective and differential media.
MacConkey agar with sorbitol	*Escherichia coli* O157:H7	Selective and differential for Shiga toxin–producing *E. coli* O157:H7, which does not ferment sorbitol, unlike other *E. coli* strains.
Regan–Lowe, Bordet–Gengou agar	*Bordetella pertussis*, *B. parapertussis*	Selective media for *Bordetella* spp., which do not grow on routine bacterial culture media.
Buffered charcoal-yeast extract (BCYE) agar	*Legionella* spp., *Nocardia* spp.	Selective and differential agar with required growth (cysteine and iron) factors for *Legionella* spp.
Cystine tellurite blood (CTB) agar	*Corynebacterium diphtheriae*	Selective and differential.

TABLE 2.3 ■ Select Culture Media for Propagation of Bacterial, Mycobacterial, and Fungal Pathogens—cont'd

	Examples of Organism(s) Recovered	Key Laboratory Pearls
Todd–Hewitt broth	Streptococcus agalactiae	Enriched selective liquid medium for isolation and cultivation of S. agalactiae (group B Streptococcus).
Mueller–Hinton agar	Variety of bacteria	Used for antimicrobial susceptibility testing of a variety of bacteria.
Brucella or CDC anaerobic agar	Anaerobic bacteria	Primary recovery of anaerobic bacteria. "Brucella" is a misnomer because Brucella spp. are aerobes and not recovered on this media.
Mycobacterial Culture Media		
Lowenstein–Jensen (LJ), Middlebrook media	Mycobacterium spp.	Enriched media for growth of both rapid- and slow-growing mycobacterial species.
Fungal Culture Media		
Inhibitory mold agar, brain heart infusion blood agar	Filamentous fungi, yeast	Contains antibiotics for suppression of bacteria; enriched and selective for recovery of filamentous fungi and yeast.
Chromogenic agar	Candida spp.	Selective and differential media; Candida albicans, C. krusei, and C. tropicalis differentiated based on colony color.
Birdseed (Niger seed) agar	Cryptococcus spp.	Selective and differential agar; Cryptococcus colonies develop brown/black color.
Potato dextrose agar, V-8 agar, cornmeal agar	Filamentous fungi	Nutritionally deficient agars that induce sporulation of filamentous fungi for microscopic identification.
Czapek–Dox agar	Aspergillus spp.	Induces sporulation of Aspergillus spp. for microscopic identification.
Mycosel agar	Dermatophytes	Selective media to suppress growth of environmental fungi and bacteria.

Given the multitude of culture media available and varying incubation conditions, it is critical that providers clearly identify the specimen source, contact the laboratory if unsure of the appropriate specimen to submit or the transport conditions (e.g., anaerobic transport vials are required if suspecting anaerobic pathogens), and prioritize testing if limited specimen is available. Additionally, if a patient is suspected to be infected with a Biosafety Level 3 (BSL3) pathogen, such as Brucella spp., Francisella spp., or Coccidioides spp., the provider should notify the laboratory immediately so that appropriate precautions can be taken to minimize the risk of laboratory personnel exposure.

One of the critical functions of the clinical microbiology laboratory is to detect circulating bacterial, fungal, or mycobacterial pathogens in blood. Multiple different continuous-reading, automated blood culture systems have been developed and are used in clinical laboratories, all alerting technologists the moment growth is detected in a blood culture bottle. Studies using these systems have demonstrated that incubation for up to 5 days is sufficient to rule out septicemia for the vast majority of pathogens, with the notable exception of Cutibacterium acnes (previously Propionibacterium acnes), which often requires up to 14 days of incubation. Bottles that flag positive on these systems are subsequently Gram stained to help guide selection of the appropriate solid media for subculture and identification. More recently, multiple different multiplex molecular panels targeting frequent causes of septicemia and a number of antibiotic-resistance genes have received Food and Drug Administration (FDA) approval for direct testing of positive blood culture bottles. These panels have significantly reduced the time to pathogen identification and, for certain pathogens, have helped guide appropriate antibiotic management and de-escalation of inappropriate antibiotics. Importantly, fungal and mycobacterial pathogens can also be isolated from blood culture; however, optimal recovery frequently requires specialized fungal and myco- bacterial blood culture bottles to promote the growth of these more fastidious or slow-growing organisms. Finally, it is important to be aware that certain organisms, such as *Coxiella burnetii* (causative agent of Q fever), *Bartonella* spp., *Treponema pallidum,* and *Borrelia* spp., cannot be recovered in routine culture and require serologic testing for definitive diagnosis.

Viral culture using mammalian cell culture lines continues to be performed in large hospital and commercial reference laboratories. Viral culture is associated with prolonged turnaround time (TAT) and requires technologist expertise to interpret cytopathologic effect (CPE). As a result, molecular assays and/or serologic methods are increasingly being applied for the detection of viral infections.

MATRIX-ASSISTED LASER DESORPTION-IONIZATION TIME OF FLIGHT MASS SPECTROMETRY

Traditionally, after growth on solid culture media, bacterial, mycobacterial, and fungal agents are identified using a combination of microscopic findings (e.g., Gram stain, lactophenol blue, etc.) and numerous biochemical reactions, which frequently require overnight incubation and may be complex to interpret (detailed discussions of these traditional methods can be found in the *Manual of Clinical Microbiology* and *Koneman's Color Atlas and Textbook of Diagnostic Microbiology*). More recently, however, the identification of cultured isolates has been dramatically accelerated using matrix-assisted laser desorption-ionization time of flight mass spectrometry (MALDI-TOF MS) (Fig. 2.2).[2] This method is based on the generation of species-specific protein profiles after ioniza- tion of the culture isolate. The generated profile is subsequently compared with a library of known protein profiles and an identification is generated. This process is rapid (<15 minutes), is high throughput, is inexpensive, and has replaced many of the classic identification techniques men- tioned earlier. Limitations of MALDI-TOF MS include up-front cost to purchase the equipment, the requirement of isolated and pure pathogen growth in culture (although direct-from-specimen testing continues to be evaluated), lack of routine antimicrobial susceptibility information, and an inability to differentiate between very closely related species or groups of organisms. Although MALDI-TOF MS is not used as a primary method of identification by all microbiology labora- tories, many use this technique rather than older biochemical-based methods.

MOLECULAR DIAGNOSTICS

Many different types of molecular assays have been developed for the identification of pathogens grown in culture and/or directly from patient specimens. These can generally be separated based on whether the nucleic acid of interest is amplified or not.

Nonamplifying Molecular Assays

These assays include peptide nucleic acid fluorescence in situ hybridization (PNA FISH) probes, ribosomal ribonucleic acid (RNA) target probes, and deoxyribonucleic acid (DNA) target probes. All of these assays share the common feature that nucleic acid from the pathogen is bound by a probe with a complementary nucleic acid sequence, which is labeled with either a chemilumines- cent or fluorescence marker. These DNA:DNA or RNA:DNA hybrids are subsequently detected using a fluorescence microscope, in the case of PNA-FISH, or using a luminometer to detect relative light units (RLUs) from chemiluminescent bound probes. An advantage of the PNA FISH technology is its ability to be performed directly from positive blood culture bottles, most commonly used for differentiation of *Candida* species in this sample type. Notably, however, due to the high cost associated with PNA FISH probes and the introduction of multiplex NAATs (see later), this method is being supplanted by alternative methods in many laboratories. A primary limitation of the DNA target probe technology is the requirement of isolate growth in culture before testing can be performed. Additionally, these hybridization probes have only been developed for certain pathogens (e.g., *Candida* spp., select *Mycobacterium* spp., *N. gonorrhoeae, Listeria monocytogenes, Blastomyces dermatitidis,* etc.) and require technologist expertise to identify which isolates should be tested by which probes.

Nucleic Acid Amplification Tests

A wide variety of different NAATs are available for diagnostic testing. Among other factors, these assays differ in their regulatory classification, being either FDA approved or cleared or are laboratory-developed tests (LDTs), validated by the individual clinical laboratory. Additionally, NAATs may differ in the probe chemistry used to detect the nucleic acid (e.g., real-time polymerase chain reaction [RT-PCR], strand displacement amplification [SDA], transcription-mediated amplification [TMA], branched DNA amplification, loop-mediated, isothermal DNA amplification [LAMP], etc.), the identity and copy number of the targeted gene, the number of pathogens able to be detected (i.e., monoplex [single pathogen target] vs. multiplex [more than one pathogen target]), whether they are qualitative or quantitative in design, and the specimen types on which they can be performed. For additional information on the specific types of NAATs, the reader is encouraged to review dedicated publications on these topics.

NAATs are increasingly preferred for the diagnosis of acute infections (e.g., influenza, *Plasmodium* spp., *Bordetella* spp., etc.), are used preemptively to monitor for primary infection

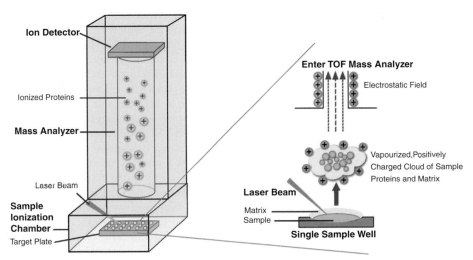

Fig. 2.2 Matrix-assisted laser desorption ionization-time of flight mass spectrometry (MALDI-TOF MS). Individual microorganisms are spotted onto the MALDI-TOF plate and placed in the mass spectrometer. Spots are shot by a nitrogen laser charging and aerosolizing individual microbial molecules from the target plate into the positively charged electrostatic field of the TOF mass analyzer. The ionized molecules travel toward an ion detector, with small analytes traveling fastest, followed by the larger molecules. These ionized particles hit the detector, which generates a mass spectrum that is compared with a library of species-specific mass spectra to identify the microorganism.

or reactivation in immunocompromised patient populations (e.g., quantitative NAAT for cytomegalovirus [CMV] in high-risk patients post-transplant), and remain the method of choice for monitoring response to therapy for certain chronic diseases (e.g., human immunodeficiency virus [HIV], hepatitis C virus [HCV]). Importantly, however, NAATs have notable limitations. First, NAATs are notoriously insensitive for the detection of certain infections, including Lyme disease (*Borrelia* spp.), syphilis *(T. pallidum)*, and latent tuberculosis infection (LTBI), due to the limited dissemination and/or low pathogenic loads in infected patients. For these infections, serologic testing remains the preferred diagnostic method. Second, for certain infections, including vector-borne viral infections (e.g., West Nile virus, Dengue virus, etc.), the clinical sensitivity of NAATs rapidly decreases 5 to 7 days after symptom onset due to immune clearance of the organism, at which point serologic testing is the preferred diagnostic method of choice. Collectively, it is important for clinicians to recognize that in certain scenarios, a negative NAAT does not definitively rule out infection and additional testing should be pursued. Third, for certain quantitative NAATs—for example, quantitative BK virus NAATs—providers should be aware that the reported values, for example, in copies per milliliter, may not be comparable across laboratories due to use of different assays at each site and the absence of a universal quantitative standard. Although universal quantitative standards exist for some viruses (e.g., CMV, Epstein–Barr virus [EBV]), there are many viruses for which such standards are not available. Therefore patients who are serially monitored for viral loads using assays that are not universally standardized should be tested by the same assay at the same laboratory in order for the quantitative results to be clinically meaningful. Finally, providers may be faced with scenarios in which a NAAT remains positive for a particular pathogen, despite completion of a standard course of antibiotics and/or clinical resolution of symptoms. In these scenarios, it is important to remember that NAATs do not distinguish between DNA/RNA released from live organisms versus killed organisms that have not yet been cleared by the host. Additionally, nucleic acid from some pathogens (e.g., EBV, human herpesvirus 6 [HHV-6], etc.) integrates into the host and may remain detectable for life. Contacting the laboratory to discuss confounding NAAT results is always recommended!

Finally, the recent introduction of multiplex, "syndromic" testing panels has led to a significant paradigm shift, both for the clinical practice and within the clinical microbiology laboratory. These multiplex panels are designed to target many different pathogens (bacterial, viral, fungal, parasitic) that are associated with causing the same clinical syndrome, including bloodstream, upper or lower respiratory, gastrointestinal, or central nervous system (CNS) infections. Additionally, some of these panels include gene targets associated with antimicrobial resistance, providing immediate susceptibility information, which can be used to guide more timely antimicrobial stewardship activities. Use of these syndromic panels is advantageous, as a single test can now be performed, rather than multiple monoplex NAATs, which removes the burden from providers to "choose the right tests." Although revolutionary, these syndromic panels have a number of key limitations that are important to consider. First, they are expensive, typically costing >$500 per test, thus necessitating implementation of appropriate test utilization management strategies, which should be established collaboratively between the laboratory and the clinical practice based on patient population. Second, the sensitivity of targeted molecular assays remains higher than that achieved by syndromic panels; thus for some targets on large multiplex panels, a negative result may not rule out infection. Additionally, the targeted pathogens in each type of syndromic panel vary based on assay manufacturer, and for some of the included targets, the clinical significance of a positive remains unclear (e.g., Enteroaggregative *Escherichia coli* detected in diarrheal stool) and may cause confusion and possibly lead to unnecessary treatment. Finally, although these are entirely closed testing systems, contamination events and false-positive results have been documented in the literature, necessitating careful clinical correlation between result and clinical presentation. Additional information on the available syndromic panels is reviewed by Ramanan and colleagues.[3]

Traditional Sequencing and Next-Generation Sequencing

Traditional sequencing using Sanger sequencing or termination sequencing involves incorporation of dideoxynucleotides (ddNTPs) in a growing DNA strand, after which addition of new deoxynucleotides cannot occur. Sequencing of targeted gene regions using this method has been applied for genotyping of microorganisms and to monitor for development of antiviral drug resistance, including most prominently for HIV, but also for CMV, HCV, and herpes simplex virus (HSV), among others. Sanger sequencing is limited by short read length, imperfect base calling, and inability to detect and distinguish mixed populations or genotypes of the same pathogen.

Increasingly, the potential of NGS or massively parallel sequencing is being harnessed by clinical microbiology laboratories to provide more detailed sequencing information beyond that available through traditional sequencing methods. NGS offers numerous advantages, including the ability to detect subpopulations of resistant variants within a single sample, which may have significant impact on treatment outcomes, particularly for HIV and HCV. Additionally, NGS technologies are poised to provide pathogen identification directly from patient specimens, particularly for rare or emerging infectious agents. Also, the ability to rapidly sequence entire genomes by NGS will significantly affect epidemiologic and outbreak studies and opens the door to new research focused on the human microbiome and its impact on health and new pathogen discovery. There are multiple NGS platforms, all differing in their sequencing chemistry, read length, depth of coverage, sequence accuracy, and cost. Although continuously improving, a number of challenges associated with NGS deserve mention, including high test cost, limited availability, and long TAT to results. This is a rapidly evolving area, however, and the reader is referred to a number of references on this topic.[4] Although Sanger sequencing is performed at some larger clinical microbiology laboratories, NGS is currently largely limited to reference laboratories.

ANTIMICROBIAL SUSCEPTIBILITY TESTING OR DRUG SUSCEPTIBILITY TESTING

After an organism is identified as a possible or definitive pathogen, susceptibility or resistance of that organism to certain antimicrobials may be measured. The goal of antimicrobial susceptibility testing (AST) is to attempt to predict the in vivo success or failure of a particular antimicrobial. This is accomplished by reporting the organism as susceptible (S), susceptible dose dependent (SDD), intermediate (I), or resistant (R). These are interpretive categories used to explain the in vitro AST results for microorganisms isolated from infected patients. An isolate that tests resistant to an antimicrobial is highly unlikely to respond to treatment with that antimicrobial, whereas an isolate that tests susceptible is likely to respond clinically. However, even when an isolate is "susceptible" to an antimicrobial agent in vitro, the ultimate outcome in the patient is dependent on the condition of the patient, the site of the infection, and use of ancillary treatment approaches, such as removal of an infected catheter source or drainage of an abscess cavity.

Interpretive categories are related to minimal inhibitory concentrations (MICs) and breakpoints (also known as *clinical breakpoints*). An MIC is the lowest concentration of an antimicrobial agent that prevents the growth of a microorganism as measured with the in vitro susceptibility test. Breakpoints are the MIC values that categorize an isolate as S, SDD, I, or R to a specific antimicrobial agent. MICs may be measured by automated or nonautomated methods, including but not limited to broth microdilution (BMD), agar gradient diffusion (e.g., Etest [bioMérieux, Marcy l'Etoile, France]; MIC Test Strips [MTS, Liofilchem, Inc., Waltham, MA]), and agar dilution. Antimicrobials are typically tested at two-fold doubling serial dilutions (e.g., 4 µg/mL, 8 µg/mL, 16 µg/mL, etc.). The BMD technique is considered the reference, international testing methodology and involves testing several antimicrobials against an organism in a microtiter plate (Fig. 2.3). Disk diffusion, another commonly used AST method, involves measuring zone diameters of organism growth around Kirby–Bauer disks and comparing to MICs to report

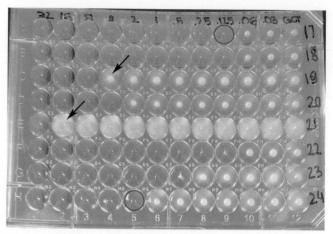

Fig. 2.3 Broth microdilution panel for antimicrobial susceptibility testing. Each row contains a different antimicrobial agent, with decreasing concentrations when read from left to right. Each well in the plate contains bacteria at a particular concentration throughout the plate. Growth of bacteria in a well is viewed as turbidity, or as a "button" of growth *(arrows)*. The minimal inhibitory concentration (MIC) is the lowest concentration of antimicrobial that inhibits bacterial growth. For instance, the MIC of the bacteria for the antimicrobial in row 17 is 0.125 µg/mL and for row 24 is 2 µg/mL *(red circles)*.

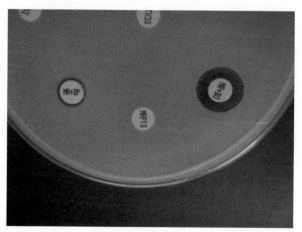

Fig. 2.4 Disk diffusion antimicrobial susceptibility testing. Disks containing certain concentrations of antimicrobials are added to a plate that has been inoculated with a particular concentration of a bacterium. Antimicrobials within the disk diffuse radially from the disk onto the plate. After overnight incubation, the zones of growth around the disks are read. In this example, bacteria grew up to the edge of the MRP10 disk *(bottom disk)*, indicating resistance to that antimicrobial. For the MR+BO antimicrobial on the right side of the plate, the zone diameter of growth *(red circle)* is measured in millimeters and compared with the MIC.

interpretive categories (Fig. 2.4).[5] Several automated FDA-cleared AST platforms are available in the United States, including BD Phoenix (Becton Dickinson, Franklin Lakes, NJ), Microscan (Siemens Healthcare Diagnostics, Deerfield, IL), and Vitek2 (bioMérieux).

The concentration ranges tested vary according to antimicrobial agent, organism, and infection site. Importantly, the drug with the lowest MIC does not necessarily mean that the organism is *most* susceptible to that antibiotic. Each organism–antimicrobial combination has its own established ranges of S, I, and R, and therapy must be tailored around each bug–drug combination. For instance, a measured MIC of 1 μg/mL for ciprofloxacin is within the resistant range for *Salmonella* spp. (R ≥ 1 μg/mL) and *Neisseria meningitidis* (R ≥ 0.12 μg/mL), is intermediate for *Pseudomonas aeruginosa* (I = 1 μg/mL), and is within the susceptible range for *Acinetobacter* spp. (S ≤ 1 μg/mL) according to current Clinical and Laboratory Standards Institute (CLSI) guidelines.

When clinical breakpoints are not available, epidemiologic cutoff values (ECVs) may be reported by clinical laboratories for certain organism–antimicrobial combinations. ECVs are used primarily for antifungal testing, but a few ECVs for bacteria exist as well. The ECV is an MIC value that separates populations of organisms into those which are wild type (WT) or nonwild type (NWT). If an isolate is reported as WT, the clinician should interpret the isolate as unlikely to carry a resistance mechanism to the antimicrobial tested. Conversely, if the isolate MIC is within the NWT range, a resistance mechanism may be present in the organism. Importantly, ECVs are less predictive of clinical response than are clinical breakpoints and so should not be given as much weight as a clinical breakpoint when determining the antibiotic course. This is because clinical outcome data are not considered when developing ECVs, whereas they are part of the process of clinical breakpoint setting.

Antimicrobial susceptibility testing is not performed on all organisms. Reasons for which an organism may not be tested include (1) predictable susceptibility or resistance against certain antimicrobials (e.g., *Streptococcus pyogenes* [group A *Streptococcus*] is predictably susceptible to penicillin); (2) lack of available AST methods based on growth requirements for certain organisms (e.g., *Malassezia furfur* requires oil for growth, but current AST methods cannot incorporate oil); (3) inability of organism to grow at all on media (e.g., *Mycobacterium leprae*); (4) lack of an isolate due to detection of the organism using antigenic, serologic, molecular, or other culture-independent methods (e.g., *Mycoplasma pneumoniae* diagnosed by multiplex molecular panel); (5) organism is a component of usual flora and/or not believed to be pathogenic; and (6) the organism is an agent of bioterrorism, to which laboratorians should not be exposed unless working in appropriate BSL conditions (e.g., *Francisella tularensis*, an agent of tularemia).

Empiric antimicrobial therapy is employed when a definitive etiologic agent has not yet been established but treatment is indicated, either because the patient is critically ill or when there is enough circumstantial evidence pointing to a potential etiology. Clinicians may refer to an institutional antibiogram (Table 2.4), which aids in selecting appropriate empiric therapy. Antibiograms display the susceptibility patterns of select organisms isolated from the local facility over a defined period. They also aid in selecting antimicrobial therapy when an etiology has been established but AST results are not yet available.

SEROLOGIC TESTING

Among the most commonly ordered tests for infectious diseases are serologic tests for detection of antibodies to and/or antigens from pathogenic agents. Serologic tests can be broadly categorized as either (1) classic reference methods, which include immunodiffusion assays, complement fixation assays, and agglutination tests, or (2) as more contemporary methods, including EIAs, lateral flow assays, multiplex flow immunoassays, and peptide microarrays. It is beyond the scope of this chapter to discuss these methods in detail, so references are provided for the interested reader. Infectious diseases serologic testing is sometimes under the technical oversight of clinical chemistry laboratory directors. Nonetheless, microbiologists may be consulted for advice concerning this area of testing.

The appropriate utilization of serologic assays is of critical importance for providers to understand in an effort to minimize the risk of missed or incorrect diagnoses. First, the clinical accuracy of serologic testing is significantly affected by the pretest probability of the patient having the disease and the positive predictive value of the test. Simply put, in individuals at low risk of infection

TABLE 2.4 ■ **Examples of Antibiograms for *Citrobacter freundii* Complex and *Enterococcus faecalis* at a Single Facility**

(A) CITROBACTER FREUNDII COMPLEX ICU (Adult) (All Sources) Antimicrobial	% Susceptible
Amikacin	100
Ampicillin	R
Ampicillin–sulbactam	R
Ciprofloxacin	94
Ertapenem	100
Gentamicin	94
Levofloxacin	94
Meropenem	100
Piperacillin–tazobactam	98
Tobramycin	96
Trimethoprim–sulfamethoxazole	89

(B) ENTEROCOCCUS FAECALIS Inpatient (All Ages) (All Sources) Antimicrobial	% Susceptible
Daptomycin[a,b]	46
Gentamicin (Synergy)[c]	79
Penicillin	99
Vancomycin	99

R, Intrinsic resistance.
[a]Restricted formulary.
[b]Limited number of isolates tested.
[c]Never use as monotherapy.

due to either lack of appropriate exposures or rarity of the disease, a positive serologic result is more likely to be falsely positive. The importance of pretest probability with respect to serologic testing was recently highlighted by the American Board of Internal Medicine (ABIM) Choosing Wisely campaign, an initiative with the goal of advancing a national dialogue to avoid unnecessary medical testing, procedures, and treatment. Second, unlike culture- and molecular-based assays, serologic tests provide supportive, but not necessarily definitive, evidence of infection, with result interpretation requiring correlation to clinical presentation and other laboratory findings, risk of infection, and timing of specimen collection. There are a few notable exceptions to this general rule, for which serologic testing remains the definitive means of diagnosis, including for Lyme disease, syphilis, EBV mononucleosis, *Cryptococcus* spp. infection, and arboviral infections such as West Nile virus (WNV). Serologic testing is the preferred method of diagnosis for these infections due to either an inability to culture these pathogens (e.g., *Borrelia* spp., *T. pallidum*) or the limited clinical sensitivity of molecular diagnostics due to the short duration of viremia (e.g., arboviruses). Additionally, for *Cryptococcus* spp., current agglutination and lateral flow assays to detect cryptococcal antigen in serum or CSF provide superior sensitivity over culture or molecular methods.

Also important to consider is that the development of an immune response takes time, with immunoglobulin M (IgM) antibodies typically detectable 5 to 10 days after symptom onset, followed closely thereafter by development of an immunoglobulin G (IgG) antibody response. Therefore in acutely ill patients (e.g., <5 days after symptom onset) for whom a high index of suspicion exists for a particular infection that cannot be routinely diagnosed using culture or molecular assays, serologic testing can be performed to establish a baseline titer, which will most likely be negative. Repeat testing on a convalescent sample collected 2 to 3 weeks subsequent to the acute specimen to show either seroconversion to IgM/IgG positive or a fourfold rise in titer levels can subsequently be used to establish a definitive diagnosis. Notably, detection of IgM-class antibodies is most helpful in cases of immune-mediated disease after a viral infection, including EBV-associated mononucleosis, measles, and parvovirus B19. Typically, for these infections, by the time patients present clinically, the viral load has declined and may be undetectable. Finally, serologic assays notoriously suffer from antibody cross-reactivity between closely related species or pathogenic groups or due to other endogenous factors in patient samples (e.g., rheumatoid factor). Although laboratories try to mitigate these confounding factors, as with other diagnostic tests, health care providers are encouraged to call the laboratory to discuss any concerning or unclear serologic result.

RAPID DIAGNOSTIC ASSAYS AT THE POINT OF CARE

Rapid diagnostic assays are increasingly implemented at point-of-care (POC) clinics, with the ultimate goal to decrease the window of time between specimen collection, pathogen identification, and antimicrobial susceptibility information. The majority of POC tests have received waivers from the Clinical Laboratory Improvement Amendments (CLIA) requirements, as they are simple to perform and the risk of an incorrect result has been deemed low to patient care. Examples of CLIA-waived POC tests include testing for heterophile antibody in cases of presumed infectious mononucleosis, certain rapid molecular assays for influenza and respiratory syncytial virus (RSV), and screening for HIV antibodies. Importantly, however, although these POC tests offer a rapid TAT for results, additional confirmatory testing may still be required for some infections, including for HIV (i.e., antibody and viral load testing) and a recently CLIA-waived first-tier screen for Lyme disease (i.e., supplemental immunoblots).

Myths and Facts in the Clinical Microbiology Laboratory

In this section, we will address commonly received questions from providers and subsequent areas of confusion regarding a variety of topics related to the clinical microbiology laboratory, including issues such as sources of error to the importance of report comments and the importance of assay validation.

Question 1: What are the possible sources of error in a clinical laboratory?
Laboratory testing procedures are split up into three phases:
1. Preanalytic: Including patient assessment and identification; test order entry; and specimen collection, labeling, and transport
2. Analytic: Defined as preparation of the specimen for testing, testing, and result interpretation
3. Postanalytic: Encompassing data entry and result reporting

Although errors can occur during any of these phases, errors most frequently occur during the preanalytical phase (46% to 68% of all errors), followed by the postanalytic phase (18% to 47% of all errors). Notably, the analytic phase of testing is associated with the fewest laboratory errors, ranging from 7% to 13% of all recorded errors.

The type of errors most frequently encountered during the preanalytic phase of testing include issues such as misidentification of the patient and mislabeling of the sample, inappropriate test orders (e.g., HSV serology ordered on dermal swab specimen), order entry errors, inadequate specimen volume, and incorrect collection and transport of samples. Prevention of such errors is most effectively minimized with targeted and ongoing health care provider training and comprehensive specimen collection and transport procedures, alongside automation of specimen receipt processes and fostering interdepartmental communication and cooperation. Specific analytical errors include instrument malfunction, undetected quality control failures, and the presence of interfering substances leading to inaccurate results. The reason that analytical errors are least common is multifold and includes the rigorous technical procedures and quality assurance controls that laboratory technologists are required to follow, the thorough up-front assay verification and validation assessments, and the blinded proficiency testing that laboratories are required to perform for each assay multiple times per year. Finally, errors occurring in the postanalytic phase include such issues as incorrect result entry (may occur if result entry is manual rather than automated) and inappropriate use or interpretation of laboratory results.

Patient safety is of utmost importance when it comes to laboratory errors, and all laboratories strive to minimize errors through implementation of total quality management systems specific to their location. These quality management systems revolve around error prevention (i.e., through procedures and training), error detection, and error management. Despite these controls, errors will likely still occur; therefore health care providers are encouraged to contact their laboratory with any concerns regarding inconsistent test results.

Question 2: What is test verification and validation, and why is it so important?

Before offering any diagnostic assay for clinical use, laboratories are required to confirm (verify) or establish (validate) the performance characteristics of FDA-cleared or -approved tests or LDTs, respectively, to ensure that results released by the assay are clinically meaningful and accurate. FDA-cleared or -approved tests are diagnostic assays for which the performance characteristics have been reviewed and approved by the FDA. In contrast, LDTs are tests produced by individual laboratories and have not undergone FDA review. Importantly, however, laboratories that produce LDTs are certified by CLIA, which outlines specific requirements for LDT validation to establish and ensure clinical utility and accuracy.

The performance characteristics that are evaluated for FDA-cleared or -approved tests and LDTs overlap significantly and include evaluation of assay accuracy, precision, reportable range, and reference range. In addition to these four factors, validation of LDTs requires establishment of analytical sensitivity and analytical specificity. Briefly, accuracy is defined as the extent to which the new test method agrees with a comparative or reference method, or with the presence or absence of the disease of interest. In contrast, precision, also referred to as *reproducibility*, can be defined as the closeness of agreement between independent measurements (i.e., a positive sample remains positive upon repeat testing). The reportable range of an assay refers to the span of test values over which the laboratory can measure an accurate response (not applicable to qualitative assays), whereas the reference range, also referred to as the *normal range*, is establishment of the expected test result in otherwise healthy individuals who do not have the disease of interest (for microbiology, the reference range is typically "negative"). The two additional metrics required for LDTs—analytical sensitivity and analytical specificity—involve determination of the lowest analyte concentration that is able to be detected in a clinical specimen by the new assay and identification of any cross-reactivity of the assay with other organisms closely related to the target pathogen, respectively. If any of these parameters do not meet acceptance criteria established beforehand, the assay is typically not implemented for routine clinical use.

A number of important points regarding assay validation/verification require comment. First, health care providers should be aware of the distinction between "clinical sensitivity" and "analytic or diagnostic sensitivity." Clinical sensitivity answers the question "What percentage of patients with the infection will test positive by Test X?" In contrast, laboratorians more frequently refer to analytic or diagnostic sensitivity, which answers the question "If the analyte (e.g., DNA, RNA, antibody, antigen) of interest is in the sample, what percentage of these samples will be positive by Test X?". To better explain this difference, consider a patient with acute Lyme disease for whom a Lyme disease NAAT on blood is ordered and results are "negative." During the validation process, let us assume that the laboratory determined that the NAAT can detect down to one *Borrelia burgdorferi* DNA copy per milliliter. Collectively, therefore, we would consider this assay to have high analytic sensitivity but low clinical sensitivity, with the reason that the patient with acute Lyme disease was negative by the Lyme NAAT being due to the absence of circulating *B. burgdorferi* DNA in the blood during acute infection. Understanding this difference between clinical and analytical sensitivity may be helpful to explain scenarios where test results and patient disease state are contradictory.

Not infrequently, clinicians will request that laboratories perform testing on specimen sources that have not been validated for a particular assay or will request that specimens be tested outside of the laboratory-validated acceptance parameters (e.g., outside of stability criteria, specimen was collected or transported incorrectly, etc.). Although exceptions may be made on a case-by-case basis by laboratory directors, this practice is strongly discouraged simply because the laboratory cannot vouch for the accuracy of the test when performed outside of the validated conditions or on inappropriate specimen types, and clinical decisions based on those results may ultimately be harmful to patient care. In addition, some institutions or regulatory bodies may discourage such testing.

Question 3: Are result reporting comments important?

Yes! Test results are typically reported as qualitatively (i.e., positive, negative, etc.) or quantitatively with a numerical value and the appropriate units (e.g., copy number, index value, titer, etc.). Although many test results are self-explanatory, such as bacterial culture results identifying a growing pathogen, accurate interpretation of other results by health care workers may require additional information provided by the laboratory. For example, as mentioned earlier, one of the limitations of NAATs for arboviruses such as WNV is the limited sensitivity >7 days after symptom onset. This fact may not be readily known by all providers ordering WNV NAAT on blood; therefore laboratories may include a comment indicating this limitation on all negative results by this assay. Alternatively, in the realm of serologic testing, there are well-known causes of cross-reactivity for certain analytes (e.g., cross-reactivity between IgG-class antibodies to *Borrelia* spp. and *T. pallidum*, IgM-class antibodies to EBV and CMV, etc.), which could affect patient diagnosis if providers are unaware. For other assays, definitions of acronyms used in the report may be provided, or if the organism name has recently changed, the previous name may be added in the reports.

These and other types of comments relevant to a test result are added to reports by laboratory directors. Importantly, however, laboratories strive to be stringent in both the number and length of these comments, which are included on test reports where they will have significant added value. Therefore health care providers are encouraged to read reporting comments, particularly for assays with which they may be less familiar, as the laboratory has determined that the information is important from a patient safety perspective in an effort to minimize misinterpretation of test results.

Question 4: What is the difference between critical and semi-urgent results?

Microbiology test results are released to clinicians as soon as possible to positively affect patient management. Some tests are performed more quickly than others in the laboratory, resulting in quicker TAT to results for some assays. Test results or laboratory values may be considered critical, semi-urgent, or routine, depending on their urgency. Critical results are those that are considered to be life-threatening unless prompt action is taken. Critical results are also referred to as urgent, panic, alert, or STAT results. Although regulatory bodies that oversee clinical laboratories have not achieved consensus on the time required to report a critical value after receipt of the specimen in the laboratory, it is generally agreed that 1 hour is desirable. Semi-urgent results, also known as *"significant risk"* values, are those that may be unexpected clinically but do not necessarily pose an immediate health risk to the patient if the result is not quickly acknowledged or treatment begun. Routine results are considered noncritical and not semi-urgent.

TABLE 2.5 ■ Examples of Critical and Semi-Urgent Results in Clinical Microbiology Laboratories

Critical Reports	Semi-Urgent Reports
Direct Gram-positive bacteria from cerebrospinal fluid (CSF), body fluid, or other sterile site	Salmonella, Shigella, or Campylobacter detected by culture or molecular methods in stool
Gram-positive bacteria from blood culture	Legionella detected by culture
Acid-fast bacilli detected on direct smear from patient specimen	Carbapenemase-producing Enterobacterales detected by culture
Malaria parasites or Babesia seen on blood smear	Clostridioides difficile in stool
Select agent (e.g., Bacillus anthracis) detected by culture	Neisseria gonorrhoeae detected by culture in genitourinary source of pediatric patient ≤15 years of age[a]
Detection of Strongyloides stercoralis larvae in nonintestinal specimen	Detection of antibodies in serum against Coxiella burnetii, Leptospira spp., measles, or mumps
Haemophilus influenzae detected by culture of cerebrospinal fluid, blood, or epiglottis	H. influenzae detected by culture of other sterile body fluid or tissue
Vibrio cholerae detected by culture	Vibrio spp. (other than V. cholerae) detected by culture
Herpes simplex virus detected from any source in neonate (<1 month)	Cytomegalovirus or adenovirus detected from any source in neonate (<1 month)
Detection of Cryptococcus spp. antigen in CSF	West Nile virus (WNV) antibodies in serum

[a]N. gonorrhoeae detected by culture in patients >16 years of age is usually considered a routine result.

Regulatory agencies require timely reporting of critical and semi-urgent results but do not provide a definition for each category, nor do they designate which assays should be categorized as critical. Institutions and laboratories develop their own lists of critical or semi-urgent tests. Distinction between critical, semi-urgent, and routine results depends on many factors, such as whether the natural course of disease due to the pathogen is rapidly progressive or indolent, whether disease at the infected site is life threatening (e.g., CNS infection), and whether a positive or negative test result may drastically change treatment or affect control precautions (e.g., detection of acid-fast bacilli on smear of direct sputum necessitates respiratory precautions). The critical status of a result may be defined by the type of organism identified, by the specimen source, or by patient age. Occasionally, the logistical necessity of moving patients through the emergency department influences the categorization of critical results. Examples of various microbiology tests that may be considered critical or semi-urgent are listed in Table 2.5.

Characterization of the critical nature of tests differs between institutions based on geographic differences in patient populations, capabilities of the electronic communication system of the laboratory, and the clinician clients of the laboratory. Laboratories and hospital information systems utilize information technology (IT) aids to encourage quick and clear communication of test results.

Question 5: What are some of the common infectious disease diagnostic algorithms health care providers should be aware of?

Diagnostic algorithms are typically established and adopted as a means to streamline testing, and for diseases that may be complicated to diagnose, ensure that the correct testing is performed in the right order. Although there are well-defined national and international diagnostic guidelines for certain diseases, it is important for health care providers to recognize and be familiar with site-specific testing algorithms for infections that lack national guidelines.

Some of the national testing guidelines to be familiar with include two-tiered testing for Lyme disease, performing either the traditional or reverse algorithm for diagnosis of syphilis, performing

TABLE 2.6 ■ Select Infectious Diseases which Warrant Algorithms and/or Recommended Testing Approaches

Infectious Agent (Disease)
Borrelia burgdorferi (Lyme disease)
Clostridioides difficile
Helicobacter pylori
Treponema pallidum (syphilis)
Plasmodium spp. (malaria)
HIV
Hepatitis B virus
Hepatitis C virus

HIV1/2 antibody/antigen testing followed by a differentiation assay and molecular testing of positive samples for HIV, and completing serial glutamate dehydrogenase (GDH) and toxin A and B EIAs for detection of *C. difficile* (Table 2.6). The Centers for Disease Control and Prevention (CDC) is an excellent resource that clearly outlines many of these algorithms, in addition to a recently published document from the Infectious Diseases Society of America (IDSA) entitled "A Guide to Utilization of the Microbiology Laboratory for Diagnosis of Infectious Diseases."[1]

Question 6: What is the future of clinical microbiology?

Over the past few decades, the practice of clinical microbiology has made significant strides in diagnostics. Molecular testing has enabled detection of viruses and other organisms that have been difficult to grow in traditional culture media. Reporting of results is faster with many molecular assays compared with slower culture-based techniques. Syndromic testing of various pathogen groups based on body site has allowed for comprehensive diagnosis from one specimen. The advancements in microbiologic diagnosis continue. Performance of tests direct from the patient specimen—without the need for incubation—is now possible for some specimen types and will continue to grow. Rapid antimicrobial susceptibility test results are available for some antibiotics the day the blood culture turns positive, which improves appropriate patient management. Although limited in clinical use currently, NGS is increasingly used. Clinical microbiology laboratories continue to pursue improved and advanced test diagnostics.

Suggested Reading

1. Miller JM, Binnicker MJ, Campbell S, et al. A guide to utilization of the microbiology laboratory for diagnosis of infectious diseases: 2018 update by the Infectious Diseases Society of America and the American Society for Microbiology. *Clin Infect Dis.* 2018;67:813–816.
2. Patel R. MALDI-TOF MS for the diagnosis of infectious diseases. *Clin Chem.* 2015;61:100–111.
3. Ramanan P, Wengenack N, Theel ES. *Clin Chest Med.* 2017;38:535–554.
4. Boers SA, Jansen R, Hays JP. Understanding and overcoming the pitfalls and biases of next-generation sequencing (NGS) methods for use in the routine clinical microbiological diagnostic laboratory. *Eur J Clin Microbiol Infect Dis.* 2019;38(6):1059–1070.
5. Jenkins SG, Schuetz AN. Current concepts in laboratory testing to guide antimicrobial therapy. *Mayo Clin Proc.* 2012;87:290–308.

CHAPTER 3

A Primer on Microbiology

Brian Schwartz ■ Erin M. Bonura

Introduction to Microorganisms That Interact with Humans

In this section, we will introduce the main categories of organisms that interact with humans both as part of the human microbiome and those that are able to cause disease. Some organisms are primarily colonizers of humans and exist in a symbiotic relationship, others are primarily pathogens that cause disease, and some are able to do both. The predominant categories of organisms that interact with humans are bacteria, viruses, fungi, protozoa, and helminths. See Table 3.1 for key features of these groups. Prions, algae, and ectoparasites are able to cause human disease as well, but are much less common. We will discuss the basic microbiology and touch on elements of the microbiome niche, epidemiology, clinical presentation, and management, though these latter elements will be discussed in greater detail in the following chapters.

BACTERIA

Bacteria are small, single-celled, prokaryotic organisms that grow in differing environments with varying levels of oxygen. Those that require oxygen are considered aerobic. Those that require oxygen but at less than atmospheric levels are microaerophilic, and those that do not require oxygen are anaerobic. Anaerobic bacteria can be either facultative anaerobes (adapt to and survive in aerobic conditions) or strict anaerobes (cannot survive in the presence of high levels of oxygen). Bacteria are typically identified according to their staining properties. The Gram stain

TABLE 3.1 ■ Key Features of Groups of Organisms That Interact with Humans

	Size (µM)	Nucleic Acid	Cell Type	Motile	Method of Replication
Virus	0.002–0.2	DNA or RNA	Noncellular	None	Nonbinary fission
Bacteria	1–5	DNA and RNA	Prokaryotic	Some	Binary fission
Fungi	3–10	DNA and RNA	Eukaryotic	None	Budding/mitosis
Protozoa	15–25	DNA and RNA	Eukaryotic	Most	Mitosis
Helminth	Can be macroscopic	DNA and RNA	Eukaryotic	Most	Mitosis

DNA, Deoxyribonucleic acid; *RNA,* ribonucleic acid.

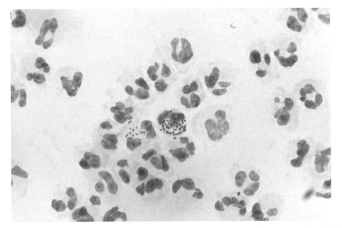

Fig. 3.1 Gram-stained smear of urethral exudates showing intracellular Gram-negative diplococci that are characteristic of gonorrhea. (From Apicella MA, Marrazzo JM. Neisseria gonorrhoeae [Gonorrhea]. In *Mandell, Douglas, and Bennett's Principles and Practice of Infectious Diseases*. 9th ed. Philadelphia, PA: Elsevier; 2020: Fig. 212.16.)

separates bacteria based on their cell wall structure in that Gram-positive organisms retain the violet color due to their thick peptidoglycan cell wall and Gram-negative organisms cannot retain the violet color after decolorization, as their peptidoglycan is much thinner. They are counterstained with safranin and appear pink instead (Fig. 3.1). Thus begins the separation of Gram-positive and Gram-negative organisms: purple and pink. Once the bacteria are stained, they can be further characterized by their shape and configurations as cocci (spheres), bacilli (rods), filamentous, beaded, and pleomorphic.

Gram-Positive Bacteria

Staphylococci. Staphylococci are Gram-positive cocci that form clusters (Fig. 3.2). They are a component of the skin microbiome and are opportunistic pathogens, in that they cause disease if given the right environment or opportunity. *Staphylococcus aureus* is the most frequent cause of staphylococcal sepsis. Infection results in severe disease in humans due to its ability to produce numerous virulence factors ranging from those causing tissue damage and disease spread to toxic

TABLE 3.2 ■ Common Species of Staphylococci Causing Human Disease

	Epidemiology	Clinical Disease
S. aureus	Colonizes nares and skin	Skin and soft tissue infections Bacteremia Endocarditis Epidural abscess
S. epidermidis	Normal flora of skin	Infection of prosthetic materials Catheter-associated bloodstream infections
S. saprophyticus	Colonizes genitourinary tract	Urinary tract infections

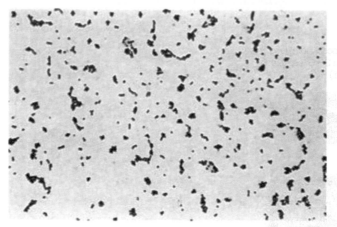

Fig. 3.2 The Gram stain shows the characteristic "bunch of grapes" appearance that gave staphylococci their name. (From Gillespie SH. Gram-positive cocci. In SH Gillespie, ed. *Medical Microbiology Illustrated*. Waltham, MA: Butterworth-Heinemann; 1994: 12–29, Fig. 2.1a.)

shock from superantigens. Given its niche, *S. aureus* is one of the leading causes of skin and soft tissue infections. However, because of its ability to spread, *S. aureus* is also a common cause of bacteremia, endocarditis, and abscesses throughout the body (Table 3.2).

Streptococci. Streptococci are Gram-positive cocci that tend to form chains rather than clusters in culture (Fig. 3.3). Once a streptococcus is identified, further speciation is warranted, given the large number of streptococci and various virulence capabilities. Traditionally, laboratories have separated streptococci via two different but useful ways: hemolysis patterns and Lancefield antigen testing. When growing on a blood agar plate, streptococci can cause three different hemolysis patterns: beta (full hemolysis), alpha (partial hemolysis), and gamma (no hemolysis) (Fig. 3.4). Beta-hemolytic species tend to cause fairly destructive clinical presentations, given their ability to destroy tissue, as evidenced by the hemolysis. However, alpha- and gamma-hemolytic species can cause human disease as well, and depending on the host factors, quite dramatically at times.

Along with hemolysis patterns, Lancefield antigens are used to name specific streptococci. *Streptococcus pyogenes* contains the "A" Lancefield antigen, and thus is also called *group A streptococci* (GAS). GAS are beta-hemolytic and well known as the agent that causes streptococcal pharyngitis. It can also cause severe skin and soft tissue infections (cellulitis and necrotizing fasciitis,

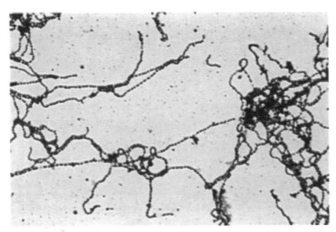

Fig. 3.3 Streptococci form long chains of cocci, as in this preparation of *S. pyogenes*. (From Gillespie SH. Gram-positive cocci. In SH Gillespie, ed. *Medical Microbiology Illustrated*. Waltham, MA: Butterworth-Heinemann; 1994: 12–29, Fig. 2.1a.)

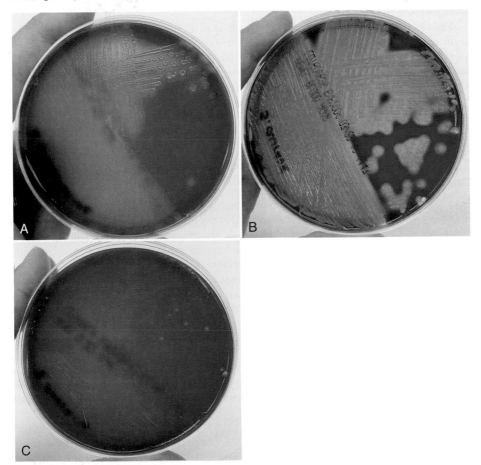

Fig. 3.4 Examples of various types of hemolysis on blood agar. (A) *Streptococcus pneumoniae* showing alpha-hemolysis (i.e., greening around colony). (B) *Staphylococcus aureus* showing beta-hemolysis (i.e., clearing around colony). (C) *Enterococcus faecalis* showing gamma-hemolysis (i.e., no hemolysis around colony). (From *Bailey & Scott's Diagnostic Microbiology*. 14th ed. St. Louis, MO: Elsevier; 2017; Fig. 5-2.)

respectively). The human immune response to GAS antigens can also be associated with disease, most commonly rheumatic fever and post-streptococcal glomerulonephritis. Group B streptococci (GBS) correspond to the *Streptococcus agalactiae* species, whose niche is the gastrointestinal (GI) and genitourinary tracts. Given this location, it is responsible for neonatal sepsis and infections. Mothers who test positive for GBS are treated with penicillin before delivery to prevent disease in the newborns.

Alpha-hemolytic streptococci known to cause disease include *Streptococcus pneumoniae*, which is typically found in the nasopharyngeal niche, and viridans group streptococci, typically found in the oropharyngeal niche. *S. pneumoniae* is a well-known cause of otitis media, lower respiratory tract infections, and disseminated infections such as meningitis and bacteremia. Patients without functioning spleens are at increased risk, given their inability to effectively clear this encapsulated organism (Table 3.3).

Enterococci are also Gram-positive cocci that form chains. It is worth noting that though they are in a separate genus from streptococci, they do have a Lancefield carbohydrate antigen (group D). This was the reason why previously, enterococci used to be included in the *Streptococcus* genus as group D streptococci. However, further identification methods led to the creation of a separate genus. The *Enterococci* niche is the GI tract, with a special predilection for the biliary tract. Thus these organisms can cause cholangitis, but are also known for bacteremia and subacute endocarditis.

Though most Gram-positive disease is caused by cocci, Gram-positive rods are components of the human microbiome and pathogens. Important elements of the human microbiome include *Cutibacterium* (formerly *Propionibacterium*) *acnes* on the skin, *Actinomyces* species in the mouth, and *Lactobacillus* species in the vagina. Gram-positive rods are more often associated with disease. *Listeria monocytogenes* can cause food-borne illnesses ranging from mild, in immunocompetent hosts, to severe disseminated disease, such as bacteremia and meningitis, in pregnant and immunocompromised hosts. Some toxin-producing Gram-positive organisms include *Clostridium botulinum*, the cause of botulism; *C. tetani*, the cause of tetanus; *C. perfringens*, the cause of food-borne illness and gas gangrene; and *C. difficile*, causing antibiotic-associated colitis. *Corynebacterium diphtheriae* causes diphtheria, and *Bacillus anthracis* causes anthrax.

Gram-Negative Bacteria

Like Gram-positive bacteria, Gram-negative organisms can be cocci or rods. Most Gram-negative bacteria are rods, but a few important species are in cocci form. *Neisseria* species are Gram-negative cocci that typically attach in pairs and are some of the most common aerobic Gram-negative cocci. *Neisseria meningitidis* is a common cause of meningitis in children and young adults. *Neisseria gonorrheae* is an important cause of urethritis and cervicitis.

Most of the Gram-negative infections encountered involve aerobic rod species, though two key anaerobic species are worth mentioning: *Fusobacterium* and *Bacteroides*. *Fusobacterium* is a filamentous Gram-negative rod typically found in the oropharynx that can cause severe head and neck infections—specifically, Lemierre syndrome. *Bacteroides*, in contrast, is typically found in the GI tract below the diaphragm and is often implicated in intraabdominal abscesses, diverticulitis, and GI tract infections.

Of the aerobic Gram-negative rods, lactose fermentation is evaluated on MacConkey agar. This selective indicator agar turns pink in the presence of a colony that ferments lactose and remains yellow for those that do not ferment lactose. Key lactose fermenters include *Escherichia coli*, *Klebsiella*, and *Enterobacter* (Table 3.4).

Bacteria Not Easily Identified by Gram Stain

Spirochetes. Spirochetes are spiral-shaped bacteria that do not stain well by Gram stain or grow on culture media. There are three main pathogenic species: *Treponema pallidum*, which

TABLE 3.3 ■ Streptococci

	Epidemiology	Clinical Disease
S. pyogenes (group A beta-hemolytic streptococci)	Colonizes skin	Cellulitis Necrotizing fasciitis Pharyngitis Rheumatic fever Post-streptococcal glomerulonephritis
S. agalactiae (group B beta-hemolytic streptococci)	Colonizes gastrointestinal and genitourinary tracts	Neonatal sepsis Peripartum infections Cellulitis
S. pneumoniae	Can colonize nasopharynx	Pneumonia Meningitis Otitis media Sinusitis
Viridans group Streptococci (e.g., S. mutans)	Normal flora of mouth and gastrointestinal tract	Caries Endocarditis
Enterococci	Gastrointestinal tract	Intraabdominal infections Bacteremia Central-line infections Endocarditis

TABLE 3.4 ■ Select Important Gram-Negative Rods

	Epidemiology	Common Infections
Pseudomonas aeruginosa	Health care setting, prior antibiotic exposure	VAP
Vibrio spp.	Brackish water	Cholera
E. coli	GI tract	UTI Intraabdominal infections Diarrheal disease
Klebsiella spp.	Hospital	UTI Health care–associated infections
Enterobacter spp.	Hospital	UTI HAP VAP
Salmonella spp.	Poultry	Gastroenteritis Typhoid fever
Shigella spp.	Human spread	Gastroenteritis

GI, Gastrointestinal; HAP, hospital-acquired pneumonia; UTI, urinary tract infection; VAP, ventilator-associated pneumonia.

causes syphilis; *Borrelia burgdorferi,* which causes Lyme disease; and *Leptospira interrogans,* which causes leptospirosis. In addition to not being picked up by Gram stain, these organisms are difficult to culture, and therefore diagnoses are usually made by serologic methods.

Mycobacteria. *Mycobacteria* are slow-growing bacteria with very thick cell walls. They do not grow on routine bacterial culture techniques, and therefore special staining and culture methods are needed to identify these organisms. *Mycobacterium tuberculosis* is the cause of

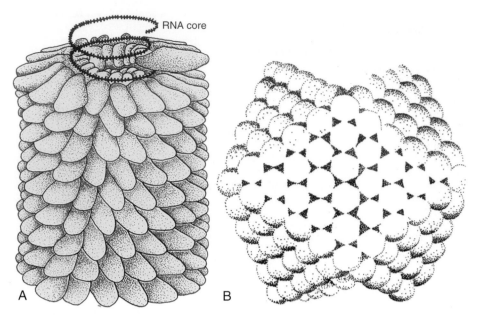

RNA core

Fig. 3.5 (A) The helical structure of tobacco mosaic virus. The nucleocapsid consists of many identical protein molecules enclosing the RNA genome. (B) The general form of an icosahedral virus capsid, illustrated by an adenovirus. The subunits of the capsid (protomers) form 20 triangular faces and thus an icosahedron. These faces meet at 12 points of fivefold symmetry, so the smallest virus of this type has a capsid of only 12 protomers. (From Guttman B. *Brenner's Encyclopedia of Genetics*. 2nd ed. Philadelphia, PA: Elsevier; 2013: Figs. 2 and 3.)

tuberculosis. *M. leprae* is the cause of leprosy (Hansen disease), and *M. avium complex* can cause pulmonary disease in normal hosts and disseminated disease in immunocompromised patients.

Other important organisms not easily identified by Gram stain. Many other bacteria are predominantly intracellular pathogens and are not easy to identify by routine staining and culture techniques. Some of the most important ones include *Chlamydia* species, which cause urethritis and cervicitis; *Mycoplasma* and *Legionella* species, which cause pneumonia; *Brucella* and *Coxiella*, which cause zoonotic infections; and *Rickettsia* species that cause insect-borne infections.

VIRUSES

Structurally, viruses are quite distinct from bacteria in that they are smaller (about ×50,000 magnification) and form either icosahedral, helical, or spherical shapes (Fig. 3.5). They contain either DNA or RNA and can be single or double stranded as well as circular or linear. Though all viruses contain a capsid, some also have a lipid bilayer membrane called an *envelope* surrounding the capsid. Viruses can spread among human hosts via respiratory droplets, airborne particles, fomites, fecal–oral contamination, and bodily fluids.

DNA Viruses

Most DNA viruses are double stranded, though parvovirus B19 is one of the main single-stranded pathogenic DNA viruses (Table 3.5). In the double-stranded DNA viruses, the capsid shape can be complex (pox viruses), helical, or icosahedral. The icosahedral viruses can either be naked or enveloped, like the linear DNA herpes viruses or circular DNA Hepadna virus (hepatitis B).

One of the most well-known double-stranded DNA virus families is the Herpesviridae. These represent the herpes viruses such as herpes simplex virus (HSV), varicella zoster virus (VZV), Epstein–Barr virus (EBV), cytomegalovirus (CMV), and others. These viruses, though in the same family, produce different clinical syndromes ranging from vesicular eruptions with HSV and VZV to mononucleosis illnesses. However, all establish latency and can resurface depending on the host immune status.

RNA Viruses (Including Retroviruses)

RNA viruses can be further classified by the number of strands (single or double) and according to the polarity of the strands: negative sense or positive sense. The polarity determines the infrastructure needed to replicate within the host. Of the RNA viruses, influenza, measles, and HIV are well known clinically. HIV, however, is distinct in that it is a retrovirus and rather than using enzymes to replicate the positive-sense RNA to a negative-sense RNA, HIV utilizes reverse transcriptase to create a DNA strand from the positive-sense RNA (Fig. 3.6 and Table 3.6).

TABLE 3.5 ■ **DNA Viruses**

Family	Example	Clinical Disease
Parvoviridae	Parvovirus B19	Exanthem "slapped cheek" Arthritis (adults)
Poxviridae	Variola	Small pox Monkey pox
Hepadnaviridae	Hepatitis B	Hepatitis Liver failure Hepatocellular carcinoma
Herpesviridae	Human herpes I and II (simplex) Human herpes 3 (varicella) Human herpes 4 (EBV) Human herpes 5 (CMV) Human herpes 6 Human herpes 7 Human herpes 8	HSV Chicken pox Shingles Mononucleosis Roseola Castleman disease Kaposi sarcoma
Papillomaviridae	HPV	Warts Cervical, genital, oropharyngeal cancer
Polyomaviridae	JC virus	PML
Adenoviridae	Adenovirus	Respiratory disease Conjunctivitis Gastroenteritis

CMV, Cytomegalovirus; *EBV*, Epstein–Barr virus; *HPV*, human papilloma virus; *HSV*, herpes simplex virus; *PML*, progressive multifocal leukoencephalopathy.

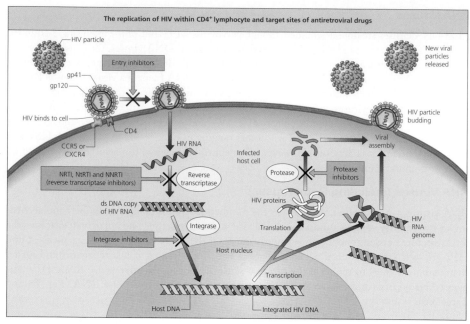

Fig. 3.6 The replication of HIV within CD4+ lymphocyte and target sites of antiretroviral drugs. (With permission from Bolognia JL, Jorizzo JL, Rapini RP, et al., eds. *Dermatology.* 2nd ed. London, UK: Mosby; 2008.)

TABLE 3.6 ■ **RNA Viruses**

Family	Example	Clinical Disease
Reoviridae	Rotavirus	Gastroenteritis
Filoviridae	Ebolavirus	Ebola
Rhabdoviridae	Rabies virus	Rabies encephalitis
Orthomyxoviridae	Influenza A and B	Flu
Paramyxoviridae	Measles morbillivirus	Measles
	Mumps rubulavirus	Mumps
	Human orthopneumovirus (human RSV)	Respiratory tract infections
Coronaviridae	SARS	Respiratory tract infections
	MERS	
	SARS-CoV-2	
Flaviviridae	Dengue virus	Dengue fever
	West Nile virus	Dengue shock syndrome
	Hepatitis C	West Nile encephalitis
	Zika virus	Chronic hepatitis
		Zika fever
Togaviridae	Rubella virus	German measles (exanthem)
	Chikungunya virus	Congenital rubella
		Arthritis
Caliciviridae	Norovirus	Gastroenteritis
Picornaviridae	Poliovirus	Paralysis
	Rhinovirus	URI
	HAV	Hepatitis
Retroviridae	HIV 1 and 2	HIV syndrome

HAV, Hepatovirus A; *HIV*, human immunodeficiency virus; *MERS*, Middle Eastern respiratory syndrome; *RSV*, respiratory syncytial virus; *SARS*, severe acute respiratory syndrome; *URI*, upper respiratory infection.

FUNGI

Unlike bacteria or viruses, fungi are eukaryotic organisms and can be single celled (yeasts) or multicellular with hyphae (septate or nonseptate) (Figs. 3.7 and 3.8). Some fungal species can also exist in multiple forms, such as a yeast form in certain environments or a mold form with hyphae in different conditions—these are called *dimorphic fungi*. For the purposes of medical mycology, it is helpful to categorize fungi into yeasts, cysts, dimorphic fungi, and molds, given their shared respective properties.

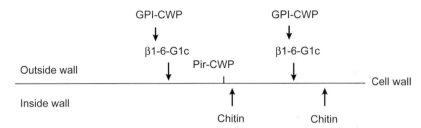

Fig. 3.7 Molecular organization of the cell wall of *S. cerevisiae*. GPI-CWP are GPI-dependent cell wall proteins, Pir-CWP are pir proteins on the cell wall, and β1-6-Glc are glucan molecules, which are highly branched. Therefore they are water soluble, which tethers GPI-CWPS to the cell wall. (From Kils, Mol, Hellingwerf, & Brul, 2002) (From A. Speers, J. Forbes. Yeast. In *Brewing Microbiology: Managing Microbes, Ensuring Quality and Valorising Waste*. Ed. Annie I Iill. New York: Elsevier; 2015: Fig. 1.2.)

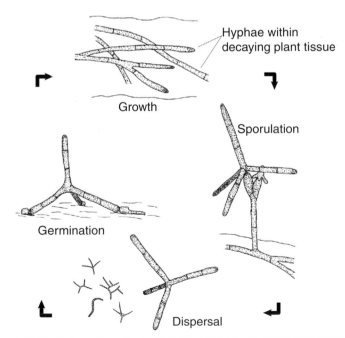

Fig. 3.8 Life cycle of a typical aquatic hyphomycete *(Lemonniera aquatica)*. Note that a few aquatic hyphomycetes may have sexual stages (not shown). Conidial shapes of several species of aquatic hyphomycetes are shown under "dispersal." Drawing by K. Suberkropp. (From Gulis V, Kuehn KA, Suberkropp K. Fungi. In GE Likens, ed. *Encyclopedia of Inland Waters*. New York: Academic Press; 2009: 233–243, Fig. 1.)

Among yeasts, the most commonly encountered pathogens are *Candida* species. *Candida* are a part of the microbiome and live on human skin and in the oropharynx, GI tract, and genital tract. Though *Candida* often exist in harmony with the human body, they are opportunistic pathogens and can cause mild disease, such as diaper rash due to cutaneous *Candida*, to severe diseases such as esophagitis, candidemia, endophthalmitis, and endocarditis.

Dimorphic fungi grow as a yeast at 37° C (body temperature) but demonstrate filamentous growth as a mold form at 28° C. This is helpful to recognize, as biologic specimens may demonstrate the spherule form of *Coccidioides*, for example, but laboratory growth would likely demonstrate the filamentous form. Dimorphic fungi are typically regional, in that they

TABLE 3.7 ■ Fungi

Species	Category	Epidemiology	Common Infections
Candida	Yeast	Skin, oropharynx, GI tract	Mucocutaneous candidiasis, catheter-related infections, candidemia
Cryptococcus	Yeast	Northwest United States Trees HIV with low CD4 count	Meningitis Pneumonia
Pneumocystis	Cyst	Ubiquitous, disease in immunocompromised	Pneumonia
Paracoccidioides	Dimorphic	Central and South America	Pneumonia Mucosa lesions
Coccidioides	Dimorphic	Southwest United States, Mexico	Pneumonia Bone and joint disease, meningitis
Blastomyces	Dimorphic	Ohio and Mississippi river valleys, northern Midwest, upstate New York, southern Canada border of Great Lakes and St. Lawrence River	Pneumonia Skin lesions Bone lesions
Histoplasma	Dimorphic	Bird/bat droppings, central and eastern United States, parts of Central and South America, Africa, Asia, Australia	Pneumonia Disseminated disease
Sporothrix	Dimorphic	Rose bushes	Lymphocutaneous disease
Dermatophytes: Trichophyton, Epidermophyton, Microsporum	Mold: septate	Skin	Tinea
Aspergillus	Mold: septate	Immunocompromised: neutropenia	Allergic aspergillosis Pulmonary disease
Mucor, Rhizopus	Mold: nonseptate	Immunocompromised, uncontrolled diabetes	Rhinosinusitis Pulmonary disease

GI, Gastrointestinal; *HIV*, human immunodeficiency virus.

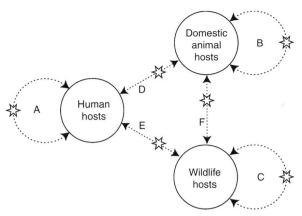

Fig. 3.9 A composite parasite web for parasite zoonoses. Solid circles represent host groups, stars represent transmission of some parasites by arthropod vectors, and dashed lines are possible transmission routes for parasites. Route *A* represents transmission among people, *B* among domestic animals, *C* among wildlife, *D* between people and domestic animals, *E* between people and wildlife, and *F* between domestic animals and wildlife. Any or all of these routes could be used in any direction, depending on parasite species, host availability, and ecosystem structure and function. (Image by Dr. Juliane Deubner. From Polley L, Kutz SJ, Hoberg EP. Parasite zoonoses. In JO Nriagu, ed. *Encyclopedia of Environmental Health*. New York: Elsevier; 2011: 325–345, Fig. 8.)

are commonly found in distinct areas of the continental United States and around the world (Table 3.7).

Molds demonstrate filamentous growth and can be septate or non/pauci-septate. Within the molds, dermatophytes and *Aspergillus* species tend to have septations, whereas zygomycetes are non/pauci-septate.

PARASITES

Similar to fungi, parasites can be classified as single-celled eukaryotic organisms (protozoa) or multicellular organisms (helminth), though the latter also contain organ systems. Both protozoa and helminths complete their life cycle within a host. However, another class of parasites can live on the host; these are ectoparasites, such as lice. Parasites often require a vector, or insect, to assist in transmission of disease, like *Plasmodia* and the *Anopheles* mosquito. Some, however, penetrate the host directly *(Ancylostoma)* or are ingested *(Entamoeba)*, leading to disease. Humans can serve as a normal intermediate host or an accidental host (Fig. 3.9).

Along with classifying parasites according to cellularity, it is helpful to consider the organ system they most often inhabit or utilize in their life cycle. *Plasmodium*, for instance, completes its life cycle in the blood and liver, though most clinical manifestations occur due to the blood phase. Leishmaniasis can present with organ involvement and is most commonly diagnosed as a mucocutaneous lesion (thus it is listed in Table 3.8 under "tissue"). Categorizing in this manner enables the provider to more readily create a differential diagnosis based on the presenting symptomatology.

Protozoa

Protozoa are most commonly classified by the type of body system where they cause disease. They can be further categorized according to structure, in that protozoa include amoebae, ciliates,

TABLE 3.8 ■ Endoparasites

Parasite	Epidemiology	Organ System	Disease
Protozoa			
Plasmodium	Mosquito vector	Blood	Malaria
Babesia	Tick vector	Blood	Babesiosis
Trypanosoma	Insect vectors	Heart, GI tract, central nervous system	Chagas disease and sleeping sickness
Entamoeba	Oral–fecal	GI tract, liver	Dysentery, liver abscess
Cryptosporidium	Oral–fecal	Intestinal	Diarrhea
Giardia	Oral–fecal	Intestinal	Diarrhea
Leishmania	Sand fly vector	Tissue	Cutaneous lesions and/or visceral lesions
Trichomonas	Sexual transmission	Tissue	Vaginitis, urethritis
Naegleria	Nasal transmission	Tissue	Acute meningoencephalitis (fatal)
Toxoplasma	Ingestion	Tissue	Fetal infection, chorioretinitis, central nervous system infection in HIV/AIDS
Helminths			
Trichuris (whipworm)	Oral–fecal	Intestinal	Diarrhea, anemia, rectal prolapse
Enterobius (pinworm)	Oral–fecal	Intestinal	Anal pruritus
Ascaris	Oral–fecal	Intestinal	Impaired growth, intestinal obstruction
Strongyloides	Skin penetration	Intestinal	Abdominal pain, disseminated infection in immunocompromised hosts
Necator/Ancylostoma (human hookworm)	Skin penetration	Intestinal	Anemia, abdominal pain
Ancylostoma braziliense (dog/cat hookworm)	Skin penetration	Tissue	Cutaneous larva migrans
Filaria	Insect vectors	Blood, lymphatics, eyes	African eye worm Lymphatic filariasis
Taenia	Ingestion of undercooked pork/ oral–fecal	Intestinal/central nervous system	Tapeworm or neurocysticercosis
Clonorchis	Oral–fecal	Intestinal/biliary	Abdominal discomfort, biliary obstruction
Schistosoma	Skin penetration	Intestinal	"Swimmer's itch," Katayama fever (systemic hypersensitivity reaction, intestinal, hepatosplenic, pulmonary, and genitourinary complications)
Echinococcus	Oral–fecal	Tissue	Liver and lung cystic disease
Trichinella	Ingestion of undercooked infected animal	Tissue	Muscle pain, swelling, and weakness

GI, Gastrointestinal; *HIV/AIDS*, human immunodeficiency virus/acquired immunodeficiency syndrome.

TABLE 3.9 ■ Ectoparasites

Common Name	Scientific Name	Human Niche	Associated Risk Factors	Transmissible Disease
Head lice	Pediculus humanus capitis	Head and neck	Homelessness, refugees, sexual contacts, head-to-head contact	None
Body lice	Pediculus humanus corporus	Torso and extremities	Homelessness, refugees, sexual contacts, head-to-head contact	Epidemic typhus, louse-borne relapsing fever
Pubic lice	Phthirus pubis	Pubic area	Homelessness, refugees, sexual contacts, head-to-head contact	None
Scabies	Sarcoptes scabiei var. hominis	Skin folds, belt line, groin area	Household or close contacts, nursing homes, extended care facilities, prisons, sexual contacts	None
Fleas	Ctenocephalides felis	N/A	Infested sleeping areas	Plague, endemic typhus, trench fever
Bed bugs	Cimex lectularius	N/A	Infested sleeping areas	None

N/A, Not applicable.

sporozoan, and flagellates (see Table 3.8), with ciliates encountered less commonly. Of the amoebae, *Entamoeba histolytica* is most well-known, which causes dysentery and can travel to the liver or lung, causing abscesses. Of the sporozoa, *Plasmodium* species, the causative organism of malaria, are the most common agents, with an estimated 219 million new cases worldwide in 2017. Lastly, with the flagellates, diseases range from diarrhea and dysuria to sleeping sickness and organ damage.

Helminths

Helminths are multicellular endoparasites that vary in size from 2 to 3 mm *(Enterobius)* to 10 m *(Taenia* species). They can be further separated into nematodes (roundworms), cestodes (tapeworms), and trematodes (flatworms). Helminths cause human disease by siphoning nutrition, obstruction, and inciting inflammation (Table 3.8).

Ectoparasites

Ectoparasites are parasites that infest the outer surface of their hosts. Some ectoparasites live exclusively on human hosts (lice, scabies); for some, humans are incidental hosts (fleas); and bed bugs live elsewhere but feed on human blood. Ectoparasite infestations can be intensely pruritic, and a few ectoparasites can transmit other diseases through their bites, such as body lice transmitting typhus and louse-borne relapsing fever, or fleas transmitting *Yersinia pestis* (the plague) (Table 3.9).

CHAPTER 4

General Principles of Antimicrobial Therapy

Jaap ten Oever ■ Inge C. Gyssens

Introduction

Antimicrobials differ intrinsically from other drugs. Antimicrobials do not aim to affect biologic processes in the patient, but instead inhibit or kill invading pathogens and commensal microorganisms. The properties of these microorganisms are crucial when choosing an antimicrobial regimen, as are the patient and drug characteristics. The pyramid of infectious diseases is a useful learning tool and illustrates the multiple interactions between the host, pathogen(s), commensals, and antimicrobial drug that should influence drug selection (Fig. 4.1).

Prescribing antimicrobial therapy is a uniform part of the clinical tasks of all physicians and nonphysician prescribers. At any given moment, 30% to 40% of the patients admitted to the hospital are prescribed systemic antimicrobial drugs, either as prophylaxis or as therapy. Many aspects need to be considered before an appropriate choice can be made, but important decisions need to be made in the following days as well. For example, what to do with a patient whose clinical situation deteriorates? Or how to streamline therapy once culture results become available? Or when those remain negative? Local guidelines support the prescriber but will never be able to cover all clinical scenarios. This chapter provides an overview of the general principles of antimicrobial therapy to help the prescriber use antimicrobials appropriately.

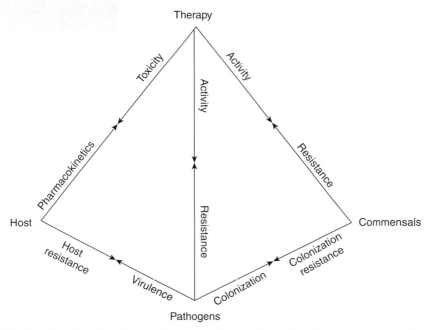

Fig. 4.1 Pyramid of infectious diseases. The arrows illustrate the multiple interactions between the host, pathogen(s), commensals, and antimicrobial drug. (From Pulcini C, Gyssens IC. How to educate prescribers in antimicrobial stewardship practices. *Virulence*. 2013;4[2]:193. Taylor & Francis Ltd. www.tandfonline.com.)

Selecting an Antimicrobial Regimen

DETERMINING THAT ANTIMICROBIAL TREATMENT IS INDICATED

In determining the indication of antimicrobial treatment, obtaining an accurate diagnosis is the first and most crucial step. It goes without saying that only bacterial infections require antimicrobial treatment. Nevertheless, (unconfirmed) viral infections are a frequent cause of antibiotic misuse, sometimes because these infections present in a similar fashion. There is a limited arsenal of antiviral drugs; for the most common viral infectious diseases (i.e., respiratory tract infections and gastroenteritis), there are no etiologic treatment options.

A high suspicion or even proof of a bacterial infection does not necessarily mean that antimicrobials are indicated. Some bacterial infections are self-limiting; antimicrobials only modestly shorten the duration of symptoms and do not reduce the complication rate. Examples include infectious diarrhea, external otitis, acute rhinosinusitis, and pharyngotonsillitis. Guidelines do not recommend systemic antimicrobial treatment for these diseases because the side effects for the patient and the risk of induction of antimicrobial resistance for the public do not justify the limited effect on clinical course. Exceptions are made for immunodeficient patients. For example, enterocolitis caused by the intracellular pathogen *Salmonella* is associated with bacteremia in patients with cellular immunodeficiency and requires treatment. Similarly, severely ill patients, such as those with bacillary dysentery presumptively due to *Shigella* or prolonged fever in rhinosinusitis, should be treated with antimicrobials. Importantly, in certain bacterial infections, other measures than antimicrobials, such as abscess drainage or removal or debridement of foreign material, are more important for cure than antimicrobial treatment.

Withholding or delaying antimicrobial treatment in patients without a certain diagnosis but in whom infection is part of the differential diagnosis can be a justifiable strategy. Obtaining a

TABLE 4.1 ■ **Criteria for Selecting an Antimicrobial Regimen**

The agent(s) should be active against the (expected) pathogen

The agent(s) should reach sufficient concentration and retain its activity at the site of infection

The agent(s) should have an appropriately narrow spectrum

The agent(s) should be suited for the preferred route of administration

The agent(s) should have the least toxicity (including allergic reactions) compared with equally effective drugs

The agent(s) should have the least costs compared with equally effective drugs

clinical diagnosis and—in case of an infection—a microbiologic diagnosis is important for management, as later attempts at identifying an etiologic agent can be obscured by administration of antimicrobials. Severity of illness and an increased risk of a complicated course are two important considerations that favor prompt initiation of antimicrobial treatment. This is discussed in more detail in the section "Timing of Administration."

The different steps of designing an antibiotic regimen are summarized in Table 4.1. Selecting an empirical regimen (i.e., treatment directed against *expected* pathogens) is based on a clinical "educated guess" and is more complex than targeted treatment in which the pathogen and susceptibility are known.

ACTIVITY AGAINST (EXPECTED) PATHOGENS

Empiric Antimicrobial Treatment

Once the decision has been made to initiate antimicrobial treatment, the next step is to choose the agent or combination of agents with activity against the purported pathogens. In case of empiric treatment (i.e., treatment given before the etiologic agent is known), this choice should be made on the integration of the relative frequency of the etiologic agent combined with its expected susceptibility. The probability that a certain antimicrobial has activity against the expected pathogens derives from the formula that adds up the incidence of the specific pathogens multiplied by the susceptibility percentage for these antimicrobials for all major pathogens. Local surveillance data on antimicrobial resistance are informative for making this determination. Risk factors for antimicrobial resistance, such as prior antibiotic use, known colonization (check prior culture results!), and exposure (e.g., hospital admission, recent travel, or antibiotic use) should be considered.

It is nearly impossible—and undesirable, as it will lead to an unjustified increase in broad-spectrum treatment—to cover all possible pathogens. The severity of illness determines which percentage of inappropriate coverage is acceptable, although clear cut-off values do not exist. It is obvious, however, that the consequences of inappropriate initial empiric treatment are far worse in the case of septic shock than in acute cystitis. Evidence-based guidelines for empirical treatment do take this principle into account. In community-acquired pneumonia, for example, the pneumonia severity index (PSI) and the CURB-65 score are commonly used to guide empirical treatment, not because of their ability to predict etiology, but because an increase in score is associated with increased mortality. Coverage of "atypical pathogens" is only indicated in patients with severe pneumonia or intensive care admission.

Targeted Antimicrobial Treatment

If microbiologic results are available, targeted treatment is given, and the choice of a specific agent is based on the criteria discussed in the following paragraphs. However, as discussed in previous chapters, a positive test result should lead to a moment of reflection: Is this isolate indeed the (only) pathogen? Is the specimen sent to the microbiologic laboratory representative? Could it be

TABLE 4.2 ■ Organs, Tissues, and Fluids That Are Difficult to Reach for (Some) Antimicrobials and the Main Causes

Difficult-to-Reach Site	Cause
Absess	Biofilm
Implant	Blood–brain barrier[a]
Brain/meninges	Epithelial barrier
Cysts	Blood–retinal barrier[a]
Eye	Blood–prostate barrier[a]
Prostate	Fibrin mass
Intravascular thrombus	Fibrin mass
Cardiac vegetation	Fibrous capsule

[a]Due to absence of porous capillary endothelium.

contaminated? And if one concludes that the isolated pathogen is relevant, one should consider the pathogenesis and consider if the infection could be polymicrobial. For example, anaerobic bacteria are more difficult and longer to culture and do play a role in infections that have an intestinal (e.g., fecal peritonitis or liver abscess) or odontogenic origin (e.g., lung abscess or brain abscess). This implies that the antimicrobial treatment of these conditions should include anaerobic coverage even if anaerobes have not been isolated.

TAILORING THE ANTIMICROBIAL SELECTION TO THE SITE OF INFECTION

Only if the antimicrobial agent reaches sufficient concentration at the site of infection can it kill an in vitro susceptible microorganism. The central nervous system is the prototypic organ that is difficult to reach. Endothelial cells within the microvasculature and the choroid plexus epithelial cells shield the central nervous system from the systemic circulation. Most large hydrophilic drugs reach low concentrations in the cerebrospinal fluid and brain tissue. This explains why the clinical breakpoint of *Streptococcus pneumoniae* for penicillin is lower for isolates cultured from cerebrospinal fluid than from other samples. The blood–brain barrier limits the therapeutic arsenal and sometimes necessitates the administration of higher doses of systemic antimicrobials or the intraventricular administration of antimicrobials. Meningeal inflammation, however, makes the blood–brain barrier more penetrable to many antimicrobials. Similarly, the posterior eye segment (blood–retinal barrier) is also poorly penetrated by most antimicrobials (Table 4.2). From a pharmacokinetic perspective, the urinary tract consists of three parts: the prostate, the urine (or bladder), and the kidney. The kidney is well perfused, and concentrations similar to plasma concentration are reached. Limited renal excretion of antimicrobial agents can lead to subtherapeutic concentrations in urine, whereas other agents are concentrated in the urine. Nitrofurantoin is the example of an antimicrobial with high urinary concentrations, which is therefore extremely suited to treat cystitis. Its low plasma—and thus renal tissue—concentration, however, precludes its use for complicated urinary tract infections. Penetration into the prostate is relatively poor for most antimicrobials. If susceptibility of the pathogen allows, preference is given to quinolones or cotrimoxazole.

Besides physiologic barriers for antimicrobial penetration, infection itself induces histologic changes that interfere with antimicrobial penetration. Biofilms are typically formed on foreign material and create three-dimensional structures of microorganisms enclosed by polysaccharides. This organization decreases both antimicrobial penetration and an effective immune response. The effect of cell wall–active agents is further diminished because biofilm-associated microorganisms are in a stationary growth phase. Rifampicin and quinolones are the prototypic antibiotics

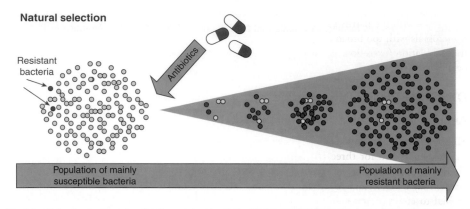

Fig. 4.2   Natural selection of antibiotic-resistant bacteria. The starting point in this example is a large bacterial population mainly consisting of bacteria that are susceptible to antibiotics and a couple of bacteria that are antibiotic-resistant by chance. A bactericidal antibiotic is added, which kills most of the susceptible bacteria in the population, whereas the resistant bacteria survive. Only the resistant bacteria will continue to proliferate in the presence of the antibiotic and increase in number over time. The end result is a population of mainly resistant bacteria. (Courtesy of ReAct – Action on antibiotic resistance. https://www.reactgroup.org/contact/.)

that that have well-established biofilm activity. Of note, many foreign body infections require surgery next to antimicrobial treatment to eradicate the pathogens. The infected platelet–fibrin deposition that forms the vegetation in infective endocarditis, for example, shows a heterogeneous diffusion of antibiotics within the vegetation that might differ between drugs. To achieve high concentrations, guidelines recommend treating infective endocarditis with high doses of intravenous antimicrobials, as in other deep-seated infections. The fibrous capsule of a mature abscess decreases permeation of the antibiotic, although most antimicrobials reach concentrations above the minimum inhibitory concentration (MIC) in small abscesses.

After reaching sufficient concentrations, retaining activity is crucial for antimicrobials to exert their effect. Antimicrobial activity can be affected by several local factors. An acidic pH increases MICs of aminoglycosides, which, together with low oxygen tension and drug-binding debris, is held responsible for their insufficient effectivity in sterilizing pus collections. Cotrimoxazole also loses its effect in pus. Another example is lung surfactant, which abolishes the antimicrobial effect of daptomycin.

Selection of resistant microorganisms can only occur if the antibiotic reaches the colonizing microorganisms. If absorption is limited, topical antimicrobial treatment only influences microorganisms at the site of application and is therefore to be chosen over systemic treatment if possible. Examples are uncomplicated cases of blepharitis, conjunctivitis, external otitis, dermatomycosis, and impetigo.

SELECTING AN APPROPRIATELY NARROW SPECTRUM

Although all bacteria need to acquire one or more resistance mechanisms—either by chromosomal mutations or by acquiring genetic elements from the environment—to become phenotypically resistant, it is the exposure to antibiotics that gives resistant subpopulations a survival benefit and the potential to proliferate and disseminate (Fig. 4.2). This is particularly relevant for the human microbiome, estimated at trillions of bacteria. The narrower the spectrum of the antimicrobial, the less selection pressure and the lower likelihood of the emergence of resistance. In empiric treatment, this means that the chosen regimen should only cover the expected pathogens, anticipating their susceptibility profile. In targeted treatment, this implicates that the agents with the narrowest possible spectrum should be chosen. The benefit of avoiding antimicrobials with too broad of a spectrum lies in the future, both for the individual patient and the population (excretion of antimicrobials in the environment and dissemination of resistant bacteria).

OTHER ASPECTS INFLUENCING CHOICE OF REGIMEN

Antimicrobial Combinations

Single-agent antimicrobial therapy often suffices, but combining two or more antimicrobials can be considered for three reasons: (1) to extend the spectrum, (2) to achieve synergy, and (3) to prevent the emergence of resistance. Extending the spectrum by combining antimicrobial agents may be necessary in cases where there is no single sufficiently broad-spectrum antimicrobial to cover the expected pathogens. Synergy implies that the effect of the combination is greater than the sum of the activities of individual agents. Synergistic combinations can be clinically indicated in serious infections for which rapid killing is required, such as endocarditis and other intravascular infections. Synergy identified in vitro may not always translate into clinical benefit. The addition of gentamicin to an antistaphylococcal penicillin is synergistic against some strains of *Staphylococcus aureus* and leads to a faster clearance of bacteria from the bloodstream in *S. aureus* endocarditis but does not improve patient survival. To the contrary, it increases the incidence of nephrotoxicity. On the other hand, a synergistic combination of a beta-lactam antibiotic and gentamicin or ceftriaxone results in a bactericidal effect and is essential for the treatment of enterococcal endocarditis. Similarly, the addition of gentamicin to penicillin can shorten the course of antimicrobial therapy in endocarditis due to viridans streptococci. The opposite of synergy is antagonism, where the addition of a second agent results in a decreased effect of the combination compared with the independent activity of the individual agents. This phenomenon has been clearly demonstrated in the combination of tetracyclines and penicillin in pneumococcal meningitis, but clinical reports on clinically significant antagonism are otherwise rare.

The emergence of resistance during treatment results either from selection of preexisting resistant clones (see Fig. 4.2) or de novo development of resistance. Provided that the resistance mechanism differs for two (or more) antimicrobial agents, the likelihood that a mutant pathogen displays both resistance mechanisms is much lower than the odds of encountering a strain that is resistant to either one. Size of the infecting population, killing rate, mutation frequency, and biologic fitness costs determine whether resistance emerging during monotherapy is occurring and if combination therapy is indicated. HIV and tuberculosis are the prototypical diseases for which combination therapy is the standard treatment.

Bactericidal Versus Bacteriostatic Therapy

Various microbiologic techniques are available to classify antimicrobial agents as bactericidal or bacteriostatic. Bactericidal agents kill microorganisms, whereas bacteriostatic agents prevent growth and as such would require an intact systemic or local immune system to effectively clear the pathogens. Aminoglycosides, beta-lactams, fluoroquinolones, glycopeptides, lipopeptides, and nitroimidazoles are considered bactericidal; tetracyclines, lincosamides, macrolides, and sulfonamides are bacteriostatic. This categorization, however, is arbitrary because a particular agent has inconsistent bactericidal or bacteriostatic effects against all bacteria. Moreover, this distinction lacks clinical relevance because most infections can be treated with similar efficacy with both groups. However, meningitis, endocarditis, and neutropenia are clinical situations in which bactericidal antimicrobial agents are preferred because in these clinical scenarios with reduced (local) phagocytic capacity, the intrinsic activity of the drug is thought to be the main determinant of clinical success.

SIDE EFFECTS OF ANTIMICROBIAL TREATMENT

The preferred antimicrobial should have the least toxic profile compared with equally effective antimicrobials. Frequent specific side effects are discussed in Chapter 5. Side effects, preferred route of administration, and costs determine the final choice of the antimicrobial and are relative. One is willing to accept (the risk of) more side effects if a certain antimicrobial results in better patient outcomes, particularly in a severely ill patient with no alternative options.

A specific group of side effects are allergic reactions, which are hypersensitivity reactions, that is, signs or symptoms provoked by exposure to a stimulus at a dose tolerated by normal persons, with a demonstrated immunologic reaction. Immediate type (occurring <6 hours) and nonimmediate type (occurring >6 hours, but often starting after 2 to 5 days) are distinguished and differ in their pathogenesis and severity. Immediate-type reactions are usually immunoglobulin E (IgE)–mediated and cause urticaria, angioedema, and sometimes anaphylaxis. Non–immediate-type reactions usually result in a maculopapular rash and are T-cell mediated. Rarely, severe cutaneous other-type IV allergic reactions occur. Around 10% of hospitalized patients report antibiotic allergies, mostly to beta-lactam antibiotics. However, only maximally 10% of the patients will have a real allergy. Allergy delabeling by taking a thorough history and eventually skin testing are increasingly being recognized as important aspects of antimicrobial stewardship programs (ASPs) to decrease the negative consequences of inexistent allergy. Incorrect allergy labeling of beta-lactams leads to the use of more broad-spectrum and less effective alternatives and is associated with more side effects, more health care–associated infections, and longer hospital stays. Cross allergies do exist, but occur less frequently than previously thought. Only 2% of the patients with a penicillin allergy show cross-reactivity to cephalosporins.

Timing of Administration

As a general rule, obtaining cultures from the blood and other expected sites of infection should precede the administration of antimicrobials, as prior antimicrobial therapy compromises the yield of microbiology tests, the results of which are necessary to guide antimicrobial treatment decisions in the days following initiation. The clinical condition of most patients with an infection allows clinical assessment and obtaining cultures before the administration of an antimicrobial. Common sense dictates that the more compromised the clinical situation of the patient, the shorter the door-to-needle time should be. For example, once a diagnosis of sepsis is made, administration of antibiotics should not be delayed.

A febrile episode without a syndromic diagnosis often creates a dilemma whether or not to start antimicrobial treatment. In practice, a febrile patient frequently evokes an antimicrobial prescription, despite the fact that fever or other signs of inflammation are not always caused by an infection requiring antimicrobials. The crux is to identify those patients whose outcome will be worse without early administration of antibiotics. Patients with organ failure, as in sepsis, without any doubt belong to this group. Patients who are prone to rapid deterioration, like patients with significant comorbidity or immunosuppression, should lead to a low threshold to initiate antibiotic treatment, although assessment should be made case by case. Otherwise, antibiotic treatment can be safely withheld or delayed while collecting and waiting for microbiologic data, such as in the patient without signs of life-threatening organ dysfunction and no clear focus of infection. Frequent reassessment may be necessary, on the one hand, to obtain a specific diagnosis and, on the other hand, to monitor for changes in vital parameters.

Dosing

As previously discussed, the selection of an antimicrobial regimen is guided by whether or not sufficient concentrations are reached at the site of infection. But what determines the concentration

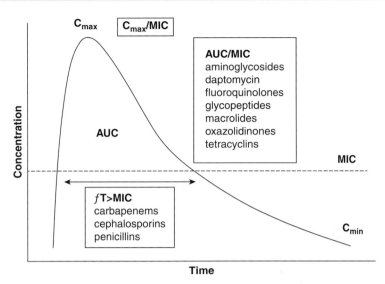

Fig. 4.3 Pharmacodynamic indices predicting efficacy of antibiotic agents.

at the site of infection? And what is a *sufficient* concentration? This is the field of pharmacokinetics and pharmacodynamics. Pharmacokinetics describes how the patient affects the antimicrobial drug. In other words, it describes the fate of the drug in the patient. Four key processes are recognized: absorption, distribution, metabolism, and excretion. Pharmacodynamics describes the effect of an antimicrobial agent on a pathogen.

TIME- AND CONCENTRATION-DEPENDENT ANTIMICROBIALS

Agents are classified either as concentration-dependent killing agents or as time-dependent killing agents. The efficacy of drugs that exhibit time-dependent killing (beta-lactam antibiotics) depends on the time that the free (unbound) concentration exceeds the MIC ($fT > MIC$). Frequent dosing, extended infusions, or continuous infusions are used for time-dependent killing agents with short elimination half-lives, because this dosing strategy increases the time the concentration is above the MIC.

Concentration-dependent agents exhibit effect once their concentration is above the MIC, but their efficacy increases with further increase of the peak concentration (Fig. 4.3). For these agents, a suppressive effect persists for a varying period after the concentration is below the MIC, the so-called *postantibiotic effect*. Efficacy of concentration-dependent agents is predicted by the ratio of the maximum plasma concentrations (peak) to the minimum inhibitory concentration (C_{max}/MIC) and the ratio of the area under the curve (AUC) of plasma concentrations to MIC (AUC/MIC). These two parameters are correlated, because the AUC increases when C_{max} increases. The total daily dose determines the AUC and thus the efficacy of concentration-dependent killing agents. The elimination half-life and the duration of the postantibiotic effect determine the dosing interval. Once-daily dosing of aminoglycosides leads to lower/undetectable trough levels, which reduces their nephrotoxicity.

SEPSIS

Volume of distribution and clearance are the two pharmacokinetic parameters that are most significantly affected by pathophysiologic state during inflammation. For hydrophilic antibiotics, an increased interstitial volume, as occurs with third spacing in sepsis, leads to a large increase in volume of distribution. The consequence might be insufficient peak concentrations of concentration-dependent killing agents like gentamicin, and insufficient time antibiotic concentrations exceed the MIC for time-dependent killing agents. Under these circumstances, higher doses would be necessary, and extended or continuous infusion for time-dependent antimicrobials (beta-lactams) are proposed. Augmented renal clearance occurs early in sepsis, whereas renal insufficiency frequently occurs in later phases. For renally excreted antimicrobial agents, this would lead to decreased and increased exposure, respectively.

PREVENTION OF RESISTANCE

Besides killing pathogens, optimal dosing has been suggested to prevent the selection of resistance. A large population of pathogens may contain a smaller population of microorganisms with increased MIC compared with the wild-type population that will grow out with a fixed dose. The mutant prevention concentration (MPC) is the lowest concentration that prevents the growth of the most-resistant single-step mutants. Dosing regimens considering this MPC have prevented the emergence of resistance in animal models, but this concept has not yet been applied in clinical practice. What has been shown is that a low daily dose of beta-lactam antibiotics and a longer duration of treatment were associated with pharyngeal carriage of penicillin-resistant pneumococci in children.

Preferred Route of Administration

The ultimate effect of the antimicrobial agent on the microorganism depends on its intrinsic properties and its concentration at the site of infection. From the microorganism's perspective, it is therefore irrelevant how the antimicrobial has been administered. Bioavailability and the available formulations primarily determine the route of administration. Because of the high bioavailability of certain antimicrobials (quinolones, clindamycin, metronidazole, fluconazole, voriconazole), these should preferentially be administered orally unless a patient vomits or has malabsorption. One should also be aware that drug–drug and food–drug interactions can decrease absorption. For example, this is the case when ciprofloxacin and iron or aluminum- or magnesium-containing antacids are taken simultaneously or when pheneticillin is not taken 1 hour before or 2 hours after a meal. Some antimicrobials only have an oral or an intravenous formulation. The latter is the case for many cephalosporins and a few penicillins. Furthermore, many penicillins cause gastrointestinal intolerance in the high doses required for severe infections, whereas these doses are well-tolerated when given intravenously. In severe or deep-seated infections or otherwise protected areas, as discussed earlier, intravenous administration is indicated to achieve adequate concentrations. The foregoing exemplifies that the preferred route of administration also affects the choice of an antimicrobial regimen.

An indication for intravenous administration is often an obstacle to outpatient treatment because this type of care traditionally requires hospital admission. However, there is a group of patients that is well enough to start or continue therapy outside of the hospital. Outpatient parenteral antimicrobial therapy (OPAT) offers an alternative to inpatient care. It is a method for delivering intravenous antimicrobials in the community or outpatient setting. OPAT was first described in 1974, and since then much experience has been gained. It is proven safe, cost-effective, and improves patient satisfaction. All types of infections can be treated outside the hospital provided that the patient does not need hospital care and follow-up is guaranteed. There are different care models within which the parenteral therapy can be provided. For example, the drugs can be administered at the patient's home, in hospital-based ambulatory care clinics, in freestanding infusion centers, or in long-term care facilities. Patients or informal caregivers—if trained—can

TABLE 4.3 ■ Aspects to Be Addressed and Associated Actions When Reassessing Antimicrobial Treatment for a (Presumed) Diagnosis of Infection

Questions	Potential Scenario	Potential Action
What is the (probable) clinical diagnosis of infection?	Unchanged	Continue treatment
	New diagnosis (if treatment was withheld/delayed or secondary infection)	Initiate treatment
	Noninfectious diagnosis	Stop treatment
What is the clinical response to empiric treatment?	Unchanged	Continue treatment. See deterioration if there is no response for a longer period.
	Improvement	Continue treatment De-escalation
	Deterioration	Reconsider diagnosis, including new diagnostics Nonpharmacologic treatment (e.g., abscess drainage) Continue treatment (if diagnosis is confirmed) Escalation, in case of anticipated resistance
What are the results of microbiologic testing?	Pending	Continue treatment
	Negative	Discontinue treatment if no infectious syndrome is present
	Microbiologic diagnosis	Targeted treatment
Are conditions present that might affect the concentration of the antimicrobial?	Yes	Therapeutic drug monitoring Dose adaptation
	No	Continue treatment in current dose
Are there signs or symptoms of side effects?	Yes	Continue plus frequent monitoring (if mild) Change treatment (if severe)
	No	Continue treatment
Is intravenous-to-oral switch possible?	Yes	Switch to oral treatment
	No	Continue intravenous administration
What is the optimal duration of treatment?	Not applicable	Determine stop date

actively participate in OPAT. A hospital should have an OPAT program that provides a framework for safe and effective care and that is preferably part of the ASP. Such an OPAT program covers all the organizational aspects, as well as the different phases of OPAT care at the patient level (initiation, follow-up, and outcome), in terms of both care at patient level and regarding responsibilities.

(Dis)continuation of Antimicrobial Therapy

Table 4.3 summarizes the questions that should be addressed in the days following the initiation of antimicrobial therapy and the potential action that might follow this assessment. Ideally, reassessment should take place daily, but an assessment on days 2 to 3 makes sense because by that

TABLE 4.4 ■ **Examples of Indications for Bedside Consultations by an Infectious Disease Specialist**

Prolonged fever without a cause
Fever in an immunocompromised patient without an obvious cause
Unexplained fever in a severely ill patient
S. aureus bacteremia
Invasive fungal infection
Infective endocarditis
Opportunistic infection
Complicated course of an infection

time, culture results will have become available and a clinical response might be expected. Some aspects will be discussed in more detail next.

THE DETERIORATING PATIENT: INTENSIFYING TREATMENT OR NOT?

In a patient whose clinical condition is deteriorating, it is of great importance to try to determine the cause, while at the same time anticipating the moment when a possible intervention might prevent further deterioration. Reconsidering the initial diagnosis and potential complications of the primary disease (e.g., formation of an abscess or empyema) is always the first step, followed by considering the occurrence of a hospital-acquired infection. Noninfectious disorders, like drug allergy, phlebitis, thrombosis, and (pseudo)gout, should be considered as well. This requires a full workup and obtaining new cultures. If the diagnosis is uncertain and the patient has had several days of treatment, cessation of the antimicrobial treatment can be justified—or even necessary— to establish a diagnosis. Under these circumstances, it is recommended to consult an infectious disease specialist (Table 4.4). Virulence of the microorganism and/or an underlying condition can also be responsible for the deterioration while the chosen regimen covers the pathogens. Escalating treatment (i.e., the change to a more broad-spectrum regimen) is not indicated at this time, but rather nonpharmacologic interventions are required: optimizing fluid management, sputum evacuation, etc. If these considerations do not apply to the patient and he or she is severely ill, escalation is indicated awaiting the results of the workup, because inappropriate empiric treatment could negatively influence outcome.

DE-ESCALATION OF TREATMENT

De-escalation, or streamlining, means changing the treatment to narrow-spectrum antimicrobials or stopping once culture results have become available. If broad-spectrum treatment was initiated anticipating antimicrobial resistance but culture results have excluded this, treatment can also be narrowed toward only covering the expected pathogens and ignoring potential multidrug resistance. Many mostly real-life studies have shown that changing to targeted and narrow-spectrum treatment is safe. Similar results have been obtained for discontinuation of empiric treatment in patients without lack of clinical or microbiologic evidence of infection. These principles of good antimicrobial prescribing are essential in diminishing selection pressure on pathogens and commensals.

THERAPEUTIC DRUG MONITORING

Changes in renal function or other biologic processes that might affect pharmacokinetic parameters can lead to ineffective or toxic concentrations (see earlier). Anticipating or

TABLE 4.5 ■ **Generally Accepted Criteria for Safe Intravenous-to-Oral Switch**

Vital signs should be good or improving.

Signs and symptoms related to the infection have to be improved.

Absence of malabsorption.

Oral intake should be possible.

Oral administration should achieve adequate antimicrobial concentrations at the site of infection. This means the following infections are contraindicated:

  Ongoing sepsis

  Necrotizing fasciitis

  Central nervous system infection

  Initial phase of *S. aureus* bacteremia

  Endovascular infection (e.g., endocarditis)

An oral formulation of the antibiotic with good bioavailability has to exist.

following these events, doses should be adapted. Therapeutic drug monitoring (TDM) aims to individualize the dose based on the concentrations measured to increase efficacy and decrease toxicity. If technically feasible, TDM should be considered if there is a large interpatient variability of pharmacokinetics, a well-characterized relationship between concentration and effect, and a small therapeutic window (i.e., the range between minimum effective concentrations and minimum toxic concentrations). Commonly used antimicrobial drugs for which TDM is generally recommended are the aminoglycosides, vancomycin, and some triazoles, such as itraconazole and voriconazole. Clinical studies have shown that performing TDM for aminoglycosides and vancomycin reduces the incidence of nephrotoxicity, whereas the effect of structural performance of TDM on mortality still remains to be shown.

INTRAVENOUS-TO-ORAL SWITCH

Oral administration has many advantages over intravenous (IV) administration and should therefore be actively pursued. A timely IV–oral switch reduces length of stay, workload of nurses, costs, and iatrogenic complications. Furthermore, it increases patient satisfaction and has been proven safe if the right patients are selected. Generally accepted criteria for IV–oral switch are presented in Table 4.5.

TREATMENT DURATION

It has become clear that for many indications, the treatment duration can be shorter than previously recommended, although for many infections high-quality studies assessing the optimal treatment duration are lacking (Table 4.6). Early treatment cessation does not select for resistance; on the contrary, it benefits the preservation of the microbiome and reduces development of collateral resistance. The course should have the length that is required for clinical success without relapse, although complete resolution of signs and symptoms is generally not obtained—nor required—before the course ends. Most guidelines give recommendations on treatment duration in days (often 5 or 7 or 14), but usually ignore the clinical response and other patient characteristics. Resolution of fever or host-derived biomarkers such as procalcitonin have already shown to be useful in guiding treatment duration in certain infections and may lead to a more personalized approach rather than indication-specific recommendations.

TABLE 4.6 ■ Summary of Optimal Treatment Duration for Infectious Diseases Derived from Randomized Controlled Trials

Infection	Comparison (days)	Shortest Effective Treatment Duration (for the whole population)
Community-acquired pneumonia in adults	3–5 versus 8–10	3–5 days
Otitis media in children 6–23 months	5 versus 10	10 days
Streptococcal pharyngitis in children	3–6 versus 10	3–6 days
Complicated urinary tract infection in adults	5–7 versus 10–14	Women: 7 days (fluoroquinolones) Men: 10–14 days
Cellulitis in adults	5 versus 10	5 days
Ventilator-associated pneumonia in adults	7–8 versus 10–15	7–8 days, except for fermenting Gram-negative bacilli
Intraabdominal infection in adults with adequate source control	4 versus 8	4 days

Data from Llewelyn MJ, et al. The antibiotic course has had its day. *BMJ*. 2017;358:j3418; El Massaoui R, et al. *BMJ*. 2006;10:322:1355; Uranga A, et al. *JAMA Intern Med*. 2016;176:1257-1265; Hoberman A, et al. *N Engl J Med*. 2016;375:2446-2456; Altamimi S, et al. *Cochrane Database Syst Rev*. 2012:CD004872; Sandberg T., et al. *Lancet*. 2012;380:484-490; Peterson J, et al. *Urology*. 2008;71:17-22; Van Nieuwkoop C, et al. *BMC Med*. 2017;15:70; Hepburn MJ, et al. *Arch Intern Med*. 2004;164:1669-1674; Pugh, et al. *Cochrane Database Syst Rev*. 2015:CD007577; Sawyer RG, et al. *N Engl J Med*. 2015;372:1996-2005.

Antimicrobial Prophylaxis

Antimicrobial prophylaxis aims to prevent infections. Three types of prophylaxis can be distinguished: perioperative prophylaxis; prophylaxis given before interventions other than surgery—for example, endoscopic retrograde cholangiopancreatography (ERCP) or certain interventions performed by intervention radiologists; and medical prophylaxis in patients at high risk of infections (e.g., transplant recipients). Weighing benefits and disadvantages (mainly selection of antimicrobial resistance and toxicity) underlies the decision-making process. For example, in perioperative prophylaxis, the type of traumatic wound determines the indication for antibiotic prophylaxis. Clean-contaminated (e.g., colectomy) and contaminated wounds (e.g., recent traumatic wounds) are associated with a risk of surgical site infection of 5% to 10% and 10% to 20%, respectively, and have thus led to the recommendation to use perioperative antibiotic prophylaxis in these types of surgery. Despite the low risk of surgical site infection (<5%) in clean wounds (e.g., hip replacement surgery), antibiotic prophylaxis is advised because of the severe impact of a postoperative infection in the presence of a prosthesis.

In prophylaxis, the agent chosen should have activity against the most common pathogens of surgical site infections. In clean procedures, the predominant causative agents of surgical site infections are skin commensals, including *S. aureus*, whereas in colorectal surgery, breaches in both skin and mucosa are made. This explains why the infecting bacteria of intra-abdominal infections after colorectal surgery are frequently part of the fecal microbiota, such as Gram-negative rods (e.g., *Escherichia coli*) and anaerobes (e.g., *Bacteroides fragilis*). A reasonable regimen in clean surgery would be a first- or second-generation cephalosporin combined with metronidazole in colorectal surgery. Preoperative *S. aureus* decolonization of the anterior nares with topical mupirocin in addition to IV antimicrobial prophylaxis reduces surgical site infections after cardiac and orthopedic procedures.

To reach adequate tissue concentrations from incision to wound closure, most antimicrobials should be given within 60 minutes before incision. Administration of antimicrobial agents that require longer administration, like vancomycin, should be started earlier. The antimicrobial's half-life and the amount of blood loss determine the need for a repeat dose. Postoperative continuation of prophylaxis is not indicated and leads to unnecessary adverse events and development of antimicrobial resistance.

Antimicrobial Stewardship Programs

Many hospitals and other health care institutions have an ASP. Antimicrobial stewardship is the persistent effort to measure and improve the appropriate use of antimicrobial agents. ASPs try to find a balance between the optimal care for the individual patient—improved outcome and reduced toxicity—and their potentially negative effect for other and future patients (i.e., the development of antimicrobial resistance). As such, antimicrobial stewardship has also been described as "a coherent set of actions designed to use antimicrobials in ways that ensure sustainable access to effective therapy for all who need them."

ASPs consist of three components: prerequisites, stewardship objectives, and improvement interventions. Prerequisites are structural conditions that should be met when initiating an ASP. Among these is a multidisciplinary stewardship team that has the mandate of the hospital board of directors, as well as financial and information technology (IT) support. An infectious disease specialist, clinical microbiologist, and hospital pharmacist generally form the core of such a stewardship team, sometimes complemented with other clinical stakeholders and a nurse. The presence of guidelines for the management of infectious diseases is another crucial aspect of ASPs. These should guide the prescribers and should at the same time function as the norm against which the stewardship team compares the actual prescriptions to measure the quality of antimicrobial use. National guidelines should form the basis for the local guidelines, but adaptations should be made based on local resistance patterns. As discussed in the section "Activity Against (Expected) Pathogens," surveillance of antimicrobial resistance is essential for translating the local epidemiology into effective treatment recommendations. Antimicrobial stewardship objectives describe the recommended use of antimicrobials at the patient level. Examples include guideline-accordant choice of empiric regimen, taking blood cultures and cultures from the site of infection, timely IV–oral switch, and correct duration of treatment. Stewardship teams make a selection from these stewardship objectives on which they will focus as a team. A systematic literature search and international consensus procedure have been performed to develop quality indicators for responsible antimicrobial use that can be used by stewardship teams worldwide to measure the quality of antimicrobial use. Unfortunately, recommended care does not automatically find its way into daily practice, and this also applies to the performance of appropriate antimicrobial prescribing. Stewardship teams have a large set of interventions at their disposal to achieve the stewardship objectives (i.e., optimizing antimicrobial use). These improvement interventions can be structural (e.g., decisional support system or the introduction of rapid diagnostic testing), persuasive (e.g., educational outreach by academic detailing), or restrictive (e.g., selective reporting of laboratory susceptibilities and formulary restriction requiring prior authorization). Any improvement intervention might work, and the challenge for the stewardship team is to select that intervention or set of interventions that is anticipated to work best in a specific setting. This means that understanding the determinants, both facilitators and barriers, of the antimicrobial is crucial in tailoring behavioral change interventions. Education will not work, for example, if lack of knowledge is not the key driver of inappropriate use. Making use of an opinion leader that promotes good clinical practice and audit and feedback to individual prescribers can be effective strategies to change a dysfunctional attitude.

Suggested Reading

Blumenthal KG, Peter JG, Trubiano JA, Phillips EJ. Antibiotic allergy. *Lancet*. 2019;393:183–198.

Drusano GL. Antimicrobial pharmacodynamics: critical interactions of 'bug and drug'. *Nat Rev Microbiol*. 2014;2:289–300.

Hulscher MEJL, Prins JM. Antibiotic stewardship: does it work in hospital practice? A review of the evidence base. *Clin Microbiol Infect*. 2017;23:799–805.

Llewelyn MJ, Fitzpatrick JM, Darwin E, et al. The antibiotic course has had its day. *BMJ*. 2017;358:j3418.

Monnier AA, Schouten J, Le Maréchal M, et al. Quality indicators for responsible antibiotic use in the inpatient setting: a systematic review followed by an international multidisciplinary consensus procedure. *J Antimicrob Chemother*. 2018;73(suppl 6):vi30–vi39.

Schuts EC, Hulscher MEJL, Mouton JW, et al. Current evidence on hospital antimicrobial stewardship objectives: a systematic review and meta-analysis. *Lancet Infect Dis*. 2016;16:847–856.

Tattevin T, Solomon T, Brouwer MC. Understanding central nervous system efficacy of antimicrobials. *Intensive Care Med*. 2019;45(1):93–96.

A Primer on Antimicrobials

Richard R. Watkins

Introduction

The serendipitous discovery of penicillin by Sir Alexander Fleming in 1928 was one of the greatest medical advances of the 20th century and marks the beginning of the antibiotic era. The term *antibiotic* originated with Selman Waksman in 1941, who defined it as any small molecule made by a microbe that antagonizes the growth of another microbe. With the widespread clinical use of antibiotics in the late 1940s came the ability to treat both minor and life-threatening infections. Antibiotics allow surgeons to perform complex procedures; have a major role in the success of organ transplantations; enable oncologists to prescribe lifesaving doses of chemotherapy, making bone marrow transplants feasible; and have greatly reduced the burden of major infectious diseases that have plagued humankind since antiquity, such as plague and tuberculosis (TB). Yet these pillars of modern medicine are threatened by the ongoing spread of antibiotic resistance, a major driver of which is the misuse of antibiotics. Thus, prescribing antibiotics judiciously is paramount to protect their long-term effectiveness and to prevent a return to the pre-antibiotic era.

The first effective antibacterial agent to be introduced was the sulfonamide prontosil in 1935, for which its discoverer, Domagk, was awarded the Nobel Prize in Medicine or Physiology in 1939. The life of Domagk's own 6-year-old daughter was saved by the drug after she developed a severe staphylococcal infection. During World War II, the industrialization of penicillin production led to major improvements in morbidity and mortality for Allied soldiers.

The period following the war until the early 1960s is often referred to as the golden age of antibiotic development, in which many new classes of antibiotics were introduced. But over the next 40 years the pace of antibiotic discovery slowed, with no new classes approved during that period. An innovation comeback in the early part of the 21st century resulted in several new agents being approved, although many of these were variants from existing classes with modified side chains.

This chapter describes our current antibacterial and antifungal armamentarium, as well as agents in late stages of clinical development, with an emphasis on mechanism of action, spectrum of activity, pharmacology, clinical indications, resistance mechanisms, and adverse events. An understanding of these principles will help the reader optimize their use of antibiotics while minimizing the risk for side effects and toxicities and limit the spread of antibiotic resistance. Antimycobacterial agents, antiparasitic agents, and antivirals are discussed in other chapters. In addition, antibiotic dosing was not addressed herein, and readers should refer to specific chapters for this information.

Antibacterial Agents

β-LACTAMS

β-lactam drugs, including penicillins, cephalosporins, monobactams, and carbapenems, are so named due to the presence of a β-lactam ring at the core of their chemical structure. They are bactericidal agents that inhibit cell wall synthesis by binding to penicillin-binding proteins (PBPs). The penicillins can be subdivided into the natural penicillins, such as penicillin G and bicillin; penicillinase-resistant penicillins, like nafcillin and oxacillin; aminopenicillins, which include ampicillin and amoxicillin; carboxypenicillins, like ticarcillin and carbenicillin; and the ureidopenicillins, which include piperacillin, azlocillin, and mezlocillin. Activity of the penicillins can be extended against aminopenicillin-resistant Gram-negative bacilli with the addition of a β-lactamase inhibitor, like tazobactam, clavulanate, or sulbactam. Cephalosporins are a diverse class of agents grouped by generations from first to fifth based on increasing activity against Gram-negative bacilli. The third-generation cephalosporin ceftazidime has been combined with the novel non–β-lactam β-lactamase inhibitor avibactam, leading to improved activity against most Enterobacteriaceae, including ceftazidime-resistant strains. Ceftazidime/avibactam also has activity against strains of carbapenemase-producing *Klebsiella pneumoniae*. Ceftolozane/tazobactam is another combination designed primarily to treat resistant Gram-negative bacilli, including *Pseudomonas aeruginosa*. The first fifth-generation drug, ceftaroline, is the only currently available cephalosporin with activity against methicillin-resistant *Staphylococcus aureus* (MRSA). Currently, aztreonam is the only available monobactam and is only effective against aerobic Gram-negative bacilli. Aztreonam/avibactam is under development primarily for carbapenem-resistant Enterobacteriaceae (CRE), and is notable for having activity against metallo-β-lactamases. Carbapenems, which include imipenem, doripenem, meropenem, and ertapenem, have the broadest spectrum activity of all the β-lactams. They have traditionally been used for polymicrobial infections and in patients with severe sepsis for whom there is a concern about antibiotic-resistant pathogens. Unfortunately, the efficacy of carbapenems has been decreasing due to the spread of carbapenemase-producing Gram-negative bacilli. Meropenem/vaborbactam was approved in 2017 for complicated urinary tract infections (UTIs) and currently is active against many CRE strains. Table 5.1 describes the most frequently used β-lactam agents in clinical practice. For a comprehensive list of all available antibiotics, the reader is encouraged to consult the latest version of the Sanford Guide.

TABLE 5.1 ■ Properties of Frequently Used β-Lactam Antibiotics

Antibiotic	Spectrum of Activity	Pharmacology	Common Clinical Uses	Mechanism of Resistance	Adverse Events
Penicillin G	Strep, *T. pallidum*, anaerobes, some enterococci	PO, IV, or IM routes	Oral infections, syphilis, pharyngitis GAS	Penicillinases	Rash in 2%–3%
Ampicillin and amoxicillin	Same as penicillin G plus some GNB	Ampicillin IV or IM, amoxicillin PO	Enterococcal endocarditis, oral infections, GAS pharyngitis	Penicillinases	Rash in 5%–9%, Increased risk with EBV
Amoxicillin/ Clavulanate	GPC as above, GNB, anaerobes	Less diarrhea with bid regimens	Mixed bacterial infections	Penicillinases	Hepatic injury, usually mild
Nafcillin	MSSA and some strep	>90% protein bound, need 12 g daily for bacteremia	Serious MSSA infections like bacteremia, endocarditis and osteomyelitis	*mecA* gene encodes the low-affinity penicillin binding protein, PBP 2a	Neutropenia, hypokalemia
Ampicillin/sulbactam	β-lactamase-producing GPC, anaerobes, GNB	IV or IM routes	Oral and neck infections, mixed skin infections; not active against *P. aeruginosa*	Not recommended for IAIs due to increasing resistance in *E. coli* caused by plasmid-mediated TEM-1 β-lactamase	GI symptoms
Piperacillin/ tazobactam	GPC except MRSA, GNB including *P. aeruginosa*, anaerobes	Use 4.5 g IV q6h for nosocomial pneumonia; prolonged infusions probably more effective	UTIs, HAP/VAP, IAIs, mixed skin infections	β-lactamases	Thrombocytopenia, increased risk of AKI with vancomycin
Cefazolin	GPC including MSSA, some GNB	Use 2 g IV q8h for serious infections, e.g., bacteremia	Skin infections, bacteremia due to MSSA	β-lactamases and altered PBPs	Increased risk of CDI
Cefoxitin	GPC, some GNB, anaerobes except *B. fragilis*	High bile concentration	Mixed infections	Avoid treating *B. fragilis* due to increasing resistance	Increased risk for CDI
Ceftazidime	Many GPC and GNB, including some *P. aeruginosa*	Can be given by prolonged infusion	Nosocomial UTIs, susceptible *P. aeruginosa* infections	β-lactamases	Increased risk for CDI
Ceftriaxone	Many GPC and GNB except *P. aeruginosa*	Good CNS penetration; use 2 g IV q12h for meningitis	CAP, UTIs, combined with ampicillin for enterococcal endocarditis	β-lactamases	Cholelithiasis

Continued

TABLE 5.1 ■ Properties of Frequently Used β-Lactam Antibiotics—cont'd

Antibiotic	Spectrum of Activity	Pharmacology	Common Clinical Uses	Mechanism of Resistance	Adverse Events
Cefepime	Many GPC and GNB, including P. aeruginosa	Use 2 g IV q8h for serious P. aeruginosa infections	Pneumonia, UTIs	β-lactamases	Delirium especially in elderly
Ceftaroline	GPC, only cephalosporin active against MRSA, some GNB but not P. aeruginosa	Use q8h for serious infections, e.g., bacteremia and endocarditis	Skin infections, pneumonia especially MRSA		Neutropenia, direct Coombs test seroconversion, eosinophil PNA
Ceftolozane/ tazobactam	GPC, GNB including MDR P. aeruginosa and ESBL producers	Decreased efficacy with CrCl <50 mL/min	MDR P. aeruginosa infections, combine with metronidazole for IAIs	AmpC and horizontally acquired β-lactamases	Cross reacts with β-lactam allergies
Ceftazidime/ avibactam	GPC, ESBL- and carbapenemase-producing GNB, MDR P. aeruginosa	Infuse over 2 hours	Pneumonia, bacteremia, UTIs, combined with metronidazole for IAIs	Not active against metallo-carbapenemases	Similar to other cephalosporins
Aztreonam	Aerobic GNB	IV and inhaled formulations	UTIs, bacteremia, nosocomial pneumonia	β-lactamases Avoid empirical use	Cross-reacts with ceftazidime allergy
Meropenem	GPC, GNRs, including P. aeruginosa, anaerobes	Use prolonged infusions in critically ill patients	Serious nosocomial infections, mixed infections, IAIs, UTIs from MDR GNB	Carbapenemases	Seizures, increased risk for CDI
Imipenem	Same as for meropenem	Use prolonged infusions in critically ill patients	Same as for meropenem	Carbapenemases	Seizures, increased risk for CDI
Doripenem	Same as for meropenem	Use prolonged infusions in critically ill patients	Same as for meropenem	Carbapenemases	Increased risk for CDI
Ertapenem	GPC except enterococcus, GNB except P. aeruginosa, anaerobes	Can be given IV or IM	Polymicrobial infections, avoid in critically ill septic patients	Carbapenemases	Increased risk for CDI
Meropenem/ vaborbactam	GPC, anaerobes, MDR GNB, including P. aeruginosa and Acinetobacter	Dose q12h with CrCl <30 mL/min	Polymicrobial infections, severe sepsis with MDR GNB	ompK36 mutations; can be used to treat ceftazidime/ avibactam-resistant isolates	Headaches, increased risk for CDI

AKI, Acute kidney injury; bid, twice daily; CAP, community-acquired pneumonia; CDI, Clostridioides difficile infection; CNS, central nervous system; CrCl, creatinine clearance; ESBL, extended spectrum β-lactamase; EBV, Epstein–Barr virus; GAS, group A streptococcus; GI, gastrointestinal; GNB, Gram-negative bacilli; GPC, Gram-positive cocci; HAP, hospital-acquired pneumonia; IAIs, intraabdominal infections; IM, intramuscular; IV, intravenous; MDR, multidrug resistant; MSSA, methicillin-susceptible Staphylococcus aureus; PBPs, penicillin-binding proteins; po; by mouth; Strep, Streptococcus spp.; UTI, urinary tract infection; VAP, ventilator-associated pneumonia.

GLYCOPEPTIDES AND LIPOPEPTIDES

Glycopeptides are bactericidal agents that inhibit cell wall synthesis by binding to precursors of the peptidoglycan chain. Vancomycin was the first glycopeptide and is one of the most commonly prescribed antibiotics for hospitalized patients. A second glycopeptide, teicoplanin, is available in Europe and Asia but not the United States. Vancomycin has activity against most Gram-positive organisms, including MRSA, with the exceptions of *Leuconostoc* spp., *Listeria monocytogenes*, and *Lactobacillus* spp. Certain species of *Enterococcus faecalis* have developed resistance to vancomycin (vancomycin-resistant *Enterococcus* [VRE]). Also, *S. aureus* isolates with intermediate susceptibility to vancomycin (vancomycin intermediate *S. aureus* [VISA]) have been reported, although fortunately they remain uncommon in clinical practice. Vancomycin is routinely used to treat serious Gram-positive infections such as meningitis, endocarditis, osteomyelitis, bacteremia, and skin infections, especially when MRSA coverage is needed or patient allergies preclude the use of β-lactam agents. The development of resistance to vancomycin is mediated in *S. aureus* by the acquisition of resistance genes, primarily *mecA*. Vancomycin trough levels should be monitored during treatment to reduce the risk for nephrotoxicity, especially for patients with underlying kidney disease or an elevated body mass index (BMI). An infusion-related reaction called *red man syndrome* can occur in some patients and is characterized by pruritus and an erythematous rash primarily on the face, neck, and upper torso. Red man syndrome can often be mitigated by slowing the infusion rate and does not indicate that the patient is allergic to vancomycin. Oral vancomycin is used to treat *Clostridioides* (formerly *Clostridium*) *difficile* infection. It is not absorbed and therefore should not be used to treat systemic infections.

The lipoglycopeptides are semi-synthetic derivatives of vancomycin that have long half-lives, allowing them to be dosed less frequently. These include telavancin, dalbavancin, and oritavancin. Only available as intravenous (IV) formulations, they have all been approved for treating skin infections, and telavancin has the additional indication for hospital-acquired and ventilator-associated pneumonia caused by *S. aureus*. Also, oritavancin is active against VRE strains that harbor the *vanA* gene, but dalbavancin and telavancin are not. QT prolongation and nephrotoxicity have been associated with telavancin, and both telavancin and oritavancin can falsely increase results of coagulation tests. The high cost of these agents remains a salient issue and has limited their use.

Daptomycin, the only lipopeptide antibiotic, is a bactericidal agent that causes rapid depolarization of the bacterial cell membrane. It has broad activity against Gram-positive organisms, including *S. aureus* (both methicillin-sensitive *S. aureus* [MSSA] and MRSA), streptococci, and enterococcus (both vancomycin-susceptible strains and VRE). Daptomycin is approved to treat skin infections and *S. aureus* bacteremia, including cases complicated by right-sided infective endocarditis. It is also commonly used to treat infections caused by VRE, such as complicated UTIs and osteomyelitis. Notably, daptomycin should not be used to treat pneumonia, as it is inactivated by pulmonary surfactant. Myositis can occur, especially with prolonged courses and concurrent statin use, and weekly monitoring of creatinine phosphokinase (CPK) is advised.

AMINOGLYCOSIDES

One of the earliest classes of antibiotics, the first aminoglycoside, streptomycin, was released in 1944 and was the first effective drug for TB. This was followed by neomycin, gentamicin, tobramycin, amikacin, and, most recently, plazomicin in 2018. Aminoglycosides are bactericidal agents that block protein synthesis using an oxygen-dependent mechanism. Thus aminoglycosides work poorly in anaerobic environments, such as abscesses. They exhibit concentration-dependent killing and have a significant postantibiotic effect. These properties have allowed the development of extended-interval dosing, which is generally perceived to be safer and possibly more effective than traditional short-interval dosing. It is recommended that drug levels be monitored during therapy to reduce the risk of nephrotoxicity. Aminoglycosides are usually used with another agent, such as a β-lactam, to prevent the development of resistance (which can occur rapidly with aminoglycoside monotherapy) and for synergistic effects. Also, when used as monotherapy, aminoglycosides are inactive against Gram-positive bacteria, as they are unable to diffuse through porins in the thick Gram-positive cell wall. They are most commonly used to treat pyelonephritis, UTIs, Gram-negative bacteremia, and in combination to treat infective endocarditis due to certain Gram-positive cocci. Plazomicin has enhanced activity against multidrug-resistant (MDR) Gram-negative pathogens, including CRE and *Acinetobacter baumannii*, and appears promising for the treatment of ventilator-associated pneumonia. It was also noninferior to meropenem for the treatment of complicated UTIs and acute pyelonephritis due to Enterobacteriaceae, including MDR strains. Bacterial resistance to aminoglycosides is due to the acquisition of aminoglycoside-modifying enzymes (AMEs). Adverse events associated with aminoglycosides include nephrotoxicity, which often improves once the drug is discontinued, and ototoxicity, which may be irreversible. Because they can cause neuromuscular blockade, aminoglycosides should be avoided in patients with myasthenia gravis and those taking calcium channel blockers. Plazomicin appears to have an improved safety profile, with a low incidence of nephrotoxicity and ototoxicity.

QUINOLONES

The first quinolone was nalidixic acid, which was discovered during the production of chloroquine and found to kill Gram-negative bacteria. The addition of fluoride to the drug gave further Gram-negative, Gram-positive, and some anaerobic activity and led to the development of the fluoroquinolones, including ciprofloxacin, gemifloxacin, levofloxacin, moxifloxacin, norfloxacin, ofloxacin, and, most recently, delafloxacin. They are bactericidal agents that block DNA synthesis by inhibiting two bacterial enzymes: DNA gyrase and topoisomerase IV. Like aminoglycosides, quinolones have a postantibiotic effect that lasts 2 to 6 hours after the dose is given. The bioavailability of quinolones is excellent, and they achieve high concentrations in the lung, kidney, bile, prostate, bone, and stool. Quinolones are available in oral, IV, and ocular formulations. The common uses for quinolones are described in Table 5.2. Bacteria can become resistant to quinolones either through target-mediated resistance, which is the most common and is caused by specific mutations in DNA gyrase and topoisomerase IV; plasmid-mediated resistance from extrachromosomal

TABLE 5.2 ■ Clinical Uses for Quinolones[a]

Drug	Common Clinical Uses	Cost
Ciprofloxacin	UTIs, IAIs, HAP and GNB pneumonia, GNB bacteremia, bacterial gastroenteritis including *Salmonella*, anthrax treatment, and prophylaxis	$
Delafloxacin	Mixed skin infections including MRSA and MSSA	$$$
Gemifloxacin	Bronchitis and CAP	$
Levofloxacin	CAP, HAP, UTIs, AECOPD, bacterial sinusitis, GNB bacteremia	$
Moxifloxacin	CAP, aspiration pneumonia, IAIs, mixed bacterial infections	$$
Norfloxacin	UTIs, prostatitis	$
Ofloxacin	Eye infections, otitis media	$

AECOPD, Acute exacerbation of chronic obstructive pulmonary disease; *CAP,* community-acquired pneumonia; *GNB,* Gram-negative bacilli; *HAP,* hospital-acquired pneumonia; *IAIs,* intraabdominal infections; *UTIs,* urinary tract infections.
[a]Because of safety concerns, other agents are now recommended as first-line therapy for several common conditions (e.g., sinusitis, UTI, pneumonia) instead of quinolones.

elements that encode proteins that disrupt quinolone–enzyme interactions, alter drug metabolism, or increase quinolone efflux; or chromosome-mediated resistance, which causes an underexpression of porins or an overexpression of efflux pumps. Some common adverse events associated with quinolones include gastrointestinal symptoms, tendonitis (for which the risk is highest in the elderly and those on corticosteroids), QT prolongation, hypoglycemia, and *C. difficile* infection. The Food and Drug Administration (FDA) has issued several black box warnings for quinolones, including to avoid them in patients with myasthenia gravis and for an increased risk for mental health side effects, serious blood sugar disturbances, tendinitis and tendon rupture, irreversible neuropathy, and (in late 2018) aortic aneurysm or dissection. *Because of the risks associated with quinolones, in 2016, the FDA recommended they should not be used for acute sinusitis, acute bronchitis, and uncomplicated UTIs when other treatment options are available.* Antacids and products containing calcium, aluminum, magnesium, iron, or zinc can reduce the oral absorption of fluoroquinolones, and patients should be advised to not take them concurrently. Finally, there are many drugs that interact with quinolones, some of which include warfarin, theophylline, nonsteroidal antiinflammatory drugs (NSAIDs), cyclosporine, phenytoin, rifampin, and cycloserine.

MACROLIDES

The currently available macrolides include erythromycin, clarithromycin, and fidaxomicin; azithromycin, an azalide, is included as a macrolide in this chapter. Telithromycin was the first ketolide, which are similar in structure to macrolides. Its use was dramatically reduced in 2007 after an FDA warning about acute liver injury, which led to the withdrawal of the drug in the United States. Macrolides inhibit protein synthesis by binding to the bacterial ribosome and blocking translocation of the growing peptide chain. Azithromycin and clarithromycin have better oral absorption and tolerability than erythromycin, which was the first of the class to be developed and is mostly used now as a prokinetic agent. Azithromycin and clarithromycin are used to treat upper and lower respiratory tract infections, group A β-hemolytic streptococcal infections in penicillin-allergic patients, and in combination therapy to treat mycobacterial infections. Azithromycin has been the most commonly prescribed outpatient antibiotic in the United States for the past several years. Fidaxomicin is approved to treat *C. difficile* infection, although it is usually limited in use to recurrent infections due to the drug's high cost. In addition to their antibacterial activity, macrolides have antiinflammatory and immunomodulatory properties. It is for these reasons that azithromycin is frequently prescribed for patients with bronchiectasis and cystic fibrosis. Resistance to macrolides most often occurs via the acquisition of methylases that change the drug-binding site on the ribosome. Adverse events include gastrointestinal symptoms and QT prolongation. QTc monitoring every 3 to 4 months is recommended for patients who are on macrolides long term.

TETRACYCLINES

Discovered over 60 years ago in soil microorganisms, tetracyclines possess many traits of an ideal antibiotic agent, including activity against both Gram-positive and Gram-negative bacteria, proven clinical safety, good tolerability, and the availability of both oral and IV formulations. The tetracyclines currently available include doxycycline, minocycline, tigecycline, eravacycline, and omadacycline. They are bacteriostatic agents that inhibit protein synthesis by binding to the 30S ribosomal subunit at a different site than the aminoglycosides. Doxycycline, minocycline, and omadacycline have high bioavailability and, like quinolones, their absorption is decreased by orally administered multivalent cations (e.g., calcium, magnesium).

There are many clinical uses for the tetracyclines. Doxycycline is effective therapy for community-acquired pneumonia (CAP); skin infections, including those due to MRSA; Lyme disease;

Rocky Mountain spotted fever; typhus; Q fever; cat scratch disease; anaplasmosis; and *Chlamydia trachomatis* infection and can be used as prophylaxis against malaria. Minocycline is often prescribed for acne and is sometimes used in combination with imipenem for serious *A. baumanii* infections. Tigecycline is a derivative of minocycline and is only available by IV. It can be used for treating skin infections, intraabdominal infections, and CAP. The FDA issued a black box warning about using tigecycline for hospital-acquired and ventilator-acquired pneumonia, as data have shown an increase in mortality compared with other agents. Tigecycline is also used in combination with colistin for MDR Gram-negative pathogens, such as *A. baumannii*. It has no activity against *P. aeruginosa*, *Proteus* spp., and *Providencia* spp. Eravacycline was recently approved for intraabdominal infections and has broad activity against a number of MDR pathogens, including extended-spectrum β-lactamase (ESBL)–producing Enterobacteriaceae, MRSA, and VRE. It is not active against *P. aeruginosa* and is only available for IV administration. Omadacycline is another recent addition to the antibiotic armamentarium. It is approved to treat CAP and skin infections and is available in oral and IV formulations. Omadacycline was designed to overcome tetracycline resistance and has broad-spectrum activity that includes Gram-positive and Gram-negative bacteria, anaerobes, atypicals, and some drug-resistant strains like MRSA. Antibiotic resistance to tetracyclines is often plasmid-mediated and attributable to efflux pumps or proteins that protect the ribosomes.

Tetracyclines are among the safest classes of antibiotics. The most common adverse events are gastrointestinal symptoms and photosensitivity. Esophagitis can occur, so patients should be encouraged to take oral formulations with a full glass of water and remain upright for at least half an hour. Minocycline has a higher risk of vestibular symptoms, such as vertigo and ataxia. Although previously it was recommended that tetracyclines be avoided in pregnancy and in those <8 years of age due to the risk of teeth discoloration, a systematic review found there was no correlation between the use of doxycycline during pregnancy and teratogenic effects or dental staining in children. The 2018 American Academy of Pediatrics *Red Book* states that "doxycycline can be used for short durations (i.e., 21 days or less) without regard to patient age." Also, the FDA issued a statement reporting that an expert review of published data on experiences with doxycycline use during pregnancy by the Teratogen Information System (TERIS) concluded that therapeutic doses during pregnancy are unlikely to pose a substantial teratogenic risk, though not zero risk. Therefore in serious infections, the benefit of doxycycline may outweigh its potential harm in pregnant women. There are few drug interactions associated with tetracyclines, although they can interfere with warfarin levels. Tetracyclines may reduce the efficacy of oral contraceptives, and additional forms of contraception should be recommended during tetracycline therapy.

CLINDAMYCIN

Derived from lincomycin, clindamycin binds to the 50S ribosomal subunit and thereby inhibits protein synthesis. It is active against many Gram-positive bacteria, including MSSA and some strains of MRSA, and anaerobes, although *Bacteroides fragilis* is becoming increasingly resistant. Available in both IV and oral formulations, clindamycin has excellent bioavailability. It has very few drug interactions. Clindamycin is used to treat skin infections, dental infections, lung abscesses when caused by susceptible pathogens, and in combination for *Pneumocystis* pneumonia and toxoplasmosis. It was shown to be more effective than metronidazole for anaerobic pulmonary infections. Topical formulations can be prescribed for acne and hidradenitis suppurativa. Clindamycin is also used as a substitution for β-lactam–allergic patients. It has toxin-binding properties and is useful add-on therapy for necrotizing skin infections caused by *Clostridium* spp., *Streptococcus pyogenes*, and *S. aureus*. Resistance is often caused by acquired methylases that modify the ribosomal drug-binding site. Gastrointestinal symptoms such as nausea and vomiting are the most common adverse events. Notably, clindamycin is one of the most frequent antibiotics associated with the development of *C. difficile* infection, which has prompted many to avoid use of this drug.

OXAZOLIDINONES

There are two oxazolidinones, linezolid and tedizolid, which are synthetic bacteriostatic compounds. They have only Gram-positive activity and inhibit protein synthesis by binding to the 50S ribosomal subunit. Both drugs have high bioavailability and are available in oral and IV formulations. Tedizolid is approved for adults with skin infections caused by MRSA and MSSA, *S. pyogenes*, *S. agalactiae*, the *S. anginosus* group (including *S. anginosus*, *S. intermedius*, and *S. constellatus*), and *E. faecalis* (both vancomycin-susceptible and VRE strains). Linezolid has additional indications for pneumonia due to *S. pneumoniae* and *S. aureus* and VRE infections, including bacteremia. Resistance to the oxazolidinones is more common in enterococci than staphylococci and is mediated by mutations in 23S transfer RNA (tRNA) genes, resulting in reduced ribosomal binding by the drug. Adverse events usually occur after long-term use (i.e., after 28 days) and include lactic acidosis, myelosuppression, and both optic and peripheral neuropathy, which unfortunately can be permanent. Tedizolid may be less likely than linezolid to cause these toxicities. Both drugs interact with serotonergic agents and can cause serotonin syndrome, although the risk is lower with tedizolid.

METRONIDAZOLE

Metronidazole is used to treat infections caused by anaerobic organisms and parasites. It is a bactericidal drug that has good oral absorption. Metronidazole is active against almost all clinically important anaerobes, including *B. fragilis*, *Helicobacter pylori*, and *C. difficile*. It used to be first-line therapy for mild to moderate *C. difficile* infection, but oral vancomycin is now recommended. Metronidazole is still given IV in combination with oral vancomycin in severe cases. Other clinical uses include bacterial vaginosis, intraabdominal infections in combination with another agent with Gram-negative coverage, oral infections and lung abscesses in combination with a Gram-positive agent, bone and joint infections due to anaerobes, and mixed infections such as those that occur in a diabetic foot or sacral pressure ulcer. Metronidazole is used for parasitic infections caused by *Giardia lamblia*, *Entamoeba histolytica*, *Blastocystis hominis*, and *Balantidium coli*. Resistance to metronidazole is rare and may result from enhanced DNA repair mechanisms, efflux pumps, or in strains that lack key endogenous enzymes. The most common adverse events are nausea, vomiting, diarrhea, and a metallic taste in the mouth. Ingestion of alcohol with metronidazole can result in a disulfiram-like reaction. Long-term use (i.e., >28 days) can result in peripheral neuropathy and bone marrow suppression. Rare cases of encephalopathy have been reported. Metronidazole can interact with warfarin, lithium, phenytoin, cimetidine, and phenobarbital.

POLYMYXINS

First developed in the 1940s for treating Gram-negative infections, colistin (polymyxin E) and polymyxin B were abandoned by 1980 due to their nephrotoxicity and the availability of safer alternatives. However, they have re-emerged in the last decade for treating infections due to MDR Gram-negative bacteria. Polymyxins are bactericidal agents that act like a detergent and damage the cell membrane. They have activity against Enterobacteriaceae, *P. aeruginosa*, and *A. baumannii* but not *Burkholderia*, *Serratia*, *Proteus*, *Providencia*, or Gram-positive organisms. Colistin is the active form of colistimethate and is available in both inhaled and IV formulations. The polymyxins are often used to treat serious health care–associated infections such as pneumonia, UTI, and bacteremia. Resistance to polymyxins is plasmid-mediated, including the recently described *mcr*-1 gene. The most common and problematic adverse event is dose-dependent nephrotoxicity, which is usually reversible. There is some evidence that polymyxin B is less nephrotoxic than colistin. Neurotoxicity from polymyxins can also occur.

SULFONAMIDES

Currently there are two sulfonamide drugs in use: trimethoprim-sulfamethoxazole (TMP-SMX) and dapsone. They are bacteriostatic agents and stop cell growth by inhibiting folic acid synthesis. Trimethoprim is a dihydrofolate reductase inhibitor that potentiates the activity of sulfamethoxazole and also has antibacterial properties. It is sometimes prescribed alone for UTI prophylaxis. TMP-SMX has activity against some Gram-positive organisms, including MSSA and MRSA, but is not reliable against streptococci. It previously had broad activity against Gram-negative organisms, but the spread of antimicrobial resistance has reduced its effectiveness. Many community-acquired strains of *Escherichia coli* remain susceptible, but most hospital strains and many strains of *Klebsiella* are resistant. TMP-SMX lacks activity against enterococcus and *P. aeruginosa*. The only nonfermentative Gram-negative organism that is susceptible is *Stenotrophomas maltophilia*. TMP-SMX is commonly prescribed for cystitis, pyelonephritis, skin infections when *S. aureus* is a concern, and treating and preventing *Pneumocystis* pneumonia. Dapsone is used to treat leprosy and for *Pneumocystis* and *toxoplasmosis* prophylaxis. It has also been developed into a gel as a treatment for acne. Recently, leukocytoclastic vasculitis has been shown to resolve with topical dapsone. Resistance to TMP-SMX arises from mutations in the target enzymes or by plasmid acquisition of resistant enzymes, such as a resistant dihydropteroate synthetase or a resistant dihydrofolate reductase.

Adverse events associated with TMP-SMX include rashes (rarely, Stevens–Johnson syndrome), hematologic abnormalities, hyperkalemia, and nephrotoxicity. Dapsone is a common etiology of acquired methemoglobinemia, so all individuals should be screened for G6PD deficiency before starting the drug. However, dapsone gel does not cause clinically significant declines in hemoglobin levels, even in those with G6PD deficiency. Many patients who develop a rash with TMP-SMX can tolerate dapsone. TMP-SMX interacts with many drugs, including warfarin, angiotensin-converting enzyme (ACE) inhibitors, antiarrhythmics like amiodarone, diuretics, and some HIV drugs. A careful review of a patient's medication list is therefore necessary before prescribing TMP-SMX. Also, it should be avoided in the third trimester of pregnancy and for patients on hemodialysis. Dapsone has fewer interactions, including with azole antifungals, clarithromycin, and several malaria drugs.

MISCELLANEOUS AGENTS

Fosfomycin is an oral agent given as a single 3-g dose that is used to treat uncomplicated UTIs. It has seen a resurgence over the last few years due to its activity against MDR pathogens. Fosfomycin is one of the first-line treatment options, along with TMP-SMX and nitrofurantoin, in the Infectious Diseases Society of America (IDSA) guidelines for uncomplicated cystitis in women. It should not be used to treat pyelonephritis or patients who are systemically ill. It is bactericidal and disrupts cell wall synthesis by inhibiting the MurA enzyme. Its spectrum of activity covers Enterococcus, including VRE, and Enterobacteriaceae, including ESBL- and AmpC-producing strains. Thus it can sometimes obviate the need for IV antibiotics. Fosfomycin lacks activity against *P. aeruginosa* and is not reliable for *Klebsiella*, for which minimum inhibitory concentration (MIC) testing is recommended, but most microbiology laboratories do not do this. In addition to UTIs, fosfomycin has good penetration into the prostate, and there are some data for its use in treating chronic prostatitis due to ESBL-producing *E. coli*. There are several mechanisms of resistance to fosfomycin, which can be plasmid or chromosomally mediated and include production of the fosfomycin-inactivating enzyme FosA, amino acid substitutions that decrease fosfomycin-binding affinity, and defects in membrane transporters. Side effects are mild and include nausea, diarrhea, and headache. Fosfomycin can interact with magnesium oxide, metoclopramide, and balsalazide. An IV formulation is available in Europe and is under investigation in the United States.

Nitrofurantoin is another oral agent used for treating and preventing uncomplicated UTIs. It is a bactericidal agent that damages bacterial DNA. Nitrofurantoin is active against many Gram-positive pathogens, including *E. faecalis*, *S. aureus*, *S. saprophyticus* (a common cause of UTIs in young women), group D *Streptococcus*, and *Corynebacterium*. It also has activity against common Gram-negative uropathogens such as *E. coli*, *K. pneumoniae*, and *Enterobacter cloacae*, including ESBL-producing strains. A 5-day course of nitrofurantoin is one of the recommended first-line empiric therapies for acute uncomplicated cystitis in otherwise healthy adult nonpregnant females. It is also a preferred drug for use in pregnancy. Nitrofurantoin has been used for over 60 years to prevent UTIs, and a recent meta-analysis of clinical trials found it remains effective for this purpose. Common side effects include nausea, vomiting, and diarrhea. Patients should be encouraged to take the drug with food to lessen these symptoms and to increase drug absorption. Long-term use increases the risk for pulmonary fibrosis and hepatitis, and nitrofurantoin was previously not recommended for elderly patients with renal impairment due to a higher risk for these events. However, more recent evidence has shown it is not associated with an increased risk of adverse outcomes in elderly patients with an estimated glomerular filtration rate (eGFR) < 60 mL/min and could be used more widely in this population.

Chloramphenicol is a broad-spectrum bacteriostatic antibiotic that has oral, IV, and ocular formulations. It inhibits bacterial growth by binding to the 50S ribosomal subunit and inhibits protein synthesis. Chloramphenicol is active against many Gram-positive organisms, including *Streptococcus* spp. and *Staphylococcus* spp., Gram-negative organisms including *E. coli* and *Neisseria meningitidis* but not *P. aeruginosa*, anaerobes including *Bacteroides* spp. and *Clostridium* spp., and atypical pathogens. It therefore has many potential clinical uses, but because of its severe toxicities chloramphenicol should only be used for severe infections when no alternative agents are available (e.g., meningitis due to *N. meningitidis* in a patent with life-threatening drug allergies). Resistance develops through reduced permeability or uptake, ribosomal mutation, or acetylation to an inactive derivative. The most serious adverse risk with chloramphenicol is aplastic anemia, which can be irreversible and fatal. It may occur even with frequent blood cell count monitoring, and it is mainly for this reason that the drug is rarely used in North America and Europe. Other potential side effects and adverse events include hypersensitivity reactions, optic and peripheral neuritis, and gray baby syndrome, which occurs with the IV form and results from an inability of newborns to metabolize the drug. An association with leukemia has also been observed.

Rifampin is a versatile drug with many clinical uses. Importantly, rifampin is almost always used in combination with other antibiotics because of the rapid development of resistance when used alone. Some exceptions include for meningitis prophylaxis and for latent TB. Rifampin is a member of the rifamycins, which also include rifabutin, rifapentine, and rifaximin. The rifamycins inhibit protein synthesis by blocking bacterial DNA–dependent RNA polymerase. Rifampin is available in oral and IV formulations. It is used in combination for staphylococcal prosthetic valve endocarditis and prosthetic joint infections, *Mycobacterium avium*-intracellulare complex (MAC) infections, active TB, as an alternative to isoniazid for latent TB, with dapsone for leprosy, and for decolonizing carriers of MRSA with a second drug, like doxycycline. Notably, in vitro data do not support the use of rifampin–vancomycin combination therapy for *S. aureus* infections. Resistance to rifampin occurs due to mutations in the gene that codes for RNA polymerase. Rifampin is antagonistic to clindamycin and TMP-SMX. Side effects include nausea, vomiting, diarrhea, and loss of appetite. Rifampin often turns urine, sweat, and tears a red or orange color, which usually resolves after a few days. It is a strong inducer of the cytochrome P450 system and has many drug interactions, some of which include warfarin, β-blockers, statins, steroids, antifungals, oral contraceptive pills, and several antiretroviral drugs. Concomitant ant-acid administration may reduce the absorption of rifampin, and antacids should be taken at least an hour after the drug.

TOPICAL AGENTS

Mupirocin was initially derived from *Pseudomonas fluorescens* in 1971. It acts by inhibiting protein synthesis through the inhibition of the bacterial enzyme isoleucyl-tRNA synthetase. Mupirocin has also been shown to reduce bacterial biofilm. It has activity against staphylococcus, including MRSA; most streptococci (with the exception of *S. bovis*); and some Gram-negative bacteria, including *Hemophilus influenzae*, *Neisseria gonorrhoeae*, *N. meningitidis*, and *Moraxella catarrhalis*. Mupirocin is commonly used for nasal decolonization of MRSA carriers who have recurrent infections. For example, data have shown mupirocin reduces the prevalence of *S. aureus* bacteremia in hemodialysis patients with nasal colonization. However, recolonization can occur after successful decolonization. Another use is for superficial skin infections such as impetigo and folliculitis. Low-level resistance to mupirocin, defined as MICs of 8 to 64 µg/mL, is due to point mutations in the *ileS* gene, whereas high-level resistance, defined as an MIC >512 µg/mL, is caused by acquisition via plasmid of the *mup*A gene. Side effects are usually mild and include pruritus, erythema, tenderness, dryness, or swelling of the treated skin.

Retapamulin is a pleuromutilin antimicrobial derived from *Clitophilus scyphoides*, an edible mushroom. It is approved in the United States for the treatment of impetigo due to MSSA and *S. pyogenes* and in Europe for impetigo and minor wound infections. Resistance is mediated by efflux pumps and may include resistance to clindamycin. Retapamulin may be an option for decolonizing patients with MRSA strains that are resistant to mupirocin.

AGENTS IN LATE STAGES OF DEVELOPMENT

There are several antimicrobial agents in late stages of development that appear promising. Arguably the most pressing need for new antimicrobials is for the treatment of MDR Gram-negative organisms. Aztreonam/avibactam is a combination of already approved agents that shows high in vitro potency against MDR Enterobacteriaceae. Imipenem/relebactam combines an older carbapenem with a novel β-lactamase inhibitor similar in structure to avibactam. It has activity against *P. aeruginosa* and ESBL-producers, including some carbapenem-resistant strains. Sulopenem is a carbapenem with both oral and IV formulations. It has a spectrum of activity similar to ertapenem, and the oral formulation is being investigated in combination with probenecid for UTIs. Cefiderocol is a cephalosporin that exhibits broad Gram-negative activity, including against metallo-β-lactamase–producing pathogens. Iclaprim is a selective bacterial dihydrofolate reductase inhibitor under investigation for skin infections. It has potent activity against a number of Gram-positive pathogens, including MSSA and MRSA. Iclaprim showed noninferiority compared with vancomycin in phase 3 trials for acute skin infections. Lefamulin is a pleuromutilin antibiotic active against respiratory pathogens. It was found to be noninferior to moxifloxacin for CAP, as well as being well tolerated. These drugs and others will be welcome additions to the antibiotic armamentarium, especially given the ongoing spread of antimicrobial resistance.

Antifungal Agents

Most fungal infections in humans are superficial, affecting the skin and nails, such as tinea versicolor and onychomycosis, or the mucosal surfaces, such as thrush of the oral cavity or vulvovaginal candidiasis. However, invasive fungal infections (IFIs) of the bloodstream and internal organs can also occur, mostly in immunocompromised patients, including those with malignancies, HIV, and organ transplants. *Candida albicans* and *Aspergillus fumigatus* have been the most common causes of IFIs, although other molds and *Candida* species (e.g., *C. glabrata*) are becoming more prevalent. The recent emergence of *C. auris* has been met with particular concern because of the difficulty identifying it using routine laboratory methods and its resistance to many antifungal drugs. Currently five classes of antifungal agents are used to treat human fungal infections: polyenes, allylamines, azoles, pyrimidine analogs, and echinocandins.

POLYENES

There are two drugs that constitute the polyene class: amphotericin B (AmB) and nystatin. AmB was isolated in 1955 from *Streptomyces nodosus*. It acts by binding to ergosterol, the principal sterol in the fungal cell membrane, and forms small ion channels that cause rapid leakage of monovalent ions (K^+, Na^+, H^+, and Cl^-) leading to fungal cell death. AmB is only available in an IV formulation. It is highly protein-bound and penetrates poorly into cerebrospinal fluid (CSF). Lipid preparations of AmB have been developed, including liposomal amphotericin B, amphotericin B lipid complex, and amphotericin B colloidal dispersion. These lipid formulations are equally effective but cause fewer adverse events and have largely superseded AmB in clinical practice. AmB is the gold-standard therapy for the treatment of IFIs, being active against most yeast (except *C. lusitaniae* and some *C. auris*) and filamentous fungi except for *Scedosporium* spp., some strains of *Fusarium* spp., and *Aspergillus terreus*. It is used to treat a wide range of fungal pathogens and infections, including cryptococcal meningitis (in combination with flucytosine), invasive aspergillosis, hepatosplenic candidiasis, mucormycosis, disseminated histoplasmosis in AIDS patients, blastomycosis, disseminated coccidioidomycosis, candidemia including endocarditis and endophthalmitis, fusariosis, *Naegleria fowleri*, and leishmaniasis. Resistance to AmB is rare but may develop in fungal strains exposed to subfungicidal plasma concentrations. A number of toxicities are associated with AmB. Nephrotoxicity occurs via a decrease in glomerular filtration rate from vasoconstriction of afferent renal arterioles. Hypokalemia is often the first manifestation of acute kidney injury, followed by a fall in serum bicarbonate and a rise in creatinine. The risk of nephrotoxicity can be reduced by administering 500 mL of normal saline before and after the dose of AmB, avoiding the concurrent use of other nephrotoxic agents, and using lipid formulations of AmB. Acute infusion reactions are common and can be reduced by premedication with acetaminophen, hydrocortisone, and diphenhydramine. Infusion reactions are also an indication for using lipid formulations, which carry a lower risk. Blood cell abnormalities (i.e., thrombocytopenia, anemia, and leukopenia) can occur, along with decreased erythropoietin production.

Nystatin was discovered in 1950 after being isolated from *Streptomyces noursei* and named after the New York State Health Department. Like AmB, nystatin binds to ergosterol and forms pores in the cell membrane leading to K+ leakage. It is available in topical forms and as an oral suspension. No IV formulation is available because high concentrations of nystatin in the blood are toxic. The oral suspension is used for prophylaxis and treatment of oropharyngeal thrush. However, fluconazole should be given to HIV patients with thrush because it has been associated with a longer disease-free interval before relapse. Nystatin cream and powder are used to treat superficial candidal skin infections. These may be more effective than fluconazole in some cases of vulvovaginal candidiasis, especially when caused by *C. glabrata* or fluconazole-resistant *Candida*. Side effects with the oral suspension include a bitter taste, nausea, diarrhea, and abdominal pain. The topical formulations may cause a hypersensitivity rash, itching, burning, and, very rarely, Stevens–Johnson syndrome.

TERBINAFINE

An agent primarily used to treat onychomycosis from dermatophytes, terbinafine is an allylamine available in oral and topical formulations. It blocks ergosterol synthesis by inhibiting the enzyme squalene epoxidase. Terbinafine has good activity against dermatophytes and some activity against nondermatophyte molds and *Candida* species. It is prescribed orally once a day for 6 weeks for onychomycosis of the fingernails and for 12 weeks for toenails. If the full course is taken, the mycologic cure for fingernails is 79% and the complete cure rate is 59%, whereas for toenails, the mycologic cure rate is 70% and the complete cure rate is 38%. Common side effects include nausea, vomiting, headache, and rash. Rarely, liver injury can occur with the oral formulation, and it is not recommended for patients with acute or chronic liver disease.

AZOLES

A versatile class of drugs, the azoles are classified into two groups. The imidazoles have two nitrogens in the azole ring and include clotrimazole, ketoconazole, and miconazole. The triazoles have three nitrogens in the azole ring and include fluconazole, itraconazole, voriconazole, posaconazole, and isavuconazole. Azoles are fungistatic agents that inhibit the cytochrome P450–dependent enzyme lanosterol 14-alpha-demethylase, which converts lanosterol to ergosterol, leading to disruption of the fungal cell membrane. Clotrimazole is available without a prescription as an antifungal cream, whereas prescription troches and throat lozenges are used for treatment and prophylaxis of thrush. Ketoconazole is available in topical and oral formulations. The topical formulation is used to treat skin infections such as athlete's foot, ringworm, tinea versicolor, and seborrheic dermatitis. It was the first orally available azole drug and was previously used to treat systemic candidal infections. However, because of poor absorption and a higher risk of toxicities, including hepatic injury, other oral azoles have replaced ketoconazole for systemic infections. Miconazole is another topical agent that is used to treat ringworm, athlete's foot, and vulvovaginal candidiasis. It is safe in pregnancy, and side effects are usually minor, such as pruritus or irritation at the site of application.

The triazoles are used to treat superficial and invasive fungal infections. Fluconazole is available in both oral and IV formulations. It has activity against most species of *Candida* except *C. krusei* and some species of *C glabrata*. Because of the concern about resistant *Candida*, many clinicians start empiric antifungal therapy with an echinocandin in patients with candidemia, then switch to fluconazole if antimicrobial susceptibilities allow. Because of its good penetration into CSF, fluconazole is used in the treatment of cryptococcal meningitis, although patients with AIDS or those with severe disease usually receive AmB and flucytosine before stepdown therapy with fluconazole is initiated. It is also used to treat coccidioidomycosis, including cases of meningitis. Resistance to fluconazole occurs through mutations in the drug target, by changes in the sterol biosynthesis pathway, and by gain-of-function mutations in transcription factors. Fluconazole is a safe drug compared with AmB, but occasionally adverse events occur, including muscle weakness, alopecia, and hepatotoxicity. Fluconazole should not be taken by pregnant women due to an increased risk for miscarriage.

Itraconazole is only available in an oral formulation in the United States. Blood levels with the oral formulation are variable, and drug level monitoring is recommended, especially when therapy is prolonged. Itraconazole has a wider spectrum of activity compared with fluconazole, which includes *Candida* spp., *Aspergillus* spp., *Histoplasma* spp., and *Blastomyces* spp. It penetrates poorly into the CSF and should not be used for central nervous system (CNS) infections. Adverse events associated with itraconazole include hepatotoxicity, heart failure, and gastrointestinal side effects like nausea and diarrhea. Itraconazole has more drug interactions than fluconazole, including several antiarrhythmics like amiodarone and quinidine (Table 5.3).

Voriconazole has broad activity against *Candida* spp., including *C. glabrata* and *C. krusei*, but is mainly used to treat aspergillosis. Available in oral and IV formulations, dosing adjustments are needed for patients with liver disease and severe renal failure. Drug levels should be monitored in these cases, especially with long-term use. Voriconazole has many drug interactions and toxicities, including rashes, photosensitivity, periostitis, hallucinations and encephalopathy, peripheral neuropathy, alopecia, nail changes, hyponatremia, and visual disturbances. An increased risk for squamous cell skin cancer has also been observed. Posaconazole is available in oral and IV

TABLE 5.3 ■ Drug Interactions of Select Antifungal Agents

Drug	Selected Interactions
Amphotericin B	Antineoplastic agents (e.g., nitrogen mustard), corticosteroids (induce hypokalemia)
Fluconazole	Decreases metabolism and increases concentration of drugs metabolized by cytochrome P450 system
Itraconazole	Reduces absorption of proton pump inhibitors, H_2 blockers, and metoclopramide
Voriconazole	Rifampin, efavirenz, ritonavir, carbamazepine, sirolimus
Posaconazole	Proton pump inhibitors, midazolam, rifampin, vinblastine, vincristine, atazanavir, efavirenz, ritonavir, cyclosporine, tacrolimus
Isavuconazole	Ketoconazole, rifampin, cyclosporine, sirolimus, tacrolimus, mycophenolate mofetil, digoxin, midazolam, bupropion, ritonavir
Flucytosine	Renal toxicity from AmB can lead to toxic flucytosine levels
Caspofungin	Cyclosporine, tacrolimus, rifampin, phenytoin, efavirenz, carbamazepine, statins
Micafungin	Sirolimus, nifedipine, itraconazole

formulations. It is approved for prophylaxis of aspergillosis and candidiasis in immunocompromised patients, such as bone marrow transplant recipients and those undergoing chemotherapy for leukemia. Posaconazole is also sometimes used as salvage therapy for invasive mold infections like mucormycosis and fusariosis. It has activity against *Candida* spp., including those that are resistant to fluconazole. This makes it an attractive alternative agent for patients with oropharyngeal candidiasis that is refractory to fluconazole. Posaconazole has several drug interactions, and reported adverse events include hepatotoxicity and QTc prolongation. Like voriconazole, drug levels should be monitored in patients with liver and kidney disease with extended use.

The newest triazole, isavuconazole, is approved for invasive aspergillosis and invasive mucormycosis. Oral and IV formulations are available. The latter can form precipitate from the insoluble drug, so isavuconazole should be administered through an in-line filter. It has broad-spectrum activity similar to that of posaconazole. Isavuconazole seems to have a better safety profile compared with voriconazole and posaconazole, with a lower risk of hepatoxicity and QTc prolongation, although gastrointestinal side effects are common. Coadministration of isavuconazole with strong CYP3A4 inhibitors and strong CYP3A4 inducers is contraindicated (see Table 5.3).

FLUCYTOSINE

Also known as *5-FC*, the clinical use of flucytosine is mostly limited to treating cryptococcal meningitis in combination with AmB. It is fungistatic and inhibits fungal DNA and protein synthesis. AmB facilitates entry of flucytosine into the fungal cell by interfering with the permeability of the fungal cell membrane. Flucytosine has activity against *Candida* spp. and *C. neoformans*. There is evidence that fluconazole and flucytosine for 2 weeks may be as effective as AmB plus flucytosine for induction therapy with cryptococcal meningitis. In addition to cryptococcal meningitis, it has been used to treat chromomycosis. Resistance develops rapidly when flucytosine is used as a single agent, but has also been observed in combination with caspofungin for treating cystitis due to *C. glabrata*. This was reported to occur due to nonsense mutations in the *FUR1* gene. Side effects are usually mild but are more common and severe when flucytosine is used in combination with AmB. These include rashes, diarrhea, hepatoxicity (usually mild), and bone marrow suppression.

ECHINOCANDINS

The echinocandins, which include anidulafungin, caspofungin, and micafungin, are fungicidal agents that block synthesis of β-glucan in the fungal cell wall by inhibiting the enzyme 1,3-β glucan synthase. They are only available in IV formulation due to their high molecular weight and poor bioavailability. Echinocandins have activity against most species of *Candida* (with the exception of *C. glabrata*) and *Aspergillus*. Although some isolates of the emerging pathogen *C. auris* have been reported as resistant to echinocandins, these agents are the empiric drugs of choice for *C. auris* infections in adults and children over 2 months of age. Echinocandins are used to treat candidemia and other invasive candidal infections, esophageal candidiasis, and invasive aspergillosis. Micafungin is sometimes used for prophylaxis in neutropenic patients when other oral options are not appropriate. Resistance to echinocandins is associated with target mutations in the hot-spot regions of Fks proteins, which are the putative binding domain for the drugs. Because they target an enzyme specific to fungi without a mammalian homolog, echinocandins are well tolerated compared with the other classes of antifungals. Side effects are usually mild and the most common include rashes, gastrointestinal symptoms, and infusion reactions. Echinocandins are neither inducers nor inhibitors of cytochrome P450 isoenzymes, thus leading to few drug interactions (see Table 5.3).

Suggested Reading

Clardy J, Fischbach MA, Currie CR. The natural history of antibiotics. *Curr Biol.* 2009;19:437–441.

Doi Y. Treatment options for carbapenem-resistant gram-negative bacterial infections. *Clin Infect Dis.* 2019;69(suppl 7):S565–S575.

Gilbert DN, Chambers HF, Eliopoulos GM, et al. *The Sanford Guide to Antimicrobial Therapy.* 49th ed. Sperryville, VA: Antimicrobial Therapy; 2019.

Hutchings M, Truman A, Wilkinson B. Antibiotics: past, present and future. *Curr Opin Microbiol.* 2019;51:72–80.

Watkins RR, Holubar M, David MZ. Antimicrobial resistance in methicillin-resistant *Staphylococcus aureus* to newer antimicrobial agents. *Antimicrob Agents Chemother.* 2019;63:e01216–e01219.

Watkins RR, Papp-Wallace KM, Drawz SM, Bonomo RA. Novel β-lactamase inhibitors: a therapeutic hope against the scourge of multidrug resistance. *Front Microbiol.* 2013;24(4):392.

Fever of Unknown Origin

Mary Jo Kasten

Introduction

Fever is a common complaint encountered by primary caregivers, internists, and surgeons. We all experience fever throughout our lives, and although frequently the cause of fever is never explained, few of us experience a true "classic" fever of unknown origin (FUO). The term *FUO* should be reserved for patients who experience all of the following:

Fever >3 weeks

Oral temperature ≥101° F (38.3° C) on several occasions

No definitive diagnosis after an evaluation that includes a comprehensive history, physical examination, and laboratory testing.

Most FUO series have required at least three outpatient visits or a 3-day hospitalization for an individual to be diagnosed with an FUO. Experienced infectious disease physicians frequently cringe when the term FUO is used for fever that does not meet the noted criteria. The concern is that the literature relevant to patients with a true "classic" FUO is not relevant to patients who have had fever for a brief time, who have "fever" but never to 101° F (38.3° C), or who have not had a competent provider consider their symptoms and conduct a thoughtful evaluation. Most cases of fever are due to self-limited viral infections, and many people experience a sensation of fever or report mildly elevated temperatures above their baseline after a major infection or other stress. Diagnosing patients with lower temperatures as having an FUO results in the inclusion of many patients with stress-related hyperthermia and chronic fatigue syndrome. Resources are wasted, and patients with benign or self-limited illnesses can be harmed by the intensive evaluation that is often required to sort out a classic FUO. Individuals with fever that does not meet the criteria for a classic FUO but with laboratory evidence of inflammation often have a similar spectrum of illness as individuals with classic FUO. Immunosuppressed patients and patients that acquire their infection in the hospital have a different set of illnesses that account for prolonged fever and will often require empiric treatment, which should usually be avoided in immunocompetent patients with a FUO. This chapter will review the evaluation and differential diagnosis for an immunocompetent patient with a classic, non-nosocomial acquired FUO.

Understanding Fever

An understanding of the basic pathophysiology behind fever is helpful in understanding the causes of FUO. Normal body temperature varies during the course of a day and is regulated by the hypothalamus. Healthy adults have temperature readings higher in the late afternoon and early evening than in the early morning. A study by Mackowiak and colleagues in 1992 of 144 healthy adults found a mean oral temperature of 36.8° C, with temperature later in the day averaging 0.5° C higher than in the early morning. There was considerable variation in temperature oscillation between subjects, with some increasing by 1.3° C and others by only 0.05° C. The highest "normal" 6 AM temperature recorded in this study was 37.2° C and highest 4 PM temperature was 37.7° C. Oral temperatures are about 0.6° C lower than rectal temperatures. Tympanic membrane temperatures are similar to oral temperatures but will be lower if the ear canal is obstructed or if the ambient air temperature is cold resulting in cooling of the tympanic membrane. Oral temperatures can be temporarily altered by eating, drinking, or smoking. Exercise and eating a large meal tend to increase core temperatures. Ideally, temperature measurements should be obtained in a relaxed state, with a comfortable amount of clothing and no sooner than 30 minutes after smoking or eating.

Chronic fever from infection or illnesses associated with inflammation is usually related to an alteration in the set point of heat-sensitive receptors in the hypothalamus. Pyrogenic cytokines include tumor necrosis factor (TNF), interleukins 1β (IL1β) and 6 (IL6), and interferon (INF)-α. When they enter the hypothalamic circulation, these cytokines stimulate the release of local prostaglandins, which activate thermoregulatory neurons of the anterior hypothalamus and reset the hypothalamic thermoregulatory set point. Some older persons may have a blunted febrile response to infections related to decreased production of or response to pyrogenic cytokines. It is not clear if this blunted response is actually due to aging, because this also occurs with other conditions, including malnutrition. Fever can also result from disruption of the autonomic system and changes in neurochemicals.

CAUSES OF FUO

The differential for an FUO is vast and includes chronic infection, malignancy, inflammatory disorders, and miscellaneous conditions, including some genetic syndromes. Worldwide, infection is the leading cause of FUO, with tuberculosis (TB) causing the highest number of cases. Infections most commonly reported to cause FUO in developing countries also include typhoid and malaria. Depending on the patient's residence and travel history, systemic fungal infection—particularly histoplasmosis or coccidioidomycosis—will be seen more commonly in the United States. Clinicians in developed countries need to remain suspicious of TB as a cause of FUO, particularly among immigrants from and travelers to developing countries where the disease is common. FUO due to TB often presents with extrapulmonary manifestations and remains quite treatable.

Recent series reveal that the frequency of infection as a cause for FUO in developed countries has continued to decrease over the past 50 years, with noninfectious, inflammatory illness now being the most common cause. FUO in community settings is more likely to be due to infection than FUO seen in academic settings. Only 12% of FUO diagnoses were caused by infection in a 2007 study from the Netherlands, whereas 36% were found to have infection in the original US study by Dr. Petersdorf and colleagues from the 1950s.

Endocarditis can be due to any bacteria or fungus and is the classic infectious cause of FUO. Abdominal abscess is the most common localized infection in many recent series. Any localized infections can cause FUO, but others frequently seen include pulmonary abscess, empyema, cholangitis, chronic cholecystitis, hepatic abscess, mycotic aneurysm, prosthetic joint infection, pelvic inflammatory disease, pelvic abscess, prostatic abscess, and chronic prostatitis. *Coxiella burnetii*, the cause of Q fever, can cause endocarditis but frequently causes FUO without endocarditis and should be considered early in individuals with FUO, particularly if they have exposure to animals. See Table 6.1 for other infections that have a propensity for causing FUO unrelated to endocarditis or localized infection.

Noninfectious systemic inflammatory and autoimmune illnesses have overtaken infection as the most common cause of FUO among adults in developed countries, particularly at tertiary care centers. Temporal arteritis is a common cause of FUO among the elderly and in several series is the most common cause of FUO in patients older than 65 years. Still's disease is an unusual illness but a common cause of FUO at tertiary care centers among those under 50 years. Because it is a clinical diagnosis and many clinicians have little experience with it, diagnosis is often delayed until patients are referred to larger centers. The constellation of daily spikes of high fever, arthritis, and transient rash, often brought on by pressure, is highly suggestive of Still's disease. Inflammatory markers (erythrocyte sedimentation rate [ESR], C-reactive protein [CRP], and ferritin) are very high with active disease. Vasculitis, including allergic granulomatous angiitis, polyarteritis nodosum (PAN), hypersensitivity vasculitis, Takayasu arteritis, and granulomatosis with polyangiitis frequently present as an FUO. Other noninfectious, inflammatory causes of FUO include antiphospholipid syndrome, Bechet syndrome, cryoglobulinemia, gout, inflammatory bowel disease, pseudogout, reactive arthritis, rheumatic fever, rheumatoid arthritis (RA), serum sickness, and sarcoid. Systemic lupus erythematosus (SLE), which was common in older series, is now an uncommon cause of FUO, most likely because its tendency to cause fever is now well recognized and antinuclear antibody (ANA) testing is done early in the evaluation of unexplained fever. It is important to remember that endocarditis can cause positive autoantibodies, including ANA, and misdiagnosis of endocarditis as lupus or another autoimmune illness can result in disastrous consequences.

Nearly every cancer has been reported to occasionally cause FUO, but hematologic cancers, particularly lymphoma, are seen most commonly. Renal cell cancer, hepatocellular cancer, and metastatic cancer to the liver commonly cause FUO. Colon cancer and breast cancer rarely cause fever, but because they are common cancers, they need to be considered when evaluating a challenging FUO.

Atrial myxomas are unusual benign cardiac tumors, but when they occur they frequently cause FUO.

Nearly every drug has been reported to cause fever. Frequently this occurs shortly after the drug is started, and when associated with rash and eosinophilia, the culprit is usually obvious and the drug is stopped. Fever can, however, start weeks, months, or even years after the initiation of a medication, and drug-associated fever is not always associated with rash or eosinophilia. The

---

TABLE 6.1 ■ Organisms and Infections Commonly Associated with FUO

Bacterial: *Bartonella* infections including cat scratch disease, brucellosis, *Coxiella burnetti* (the cause of Q fever), *Salmonella* infections, *Streptobacillus moniliformis, Streptobacillus notomytis* or *Spirillum minus* (causes of rat bite fever), *Tropheryma whippelii* (the cause of Whipple disease), *Mycobacterium tuberculosis* (the most commonly cultured organism from patients with classic FUO), and *Yersinia* infection

Spirochetes: Leptospirosis, Lyme (rare), *Borrelia* species (which cause relapsing fever), and syphilis

Fungal: Blastomycosis, coccidioidomycosis, cryptococcosis, and histoplasmosis in the Midwest

Parasitic Infections: Babesiosis, *Entamoeba histolytica* (cause of amebic liver abscess), *Leishmania* species (primarily *L. donovani* and *L. infantum*, which cause the majority of visceral leishmaniasis), malaria, toxoplasmosis, trichinosis, and trypanosomiasis

Viral Infections: Cytomegalovirus (CMV); Epstein–Barr virus (EBV); hepatitis B, C, and E; human immunodeficiency virus (HIV); parvovirus

TABLE 6.2 ■ Drugs Commonly Associated with Fever

Allopurinol	Iodides
Aminoglycosides	Isoniazid
Angiotensin enzyme inhibitors	Macrolides
Antihistamines	Methyldopa
β-Lactam antibiotics	Nitrofurantoin
Clindamycin	Phenytoin
Heparin	Procainamide
Hydralazine	Quinidine
Hydrochlorothiazide	Sulfonamides
	Vancomycin
	Many others reported

From Kasten MJ. Fever of unknown origin. In Z. Temesgen, ed. *Mayo Clinic Infectious Diseases Board Review.* Oxford: Oxford University Press; 2012: Chapter 23.

relationship of fever to the drug can be challenging in these situations, and a FUO may develop if the drug is continued. Antimicrobials, antiepileptic drugs, and antiinflammatory drugs are the classes of drugs that most frequently cause fever. Drugs that should be viewed with significant suspicion and considered a potential cause of fever in a patient with FUO are listed in Table 6.2.

The miscellaneous causes of FUO are vast and varied. Pancreatitis, alcoholic hepatitis, and alcohol withdrawal are common problems that occasionally cause intermittent FUO. Cirrhosis can also cause FUO. Clots, particularly retroperitoneal hematomas, and pulmonary emboli can cause fever and occasionally FUO. Kikuchi disease is an unusual illness, causing fever and necrotizing, histiocytic lymphadenitis and is thought to be triggered by an infection. Endocrine causes of FUO include both adrenal insufficiency and pheochromocytoma in addition to hyperthyroidism and thyroiditis. Genetic causes include familial Mediterranean fever, TNF-1 receptor antibody syndrome (TRAPS), porphyria, Fabry disease, and periodic fever syndromes, which are most commonly seen in children. Factitious fever is an unusual cause of FUO that is seen more often at tertiary referral centers than by primary care clinicians.

Depending on the population, between 10% and 50% cases of FUO are never diagnosed despite an exhaustive workup. Diagnosis is more likely for the elderly and when fever is high and persistent. Fifty percent of the patients in the 2007 Netherlands study did not receive a diagnosis, whereas only 7% of patients were undiagnosed in Dr. Petersdorf's original 1950s series. Fortunately, patients with an undiagnosable FUO generally have a good prognosis, and fever usually spontaneously resolves.

HISTORICAL CLUES

A detailed history is critical in determining how to proceed with evaluation of a classic FUO. This starts with understanding the intensity and duration of the fever. Fever that has been present for less than 6 weeks is highly likely to be due to an undiagnosed infection. The longer the duration of the illness, the less likely infection is to be the cause of FUO, especially in developed countries. Fever >39° C is suggestive of lymphoma, Still's disease, infection, or vasculitis. The pattern of fever is occasionally helpful, particularly if it is episodic with spells of fever separated by weeks or months. See Table 6.3 for specific illnesses that frequently cause episodic fever. Intermittent high spiking fever suggests an abscess, miliary TB, malaria, Still's disease, or lymphoma. A double quotidian fever (two fever spikes daily) is suggestive of infection, including typhoid, malaria, visceral leishmaniasis, miliary TB, legionellosis, or Still's disease.

TABLE 6.3 ■ **Causes of Episodic FUO**

Adult Still's disease

Atrial myxoma

Castleman disease

Crohn disease

Chronic prostatitis

Cyclic neutropenia

Dental abscess

Drug-induced fever

Subacute bacterial endocarditis (when inadequate empiric antibiotics given)

Fabry disease

Factitious fever

Periodic fever, aphthous ulcers, pharyngitis, and adenitis syndrome (PFAPA)

Familial Mediterranean fever

Granulomatous hepatitis

Hyper-IgD syndrome

Hypersensitivity pneumonitis

Hypertriglyceridemia

Malignancy (particularly lymphoma, but also occurs with solid tumors, including colon and breast cancer)

Pulmonary embolism

Subacute cholangitis

Tumor necrosis factor receptor–associated periodic syndrome (TRAPS)

From Kasten MJ. Fever of unknown origin. In Z. Temesgen, ed. *Mayo Clinic Infectious Diseases Board Review.* Oxford: Oxford University Press; 2012: Chapter 23.

Understanding the course of a patient's illness and obtaining a detailed review of symptoms can often lead to the revelation of a symptom or clue that the patient did not believe was important and was therefore missed. Searching for diagnostic clues also means investigating what the patient was doing and where they were before the onset of their illness. Past medical history, medications, and surgical history occasionally provide critical clues to determining the etiology of an FUO. Travel, occupational exposures, animal contact, sexual practices, recreational drug and alcohol use, and recreational activities can also occasionally provide important clues. Although clues frequently lead to dead ends, they are at other times the key to a diagnosis.

See Table 6.4 for examples of historical clues that can be crucial in determining what evaluation is likely to be fruitful in determining the etiology of an FUO.

PHYSICAL EXAMINATION CLUES

A comprehensive physical examination is also critical when evaluating a patient with a classic FUO. A careful skin, eye, lymph node, mouth, abdominal, cardiac, and genital examination can at times provide clues that have been missed by other clinicians. Many primary care physicians and internists are challenged by the funduscopic examination, and a formal funduscopic examination by an ophthalmologist looking for clues can occasionally lead to the diagnosis. Examples include Roth spots suggesting endocarditis or stellate neuroretinitis due to cat scratch disease. Careful cardiac auscultation can reveal fleeting murmurs of endocarditis or rheumatic fever. Fever can precede lymphadenopathy and other findings by weeks to months in some patients later found to have lymphoma. Skin findings can evolve, and the rash in Still's disease can be fleeting, so repeating

TABLE 6.4 ■ Historical Clues and Diagnostic Evaluation of FUO

Clue	Potential Diagnosis	Testing Considerations
Travel		
Area endemic for malaria	Malaria	Thick and thin smears for malaria
Prolonged contact or health care with population in developing world	Tuberculosis, typhoid	CXR. Sputum and urine cultures for *Mycobacteria*, biopsy of any areas worrisome for TB with PCR testing for TB, acid-fast staining and mycobacterial cultures, blood cultures
All travelers without usual partner or single	HIV	HIV screening test and viral load
Southwest United States	Coccidioidomycosis	Coccidioidomycosis serology, fungal cultures
Mississippi River Valley	Histoplasmosis	Histoplasma serology, histoplasma antigen testing blood and urine, fungal cultures
Animal Contact (direct or indirect, including contact with droppings)		
Cats	Cat scratch disease, toxoplasmosis	*Bartonella* serology, toxoplasmosis serology
Horses, cows, sheep, or goats	Brucellosis, Q fever	*Brucella* and *Coxiella* serology, specialized *Brucella* cultures
Birds	Psittacosis	*Chlamydia psittici* serology
Bats	Histoplasmosis	See above and Travel: Mississippi River Valley
Rodents	Rat bite fever	Clinical diagnosis and should treat empirically. Microbiology laboratory can be asked to do special cultures for *Streptobacillus moniliformis* or *Streptobacillus notomytis*. *Spirillum minus* is not able to be cultured.
	Lymphocytic choriomeningitis virus (LCMV)	Serologic testing for suspected diagnosis
Social History		
Sexually active—not monogamous or new partner	CMV, hepatitis, HIV	Serologic testing for suspected diagnosis
Injection drug use	Hepatitis, HIV, right-sided endocarditis	Serologic testing, blood cultures, echocardiogram
Alcohol use	Alcoholic hepatitis, cirrhosis	Liver function testing, liver ultrasound
Tick exposure	Babesiosis, ehrlichiosis, anaplasmosis	Serologies for *Babesia, Ehrlichia, Anaplasma,* and Lyme
	Lyme, Relapsing Fever	Special smear to look for *Babesia, Ehrlichia*, and spirochetes
Family History of Similar Illness	Familial Mediterranean fever (FMF), Fabry disease, hypertriglyceridemia, TRAPS	Genetic testing
	Strong family history of cancer	CT abdomen/pelvis, colonoscopy
Medical/Surgical History		
Recent colonoscopy, sigmoidoscopy	Abdominal abscess	CT scan abdomen/pelvis or abdominal procedure
Recent surgical procedure	DVT, PE, hematoma	Ultrasound of legs, CT pulmonary angiogram, CT abdomen/pelvis

TABLE 6.4 ■ Historical Clues and Diagnostic Evaluation of FUO—cont'd

Clue	Potential Diagnosis	Testing Considerations
Recent blood transfusion	CMV	CMV serology
Recent trauma	Hematoma	CT imaging
History of inflammatory bowel disease, diverticulitis, or other abdominal pathology	Abdominal abscess	CT abdomen/pelvis
Known valvular heart disease	Endocarditis	Transesophageal echocardiogram (TEE)
ROS Clues		
Abdominal pain	Polyarteritis nodosa (PAN), FMF	Abdominal angiogram if considering PAN, genetic testing for FMF
Back pain	Endocarditis, brucellosis, vertebral osteomyelitis	TEE, *Brucella* serology, imaging (MRI)
Headache	Psittacosis, malaria, brucellosis, Q fever, rickettsial illness, relapsing fever, chronic meningitis	Appropriate serology, thick and thin smears, LP
Flank pain or hematuria	Renal cell carcinoma	CT abdomen
Jaw claudication	Temporal arteritis	Temporal artery biopsy
Neck/throat pain	Subacute thyroiditis, Still's disease	Thyroid function testing, thyroid ultrasound, ferritin
Testicular pain	PAN, brucellosis, TRAPS	CT angiogram, biopsy of any suspicious skin lesions, *Brucella* serology, genetic testing
Pleurisy	FMF, PE, TB, SLE	Genetic testing, CT angiogram chest, CXR, sputum cultures and PCR for TB, ANA
Rash (transient)	Still's disease or other collagen vascular disease	Ferritin, inflammatory markers, ANA, other autoimmune serologic testing
Scalp pain	Temporal arteritis	Temporal artery biopsy

ANA, Antinuclear antibody; *CMV*, cytomeglavirus; *CT*, computed tomography; *CXR*, chest x-ray; *DVT*, deep venous thrombosis; *FMF*, familial Mediterranean fever; *FUO*, fever of unknown origin; *HIV*, human immunodeficiency virus; *LP*, lumbar puncture; *MRI*, magnetic resonance imaging; *PCR*, polymerase chain reaction; *PE*, pulmonary embolism; *RA*, rheumatoid arthritis; *ROS*, review of systems; *SBE*, subacute bacterial endocarditis; *SLE*, systemic lupus erythematosus; *TB*, tuberculosis; *TEE*, trans-esophageal echocardiogram; *TRAPS*, TNF-1 receptor antibody periodic syndrome.

a careful skin examination can be critical to making a diagnosis. Other skin findings that may provide a critical clue include palpable purpura suggestive of vasculitis, thrombotic thrombocytopenia purpura, meningococcemia, or rickettsial infection. Dome-shaped papules on the face or neck are suggestive of sarcoid. Classic skin findings of endocarditis are Janeway lesions and Osler nodes, although most patients with endocarditis do not have these findings. More commonly seen and less specific for endocarditis are splinter hemorrhages and purpura. Vitiligo is suggestive of an autoimmune illness. Livedo reticularis, especially when persistent, is suggestive of an underlying autoimmune illness or cryoglobulinemia. Erythema nodosum (EN) can be secondary to Epstein–Barr virus (EBV), TB, granulomatous infections (particularly histoplasmosis), Crohn disease, sarcoidosis, collagen vascular disease, and drug fever. See Table 6.5 for additional physical examination clues in an FUO evaluation. New examination findings can develop over the course of an illness, so a comprehensive physical examination should be repeated every few days during the evaluation and on a periodic basis if the patient remains undiagnosed.

TABLE 6.5 ■ **Physical Examination Clues to the Etiology of FUO**

Relative bradycardia: Typhoid, malaria, leptospirosis, *Legionella, Ehrlichia, Babesia*, psittacosis, drug-induced fever, factitious fever, lymphoma

Cerebellar ataxia: Whipple disease, malignancy

Conjunctival hemorrhages: Endocarditis

Conjunctival suffusion: Leptospirosis, relapsing fever

Decayed or tender teeth: Dental abscess, endocarditis

Heart murmur: Endocarditis, atrial myxoma, rheumatic fever

Hepatomegaly: Lymphoma, metastatic cancer, alcoholic hepatitis, granulomatous hepatitis, Q fever, typhoid fever

Joint effusion: Rheumatoid arthritis, SLE, pseudogout, gout, familial Mediterranean fever, Lyme disease, Whipple disease, TRAPS, rheumatic fever, Still's disease

Lymphadenopathy: Lymphoma, Still's disease, granulomatous infections, sarcoidosis

Mononeuritis: PAN, sarcoidosis

Myoclonus: Whipple disease

Oral ulcers: Bechet syndrome, histoplasmosis

Roth spots: Endocarditis

Skin findings: See text for discussion

Splenomegaly: CMV, EBV, endocarditis, hematologic malignancy, sarcoidosis, brucellosis, TB, malaria, Q fever, histoplasmosis, typhoid, relapsing fever, cirrhosis

Spinal tenderness: Vertebral osteomyelitis, endocarditis, brucellosis, typhoid

Sternal tenderness: Hematologic malignancy

Temporal artery tenderness: Giant cell arteritis

Thyroid enlargement or tenderness: Thyroiditis

Testicular tenderness: PAN, brucellosis, TRAPS

CMV, cytomeglavirus; *EBV,* Epstein–Barr virus; *FUO,* fever of unknown origin; *PAN,* polyarteritis; *SLE,* systemic lupus erythematosus; *TRAPS,* TNF-1 receptor antibody periodic syndrome.

Laboratory Testing and Imaging

Because patients with FUO by definition have been ill for at least 3 weeks and have been seen on several occasions by a clinician, they will generally have had a complete blood count (CBC), inflammatory markers, a urinalysis (UA), a chest x-ray (CXR), and routine chemistries, including liver function tests. These basic tests, clues in the history and clues on the physical examination, should guide additional testing. When clues are not helpful, other tests that should be considered early in the course of evaluation are listed in Table 6.6. Diagnoses that should be considered based on abnormalities from tests commonly performed in an FUO evaluation are reviewed in Table 6.7. There is no test that must be performed in every case of FUO. Testing should be guided by clues and the diagnoses that are deemed most likely for the individual patient.

DIAGNOSTIC STRATEGY

The nearly endless differential of illnesses that cause FUO makes a simple diagnostic algorithm that is inclusive of all FUO patients not possible. The diagnostic strategy should focus on identifying abnormal symptoms, significant exposures, and abnormalities of basic laboratory testing that can be a basis for targeted testing. Because many cases of classical FUO are due to unusual illnesses or are due to an unusual presentation of a common illness, most tests will have a low positive predictive value. Positive predictive value increases with the prevalence of an illness. All positive tests need to be interpreted with skepticism, particularly positive serologic tests for infection.

TABLE 6.6 ■ **Testing to Consider Early in an FUO Evaluation**

Complete blood count with differential

Blood smear

Routine blood chemistry, including lactate dehydrogenase (LDH), creatinine, bilirubin, and liver enzymes

Creatine kinase

Urinalysis, including microscopic examination

Urine culture

Chest radiograph (CXR)

Erythrocyte sedimentation rate (ESR)

C-reactive protein (CRP)

Antinuclear antibodies (ANA)

Antineutrophilic cytoplasmic antibody (ANCA)

Rheumatoid factor (RF)

Angiotensin-converting enzyme (ACE)

Tuberculosis (TB) skin test or interferon gamma release assay for TB

Routine blood cultures (three times) while not receiving antibiotics

Fungal blood cultures

Human immunodeficiency (HIV) screen (ideally fourth-generation antibody/antigen assay)

Cytomegalovirus (CMV) immunoglobulin M (IgM) or polymerase chain reaction (PCR) testing of blood

Epstein–Barr Virus (EBV) immunoglobulin G (IgG) and IGM serology

Tuberculin skin testing (purified protein derivative [PPD]) or interferon gamma release assay for TB

Computerized tomography (CT) of abdomen and pelvis

Cryoglobulins

Temporal artery biopsy in adults >75 years

Further evaluation of any abnormalities detected by previous tests and history and examination

Adapted from Arrow PM, Flaherty JP. Fever of unknown origin. *Lancet.* 1997;350:575–580.

TABLE 6.7 ■ **Clues to FUO from Routine Laboratory Tests**

Erythrocytosis	Renal cell cancer
Leukocytosis	Infections, drug fever
Neutropenia	TB, lymphoma, leukemia, brucellosis, typhoid, psittacosis, drug reaction, SLE, cyclic neutropenia, Whipple disease
Lymphopenia	Ehrlichiosis, HIV, SLE, TB, Whipple disease, sarcoidosis, malignancy (especially Hodgkin disease)
Monocytosis	TB, PAN, temporal arteritis, brucellosis, sarcoidosis, leukemia, typhoid, malaria, leishmaniasis, SLE, SBE
Eosinophilia	Trichinosis or other parasite infection, lymphoma, drug-induced fever, PAN, SLE, hypersensitivity vasculitis, myeloproliferative disease. Unlikely to be bacterial infection
Lymphocytosis	CMV, EBV, toxoplasmosis, TB, lymphoma, drug hypersensitivity (particularly phenytoin)
Basophilia	Leukemia, myeloproliferative disease, lymphoma
Atypical Lymphocytes	CMV, EBV, acute HIV, toxoplasmosis, syphilis, brucellosis, drug reactions (including serum sickness), leukemia

Continued

TABLE 6.7 ■ Clues to FUO from Routine Laboratory Tests—cont'd

Thrombocytopenia	Hematologic malignancy, myeloproliferative diseases, HIV, SLE, vasculitis, EBV, drug-induced fever
Iron-deficiency anemia	Colon cancer, Crohn disease, Whipple disease
Sedimentation rates >100 mm/hr	Vasculitis, hematologic malignancy, metastatic cancer, subacute bacterial endocarditis (SBE)
Elevated transaminases with AST:ALT >2	Alcoholic hepatitis
Elevated alkaline phosphatase	Hepatic infiltration from infection or cancer, osteomyelitis, biliary disease, lymphoma
Elevated bilirubin	Cholangitis, cholecystitis
Microscopic hematuria	Renal cell cancer, SLE, TB, SBE, PAN
Strongly positive ANA	SLE, RA, SBE
Rheumatoid factor	RA, SBE, malaria, hypersensitivity vasculitis
Blood cultures (unexplained polymicrobial bacteremia)	Factitious
Elevated LDH	Malignancy, particularly lymphoma, PE, SLE
Elevated ACE	Sarcoid, TB, leprosy, DVT, bronchogenic cancer

ACE, Angiotensin converting enzyme; *ANA,* antinuclear antibody; *AST:ALT,* aspartate amino transferase:alanine aminotransferase; *CMV,* cytomeglavirus; *DVT,* deep venous thrombosis; *EBV,* Epstein–Barr virus; *FUO,* fever of unknown origin; *HIV,* human immunodeficiency virus; *LDH,* lactate dehydrogenase; *PAN,* polyarteritis; *PE,* pulmonary embolism; *RA,* rheumatoid arthritis; *SLE,* systemic lupus erythematosus; *TB,* tuberculosis.
From Kasten MJ. Fever of unknown origin. In Z. Temesgen, ed. *Mayo Clinic Infectious Diseases Board Review.* Oxford: Oxford University Press; 2012: Chapter 23.

Antibody tests, particularly IgM antibody tests, frequently cross react with other antibodies or proteins causing a high rate of false positivity. Computed tomography (CT) scans and other imaging can reveal incidental findings unrelated to the etiology of fever. Clinicians should keep in mind that common illnesses that rarely present as an FUO (e.g., colon cancer) are more likely to be found as a cause for FUO than uncommon infections that, when present, commonly cause FUO (for example, brucellosis in the United States). The rapid response of fever to naproxen is suggestive of a noninfectious cause, particularly malignancy, and can be helpful in guiding next steps in the evaluation when the differential remains broad. Studies suggest that clues to an FUO's etiology are often critical to making a diagnosis but can be misleading up to 65% of the time. Repeating the history, examination, and simple laboratory tests frequently provides clues that are more rewarding than additional exotic testing. Discontinuation of all nonessential drugs is recommended to help exclude the possibility of drug-induced fever. All potential clues need to be fully explored. Clinicians should realize that nonspecific elevation of liver function tests occur in 50% of patients with FUO, and liver biopsy is therefore not usually recommended early in the evaluation. Liver biopsy can occasionally be diagnostic in patients with abnormal liver function tests once all other potential clues have been explored and the less invasive testing outlined in Table 6.6 has been exhausted. Liver biopsy is unlikely to be useful when there is no evidence of liver abnormality either biochemically or on imaging. Bone marrow biopsy should be considered early for patients with persistent fever, anemia, or thrombocytopenia. Bone marrow cultures have a low yield but should be done when granulomas are seen on the biopsy or if brucellosis is suspected. *Brucella*, mycobacterial, and fungal cultures should be obtained when granulomas are found on biopsy of bone marrow or other tissue. Bacterial cultures should be held for 3 to 4 weeks to increase the sensitivity for brucellosis. Cervical and inguinal adenopathy are common, and biopsy of these nodes is often unrevealing. More generalized adenopathy suggests that a biopsy may be diagnostic. Biopsied lymph nodes and other tissue needs to be examined for cancer and if negative for malignancy, cultured and stained for infectious organisms. Cultures should generally include routine bacterial, fungal, and mycobacterial cultures. Polymerase chain reaction (PCR) testing of lymph nodes and other tissue can on occasion be diagnostic. Biopsy of abnormalities found on imaging is often critical to making a correct diagnosis. The Sutton's law—"Go where the money is"—remains wise advice when evaluating an FUO.

Despite thoughtful evaluation of all clues, some individuals with FUO remain undiagnosed. The clinician and patient must then decide on additional evaluation versus observation with additional testing if fever does not resolve at a predetermined time, if new symptoms develop, or if deterioration occurs. A normal ESR and CRP are reassuring and suggest that additional evaluation is unlikely to be helpful. A wait-and-see strategy is reasonable for patients who believe they are improving on their own and those who appear stable and not seriously ill. Most well-appearing patients with undiagnosed FUO who have had a thoughtful evaluation do well, and their fever often spontaneously resolves. Individuals who are seriously ill deserve additional evaluation despite having exhausted the clinicians' ability to evaluate historical, examination, and laboratory clues. These individuals may benefit from referral to a tertiary center with experience in challenging FUO cases.

A whole-body test for inflammation can be useful; however, the best test is debated. Some clinicians prefer 18-fluoro-deoxy-glucose positron emission tomography (FDG-PET), which appears to be more specific and sensitive than gallium-67 scintigraphy (Ga-67) and indium-111–labelled white blood cell (indium–WBC) scans for the cause of fever; however, in the United States in 2019 insurance will frequently not cover FDG-PET for the indication of a FUO. FDG-PET scans have the advantage of being frequently positive with infection, cancer (particularly lymphoma), and inflammation due to vasculitis or other noninfectious inflammatory conditions. Indium–WBC and Ga-67 scans are also usually positive with infection. The indium–WBC scan requires at least 2000×10^9 leukocytes/µl. Indium–WBC scans are most likely to be useful when there is a strong suspicion for an acute bacterial infection and the patient has leukocytosis. Ga-67 scans are more sensitive for spinal osteomyelitis than indium–WBC scans. Ga-67 scans are often positive with lymphoma and will be more sensitive than indium–WBC scans in this situation. Indium–WBC and GA-67 scans are less likely to be positive in inflammation due to vasculitis and other noninfectious inflammatory conditions that cause FUO compared with FDG-PET scans. A triple-phase technetium-99 bone scintigraphy (Tch-99) can be useful when osteomyelitis or bone metastasis is suspected as the cause of fever and is frequently combined with an indium–WBC scan. Tch-99 is rarely useful in patients with a FUO who do not have a clue pointing toward a possible bone disorder. The choice of a nuclear imaging test should consider all of these factors in addition to the expertise of the radiologist performing the test.

TREATMENT

An empiric trial of steroids or antibiotics is only indicated with clinical deterioration. Many patients with fever and infection will temporarily improve but will be ultimately harmed by steroids. Patients with undiagnosed endocarditis may improve with empiric antibiotics but will often not completely respond and will have symptoms quickly recur when antibiotics are discontinued. If an undiagnosed but atypical infection is thought to be likely and a patient is seriously ill or deteriorating, an empiric trial of doxycycline after obtaining blood cultures and cultures from all appropriate tissue is reasonable. Tetracyclines are effective against many atypical organisms, including organisms that are difficult to grow in culture. Tetracyclines also have an excellent safety record.

Summary

In summary the pursuit of an FUO diagnosis tests even the keenest clinicians' diagnostic abilities. The vast differential can frequently be narrowed following a careful history, examination, and basic laboratory testing. An accurate diagnosis can at times be crucial for a patient's recovery; however, at other times, continued diagnostic pursuit can be more harmful than a wait-and-see approach.

Suggested Reading

Cunha BA, Lortholary O, Cunha CB. Fever of unknown origin: a clinical approach. *Am J Med.* 2015;128:
1138.e1–1138.e15.

Knockaert DC, Vanderschueren S, Blockmans D. Fever of unknown origin in adults: 40 years on. *J Intern Med.* 2003;253:263–275.

Wright WF, Mackowiak PA, FUO. *Mandell, Douglas, and Bennett's Principles and Practice of Infectious Diseases.*
Philadelphia, PA: Elsevier; 2015:721–731.

CHAPTER 7

Fever and Rash

Diana Vilar-Compte ■ Patricia Cornejo-Juárez ■ Elizabeth Salazar Rojas

Overview

Generalized rashes with fever are among the most frequent conditions seen by primary care physicians, and are a common reason for patient visits to the emergency department and dermatologists. The majority of cases do not represent an immediate danger, but some patients may have a life-threatening diagnosis, and a prompt and accurate approach is warranted.

Diagnosing fever and rash is frequently challenging, because there is a wide variety of clinical presentations and etiologies. Although infections are the most common causes, the differential diagnosis remains wide; accurate history and physical examination are necessary to rule out other causes, such as drug reactions (which occurs in approximately 5% of patients), immunologic and rheumatic diseases, allergens, neoplasia, and sometimes idiopathic causes.

An increasing number of emerging infectious diseases can present with fever and rash, and with climate change, migration, and a higher number of individuals traveling to tropical and exotic destinations, physicians will probably see more patients with this syndrome.

Approach to the Patient with Fever and Rash

The epidemiology and presentation of the patient with fever and rash vary according to each category. A comprehensive history and physical examination are the cornerstones in establishing the diagnosis.

HISTORY

Key elements from the history include the distribution and progression of the skin lesions and associated symptoms, recent exposures, vaccination status, travel history, pets and habits, occupational exposures, season of the year, drug ingestion within the past 30 days, sun exposure, and history of drug or food allergies.

When asking for recent exposures, it is important to gather precise information on:
- Contact with wild animals.
- Exposure to vector-borne and zoonotic infections, including exposure to specific vectors such as ticks, louses, fleas, and mites. Possible exposure to these infections should be sought by direct questioning, but also through determining indirect exposure, as is not infrequent that individuals do not remember seeing the ticks or mites attached, but a history of activities (e.g., walking in wilderness or rural areas) may reveal valuable information.
- Detailed history for sexually transmitted diseases, including HIV.
- Exposure to febrile ill persons within the recent past.

INITIAL ASSESSMENT AND PHYSICAL EXAMINATION

When seeing patients with fever and rash, is of utmost importance to initially evaluate if:
- The patient shows signs of severe sepsis or organ failure requiring urgent medical care, cardiopulmonary resuscitation, and antibiotic therapy.
- The patient has exposure to pathogens causing serious illness with a risk of nosocomial transmission, requiring immediate isolation with barrier precautions.

A physical examination of the skin, eyes, oropharyngeal mucosa, lymph nodes, abdomen (with special attention to hepatosplenomegaly), and genitalia should be conducted, with particular attention to conjunctivitis, jaundice, erythema, petechiae, exudates, and ulceration. Cerebral impairment and meningism should also be evaluated.

Skin Evaluation

Full exposure of skin is necessary, including the abdomen, back, chest, axilla, palms, soles, and mucous membranes. Palpation of skin lesions with a gloved hand must be conducted to determine if the lesions are flat or raised and the presence of blanching. It should also be assessed if epidermal sloughing with lateral pressure is present.

Based on visual and tactile characteristics of the eruption, skin lesions can be grouped into macules, papules, nodules, plaques, vesicles and bullae, pustules, purpura, ulcers, or eschars. In Table 7.1, a morphologic description of the skin lesions is provided to help the reader differentiate between the lesions. It is important to mention that exanthem, defined as a widespread, nonspecific rash characterized by a generalized eruption of little erythematous macules and papules, is frequently used as a synonym for rash.

On examination, the distribution and direction of spread (centrally distributed and peripheral eruptions), along with the type of lesions, help narrow the diagnosis. For an organized and systematic approach, we have grouped the rashes into six different categories: (1) central distributed maculopapular eruptions; (2) confluent desquamative erythema; (3) vesicobullous eruptions; (4) nodular eruptions; (5) petechial/purpuric eruptions; and (6) eruptions with ulcers and/or eschars.

TABLE 7.1 ■ Morphology and Skin Lesions

Type of Lesion	Description
Macules	Flat, nonpalpable lesions above the skin surface (see Figs. 7.6, 7.12, and 7.13).
Papules	Small, superficial, and solid palpable lesions elevated above the skin surface (<5 mm) (see Figs. 7.4, 7.5, and 7.9).
Nodule	Deep-seated, indurated, roundish lesion ≥5 mm in diameter that can involve the epidermal, dermal, and/or subcutaneous tissue (see Figs. 7.14 and 7.15).
Plaques	Palpable lesions with elevation above the skin surface >5 mm (see Fig. 7.5).
Vesicles (<5 mm) Bullae (>5 mm)	Circumscribed, elevated lesions containing fluid (see Fig. 7.3, 7.10, and 7.11).
Pustules	Small, palpable lesions filled with purulent exudates.
Nonpalpable purpura	Flat lesion due to bleeding into the skin. If <3 mm, the purpuric lesion is called petechiae. If >3 mm, are called *ecchymosis* (see Fig. 7.6).
Palpable purpura	Raised lesion secondary to an inflammation of the vessel wall with subsequent hemorrhage.
Ulcer	Defect in skin extending at least into the upper layer of the dermis. The superficial lesions are called *erosions*.
Eschar	Necrotic lesion covered with a black crust.

For easier reading, the most frequent causes of fever and rash are found in each corresponding vignette. Information on epidemiology, clinical presentation, diagnostic tests, and treatment is provided. A list of common causes of fever and rash according to the type of skin lesions is presented in Table 7.2. The most important infections and syndromes are described according to the type of rash. For better presentation and comprehension, we designed an acronym, including: **I:** Important characteristics/epidemiology; **C:** Clinical-related data; **R:** Rash characteristics; **A:** Ancillary diagnostic studies; **T:** Treatment; and **O:** Other recommendations.

MACULOPAPULAR RASH

These are the most common types of rashes, with the broadest differential diagnosis. These rashes are characterized by a combination of two types of lesions: macules, defined as a nonpalpable, circumscribed lesion that is flat, with any size; and papules that are palpable solid lesions, elevated, and the size is ≤0.5 cm in diameter. It is also known as *morbilliform exanthem*.

These lesions are usually seen in viral illnesses, including the classic childhood viral diseases such as rubella, measles, roseola subitum, and erythema infectiosum, but can also be seen in bacterial infections, drug eruptions, and immune complex–mediated syndromes. The presence of fever and systemic illness or toxic appearance suggests a potentially deadly condition. An important consideration is the location of the lesions: central (chest, abdomen, or back) or peripheral (extremities).

1. Febrile/toxic and central: Includes many benign viral exanthems and some dangerous causes.

MEASLES

I: Most common in children. Highly contagious: 90% of susceptible individuals will present the disease after exposure. Case-fatality rate: 4% to 10%.
C: Incubation: 6 to 21 days. Prodromes: 2 to 4 days, fever, malaise, anorexia, cough, coryza, conjunctivitis, Koplik spots (white, gray, or blue elevated lesions with an erythematous base, usually

TABLE 7.2 ■ Classification of Rashes and Frequent Causes

Maculopapular Rash

Febrile/Toxic and Central Distribution	Febrile/Toxic and Peripheral Distribution	Afebrile/Nontoxic, Central or Peripheral
Measles Rubella Roseola subitum Infectious mononucleosis Primary HIV infection Ehrlichial diseases Typhoid fever Leptospirosis Murine (endemic) typhus Lyme disease Relapsing fever Arbovirosis (dengue, Chikungunya, Zika) Ebola	Erythema infectiosum Secondary syphilis Stevens–Johnson syndrome	Drug reactions Pityriasis Scabies Eczema Psoriasis Erythema multiforme

Erythematous Rash

Febrile and Positive Nikolsky Sign	Febrile and Negative Nikolsky Sign	Afebrile with Nikolsky Sign	Afebrile Without Nikolsky Sign
Staphylococcal scalded skin syndrome Toxic epidermal necrolysis	Toxic shock syndrome Streptococcal toxic shock syndrome Kawasaki disease Scarlet fever	Drug-induced Associated with *Mycoplasma pneumoniae*, herpes virus infection	Anaphylaxis Scombroid Alcohol flush Medications

Purpuric/Petechial Rash

Febrile and Palpable	Febrile and Nonpalpable	Afebrile and Palpable Lesions	Afebrile and Nonpalpable Lesions
Acute meningococcemia Rocky mountain spotted fever Disseminated gonococcal infection Bacterial endocarditis Henoch–Schönlein purpura	Disseminated intravascular coagulation and purpura fulminans Viral hemorrhagic fever Enteroviral rash	Autoimmune vasculitis (lupus erythematosus, rheumatoid arthritis, systemic vasculitides) Chronic hepatitis B or C Medications	Idiopathic thrombocytopenia purpura

Vesiculobullous

Febrile with Diffuse Distribution	Febrile and Localized Distribution	No Fever and Diffuse Distribution	No Fever and Localized Distribution
Varicella Smallpox Disseminated intravascular coagulation	Necrotizing fasciitis Hand–foot–mouth disease	Bullous pemphigoid Pemphigus vulgaris	Herpes zoster (shingles)

Nodular, Ulcers, and Eschar Forming

Nodular Eruptions	Eruptions with Ulcers and/or Eschars
Disseminated infections Erythema nodosum Bacillary angiomatosis Sweet syndrome (see Fig. 7.12)	Tularemia Anthrax Ecthyma gangrenosum Rickettsial pox

on the buccal mucosa opposite the molar teeth). Exanthem: 2 to 4 days. Recovery and immunity: Cough persists 1 to 2 weeks after rash. Complications: diarrhea, respiratory tract, deafness, encephalitis.

R: Discrete blanching, erythematous, "brick-red" lesions; confluent rash spreads from face, neck, trunk, and lastly, the extremities.

A: Thrombocytopenia, leukopenia, lymphopenia. Complicated measles, head computed tomography (CT) and/or brain magnetic resonance imaging (MRI). Diagnosis by serologic antibody testing.

T: Supportive: antipyretics, fluids, and treatment for superinfections. Vitamin A could reduce morbidity and mortality.

O: Patients should be isolated and placed on airborne precautions. Vaccination interrupts transmission and affords protection to unvaccinated individuals.

With the increasing cases of measles across the United States and some countries in Europe and South America, additional epidemiologic information and current immunization recommendations are provided.

Measles was eliminated from the United States and many countries in the Americas in the early 2000s thanks to national vaccination policies. Despite the overall control, small numbers of cases continued to occur annually related to exposure to cases imported from areas of the world where measles is still endemic.

Within 2018 and 2019, localized measles outbreaks have occurred by travel-related introduction of the virus by infected persons, with subsequent spread through groups of undervaccinated subpopulations in the United States and Europe. By mid-June 2019, more than 1000 individual cases of measles have been confirmed in the United States, and countries such as Venezuela and Ukraine experienced important outbreaks in 2019.

Measles can be prevented with a measles-containing vaccine, which is usually administered as the combination measles–mumps–rubella (MMR) vaccine. One dose of MMR vaccine is approximately 93% effective at preventing measles; two doses are 97% effective, and children who received one dose of the live-attenuated measles vaccine between 12 and 15 months of age and a second dose between 4 and 6 years of age are considered fully immunized. People born before 1957 and those who had measles are also considered protected against the measles virus.

Risk Groups for Acquiring Measles

People not vaccinated because of religious or personal beliefs, pregnant women, and immunosuppressed individuals.

People born after 1957 who were not vaccinated or only received one dose of an inactivated measles vaccine and do not have evidence of immunity.

Students in postsecondary educational institutions, international travelers, and households or close contacts of immunocompromised persons with no evidence of immunity.

Vaccination Recommendations

MMR vaccination is the most effective way to prevent spread of the virus, and in the midst of an outbreak with increased public awareness, health care workers need to be updated on the policies and recommendations of measles vaccination. Table 7.3 summarizes the most current recommendations, but we encourage the reader to keep updated on the topic, as the current measles outbreak in the United States and other parts of the world is rapidly changing.

Can we still vaccinate individuals after contact with measles? People exposed to measles who are not able to show evidence of immunity against the disease should be offered postexposure prophylaxis (PEP) and/or be excluded from the setting (hospital, school, nursery) for 3 weeks

TABLE 7.3 ■ Recommendations on Measles, Mumps, and Rubella Vaccination According to the CDC

Patient Category	First Dose	Second Dose
Children between 12 months and older If traveling[a]	Age 12–15 months Get the first dose immediately	Age 4–6 years Get a second dose 28 days after the first dose
Teenagers and adults with no evidence of immunity If traveling[a]	As soon as possible	Four weeks apart from the first dose Get a second dose 28 days after the first dose[a]
Students in postsecondary educational institutions, international travelers, and household or close personal contacts of immunocompromised persons with no evidence of immunity to measles, mumps, and rubella	As soon as possible	Only consider a second dose at least 4 weeks apart from the first dose if previously did not receive any MMR or measles/rubella vaccine
Health care workers born in 1957 or later with no evidence of immunity to measles, mumps, or rubella	As soon as possible	Four weeks apart from the first dose

[a]We encourage the reader to review the Global Travel Notice from the CDC for patients traveling internationally, as several popular travel destinations are experiencing measles outbreaks.

from the exposure. To potentially provide protection to these susceptible persons, the current recommendations are:

1. Administer the vaccine within 72 hours of initial measles exposure.

OR

2. Immunoglobulin (IG) within 6 days of exposure. Do not administer the MMR vaccine and IG simultaneously, as this practice invalidates the vaccine.

According to the Centers for Disease Control and Prevention (CDC), if many cases of measles are occurring in infants younger than 12 months of age, vaccination of infants >6 months may be used as an outbreak control measure.

Individuals at high risk of severe illness and complications from measles, such as infants younger than 12 months of age, pregnant women without evidence of measles immunity, and severely immunocompromised individuals, should receive IG.

Individuals receiving the vaccine within the first 72 hours of measles exposure, and after an individualized analysis, may return to child care, school, or work. Health care workers cannot return to work immediately, and they should wait a 3-week period to go back to health care–related activities. If the IG was given, people cannot return to health care settings, and if possible, persons working in child care, school, or other settings should not return to work before a 3-week period. An individualized analysis is suggested.

CONTRAINDICATIONS TO MMR VACCINATION

When being consulted on MMR vaccination, it is of utmost importance to undertake a detailed past medical history and a review of childhood and adult vaccinations. MMR is a live-virus-attenuated vaccinate and *should never be prescribed* to pregnant women, those with HIV infection with CD4 <200 cells/mL, or any condition that causes immunosuppression (e.g., cancer patients on chemotherapy or primary immunodeficiencies).

MMR is currently not recommended for children younger than 6 months of age, regardless of the risk of exposure.

If you see or suspect a case of measles, the individual must be isolated and placed on respiratory precautions. Their contacts should be followed for at least 21 days, and notification to local public health authorities should be made immediately.

Rubella

I: Usually a childhood disease. Virus may be shed for 1 to 2 weeks before rash, and patients are contagious.
C: Incubation period: 2 weeks. Usually no serious systemic symptoms. Prominent postauricular, posterior cervical, and/or suboccipital adenopathy. Forchheimer spots (red spots on the soft palate).
R: Spreads caudally, usually disappears in 3 days.
A: Serologic assays.
T: Supportive care.
O: The goal of vaccination is to prevent congenital rubella infection. In pregnancy, rubella can lead to fetal death, premature delivery, and congenital abnormalities.

Roseola Subitum

I: Also known as *exanthema subitum* or *sixth disease*. Young children, peak prevalence 7 to 13 months. Most cases have known exposure. It is mainly caused by human herpes virus 6 (HHV-6). Also by HHV-7, enterovirus, parainfluenza-1, and adenovirus.
C: Classically starts with 3 to 5 days of high fever >40° C. When the fever abates, the rash begins. Patients can present with seizures. In adults, arthralgias are common.
R: Blanching macular or maculopapular rash; begins in trunk, neck, and extremities and can spare the face. Resolves within 2 days.
A: Neutropenia and mild lymphocytosis.
T: Symptomatic treatment.
O: Supportive, standard hygienic measures, such as handwashing, may prevent its spread.

Infectious Mononucleosis

I: Acute illness due to Epstein–Barr virus (EBV) infection. Most frequently occurs in adolescents and young adults.
C: Malaise, sweats, anorexia, nausea, chills, pharyngitis, palatal petechiae, splenomegaly, and lymphadenopathy (tends to involve posterior cervical nodes).
R: A diffuse maculopapular eruption, urticarial or petechial (more common after the administration of amoxicillin or ampicillin).
A: Lymphocytosis, atypical lymphocytes, and elevated aminotransferases. Heterophile antibody and EBV-specific antibodies. If these studies are negative, consider an alternative cause for mononucleosis-like illness, such as cytomegalovirus, toxoplasmosis, and primary HIV infection.
T: Supportive therapy.
O: For people who regularly exercise, training can be gradually restarted 3 to 4 weeks after the onset of symptoms.

Primary HIV Infection

I: Occurs approximately 2 to 4 weeks after HIV infection.
C: Acute antiretroviral syndrome: sore throat, lymphadenopathy, arthralgias, myalgias, fatigue, headache, and gastrointestinal symptoms. Painful mucocutaneous ulceration is one of the most distinctive manifestations.
R: Nonspecific macules and papules, well circumscribed, oval or round pink to deeply red colored. The rash persists for 5 to 8 days, nonpruritic, trunk or facial in localization.

A: Antigen/antibody immunoassay plus quantitative plasma HIV-1 RNA levels (viral load); it is usually >100,000 copies/mL. Transient CD4 lymphopenia. HIV serology (delay at least 1 month after acute illness).

T: Prompt initiation of antiretroviral therapy reduces the likelihood of HIV transmission to others and can reduce the size of the latent HIV reservoir.

O: High level of suspicion. Patients should be referred promptly to an infectious diseases specialist to review treatment options. Counseling to adopt behaviors that guard against HIV transmission.

Erlichial Diseases

I: Human monocytic ehrlichiosis (HME), caused by *Ehrlichia chaffeensis*, and human granulocytic anaplasmosis (HGA), caused by *Anaplasma phagocytophilum*. Most cases occur in spring and summer in the United States. Vector ticks. Mortality rates are between 2% and 5% in HM, and 7% to 10% in HGA.

C: Acute illness. Incubation period of 1 to 2 weeks. Nonspecific symptoms (headache, myalgias, nausea, chills, diarrhea, malaise, altered mental status).

R: HME presents with a central maculopapular eruption sparing the extremities, palms, and soles (30% of patients). HGA: rash is rare.

A: Leukopenia, thrombocytopenia, elevated counts of aminotransferases, hyponatremia. Diagnosis is made by paired acute and convalescent serology.

T: Initiate treatment based upon a presumptive diagnosis. Treatment for adults and children (including pregnant women), is doxycycline 100 mg twice daily for 5 to 10 days. Alternatives: Rifampin has been used successfully in children.

O: Preventive measures include the use of tick repellents or permethrin and removal of ticks after exposure.

Leptospirosis

I: Zoonosis caused by pathogenic spirochetes *(Leptospira)*, distributed worldwide. The organisms infect mammals, especially rodents, cattle, swine, dogs, horses, sheep, and goats. Exposure to contaminated water or soil with animal urine.

C: Variable clinical course; most cases are mild to moderate (fever, rigors, myalgias, headache, conjunctival suffusion). Severe and complicated: renal failure, uveitis, hemorrhage, acute respiratory distress syndrome with pulmonary hemorrhage, myocarditis, and rhabdomyolysis.

R: Maculopapular eruption; conjunctivitis, sclera hemorrhage in some cases.

A: Serologic testing is the most common. Molecular diagnosis is a good option. The microscopic agglutination test is a reference standard assay.

T: Antimicrobial use shortens the duration of illness and reduces shedding of the organism in the urine. Mild: doxycycline 100 mg bid PO or ampicillin 500 to 750 mg q6h PO or amoxicillin 500 mg q6h PO. Severe: parenteral penicillin 1.5 MU intravenously (IV) q6h, doxycycline 100 mg IV twice daily, or ceftriaxone 2 g IV q 24 h or ampicillin 0.5 to 1 g IV q6h. The duration of treatment in severe disease is usually seven days.

O: The majority of infections are self-limiting. Prevention includes avoiding potential sources of infection, prophylaxis (doxycycline) for individuals at high risk of exposure, and animal vaccination.

Murine (Endemic) Typhus

I: Disease caused by *Rickettsia typhi*. Primarily transmitted by the rat flea (also by cats, opossums, and others). Humans are infected by inoculation of infective flea feces within bite wounds.

C: Mild illness. Incubation period between 8 and 16 days. Onset is abrupt, with nonspecific signs (headache, myalgias, fever). In severe cases, hepatic, renal, cardiac, neurologic, and pulmonary dysfunction can occur.

R: Maculopapular eruption is most commonly observed in the trunk, sparing the face, palms, and soles.
A: Thrombocytopenia (50% of patients). Serologic and indirect fluorescent antibody tests. A fourfold rise in immunoglobulin G (IgG) titer from acute illness to convalescence confirms the diagnosis.
T: It should be initiated even if laboratory confirmation is not available to avoid severe or potentially fatal infection. Doxycycline 100 mg twice daily for 7 to 10 days is the treatment of choice. Chloramphenicol 12.5 mg/kg q6h PO or IV (maximum 4 g daily) is the alternative treatment in pregnancy.
O: Prevention is directed to control the flea vectors and potential flea hosts. Advanced age and deficiency of glucose-6-phosphate dehydrogenase (G6PD) are associated with severe or fatal disease.

Lyme Disease

I: Tick-borne illness caused by a spirochete, *Borrelia burgdorferi.*
C: Three phases: (1) Early localized (erythema migrans) with nonspecific findings, headache, myalgias, chills, photophobia. (2) Early disseminated (acute neurologic or cardiac involvement usually weeks to months after the bite). (3) Late disease, months to years after the onset of infection (arthritis as the main manifestation).
R: Large papule, with central clearing at the site of the tick bite ("bull's eye"), often found in the axilla, inguinal region, popliteal fossa, or at the belt line. It may burn or itch and is hot to the touch. Sometimes concentric rings, or indurated, or vesicular center, or multiple secondary lesions are observed.
A: Serologic testing should be performed in patients with a recent history or traveling to an endemic area and the presence of risk factors and symptoms consistent with Lyme disease. Recommendation is a whole cell–based enzyme-linked immunosorbent assay (ELISA) followed by a Western blot testing.
T: Early localized: Doxycycline 100 mg bid, amoxicillin 500 mg three times a day (tid) for 10 to 14 days. Early disseminated: same treatment or ceftriaxone 2 g bid for 14 to 28 days. Late disease: Ceftriaxone for at least 28 days. Extended courses of antibiotics are not recommended (lack of evidence for benefit and the potential of adverse effects).
O: Personal protection to avoid tick bites and tick checks after exposure in endemic areas.

Relapsing Fever

I: Caused by spirochetes of the *Borrelia* genus. Arthropod-borne infection that occurs in two forms: tick-borne relapsing fever (TBRF) and louse-borne relapsing fever (LBRF). Mortality is 4% to 10% in TBRF and 10% to 70% in LBRF.
C: Recurrent fever above 39° C (fever is present for 3 days, alternating with afebrile periods lasting about 7 days), nonspecific symptoms (headache, myalgias, arthralgias, shaking chills, abdominal complaints), and hepatosplenomegaly.
R: Central rash at the end of febrile episode; sometimes petechial.
A: Thin and thick smears of blood should be performed during the febrile period. Polymerase chain reaction (PCR) test can be performed if the organism is not identified on smear.
T: Severe: Ceftriaxone 2 g IV once per day or doxycycline 100 mg bid for 10 to 14 days. Jarisch–Herxheimer reactions are common, and the patient should be observed for about 3 hours after starting antibiotics.
O: Decrease louse and tick exposures. PEP with doxycycline should be administered after tick exposure in an endemic area.

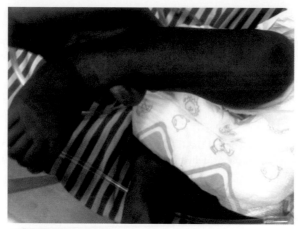

Fig. 7.1   Maculopapular rash caused by Chikungunya virus in an 8-month child. (Courtesy Dr. Teresa Gadsden.)

ARBOVIROSIS (DENGUE, CHIKUNGUNYA, ZIKA)

I: Travel to endemic areas. Arthropod-borne infection transmitted by mosquitoes. Humans are infected after being bitten by an infected female *Aedes* mosquito (*aegypti* and *albopictus*). Mosquito usually bites during the daytime and breeds in standing water.

C: Incubation period: 3 to 7 days. Dengue is characterized by retro-orbital, muscle, and joint pain. Chikungunya is characterized by long-standing polyarthralgias, arthritis, and tenosynovitis. Arthralgias are bilateral and symmetric, involving distal and proximal joints. Severe forms: meningoencephalitis, cardiopulmonary decompensation, acute renal failure, and death. Zika virus is mild and self-limited, often with pruritus, dysesthesias, conjunctivitis (nonpurulent), and arthralgia (notably in small joints of the hands and feet).

R: Maculopapular pruritic rash; intense itching may be observed toward the end of the febrile period. Rash may be present on the face, trunk, extremities, palms, and soles (Figs. 7.1, 7.2, and 7.3). The rash of dengue may become petechial or hemorrhagic.

A: Thrombocytopenia, abnormal liver function tests, reduced lymphocyte counts, and increased prothrombin time. Diagnosis is made by serology for each of the three infections; also PCR can be done.

T: Treatment consists of supportive care, plenty of fluids, antiinflammatory drugs, and analgesics. Outpatient management in the absence of warning signs or coexisting condition (pregnancy, old age, diabetes, renal failure, underlying hemolytic disease, obesity, or poor social situation). Hospitalization for severe infection and/or coexisting conditions. Assess for signs of shock.

O: Prevention: Mosquito control. For dengue, there is a vaccine that might be used in certain conditions.

There is an association between Zika virus and maternal infection, with adverse fetal outcomes, such as congenital microcephaly, fetal loss, and Guillain–Barré syndrome.

2. Febrile/toxic and peripheral.
These patients can be further differentiated based on the presence or absence of a characteristic targeted lesion. It is important to note that patients who are febrile with peripheral lesions without a target lesion require urgent evaluation for meningococcemia and Rocky Mountain spotted fever. In this classification erythema multiform, Stevens–Johnson syndrome, and syphilis are the main conditions.

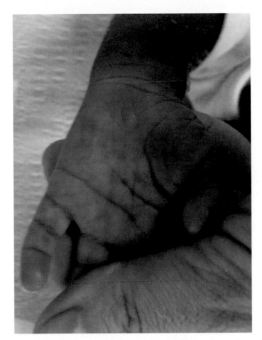

Fig. 7.2 Maculopapular rash caused by Chikungunya virus affecting the palms of an 8-month-old child. (Courtesy Dr. Teresa Gadsden.)

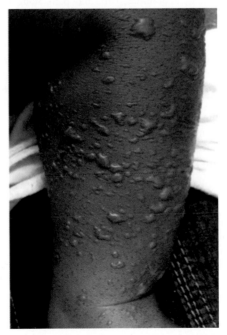

Fig. 7.3 Atypical presentation of Chikungunya virus infection with vesicles in lower extremities. (Courtesy Dr. Teresa Gadsden.)

ERYTHEMA INFECTIOSUM

I: Caused by parvovirus B19. Common in children 3 to 12 years. In adults, exists a history of exposure to an affected child. It is most contagious during the phase of active viral replication and viral shedding (5 to 10 days after exposure and lasts around 5 days). Transient aplastic crisis in patients with underlying hematologic abnormalities; causes severe anemia that resolves spontaneously within a few days to weeks.
C: Mild fever. In adults, arthralgias involving symmetric and small joints are characteristic (more common in women).
R: "Slapped cheek" appearance. The rash is spread from arms to trunk and follows a reticular pattern. Bright-red appearance, followed by diffuse, lacy, reticular rash that waxes and wanes over 3 weeks.
A: Serology: Immunoglobulin M (IgM) for acute and IgG for past infection. Levels of parvovirus B19 DNA are indicated in aplastic anemia.
T: There is no specific therapy. IV IG in addition to red blood transfusion can be helpful in patients with chronic infection and anemia.
O: Prevention depends on good infection control practices targeted toward the modes of transmission: handwashing, not sharing food or drink, and droplet precautions. During pregnancy, this infection can result in fetal complications.

ROCKY MOUNTAIN SPOTTED FEVER

I: Tick vector caused by *Rickettsia rickettsii*. It occurs in the United States, Canada, Mexico, Central America, and parts of South America. Seasonal outbreaks (spring and summer), when outdoor activities are more frequent. The case fatality rate is 25% to 30% without treatment and 4% with appropriate antimicrobials.
C: Short incubation period. Patients are febrile and toxic appearing. Headache, fever, malaise, conjunctival suffusion, myalgias, abdominal pain, and pain along the gastrocnemius muscle. Complications: skin necrosis, gangrenous digits, azotemia, pulmonary edema, acute respiratory distress syndrome, and neurologic complications.
R: Rash is common but may not occur in the first days of illness. It begins on wrists and ankles before becoming palpable petechiae and spreads to the rest of the body. In later phases, palms and soles are involved. Approximately 10% to 15% of patients will not present with skin lesions.
A: Indirect immunofluorescence assay: A fourfold rise in IgG titer from acute illness to convalescence confirms the diagnosis. PCR amplification in blood, skin, or eschar is useful.
T: Start empiric antimicrobial treatment if high suspicion. Doxycycline 100 mg bid for 7 days or for 2 days after temperature becomes normal in all nonpregnant patients, even children. In pregnancy, use chloramphenicol 50 to 75 mg/kg/day divided in four doses (maximum, 4 g/day).
O: Avoidance of contact with ticks through the use of repellents and protective clothing.

SECONDARY SYPHILIS

I: Sexually transmitted infection caused by *Treponema pallidum*. During the initial phase of the infection, the organism disseminates widely. The median incubation period is 21 days before a chancre appears (25% of individuals). Within weeks to a few months, 25% of individuals develop a systemic illness that represents secondary syphilis.
C: Constitutional symptoms (fever, headache, malaise, anorexia, myalgias, sore throat, and weight loss), lymph nodes enlargement, hepatitis, synovitis, osteitis, acute nephritis, nephrotic syndrome, meningitis and ocular findings.
R: Classically diffuse; copper, red, or reddish-brown; 0.5 to 2 cm in diameter; macular or papular lesions involving the trunk and extremities, including palms and soles, and can include mucosal surfaces. Nodules, pustules, or ulcerative forms can present (Figs. 7.4 and 7.5).

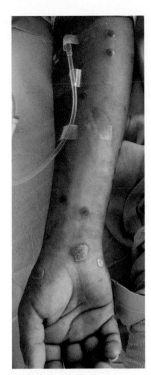

Fig. 7.4 Maculopapular caused by secondary syphilis in patient with HIV. (Courtesy Dr. Elizageth Salazar-Rojas.)

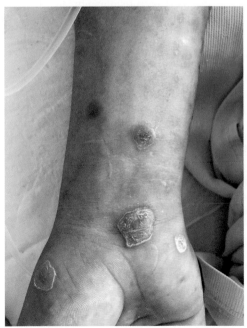

Fig. 7.5 Close-up of papules grouping together in small squamous plaques in the patient with HIV and secondary syphilis. (Courtesy Dr. Elizageth Salazar-Rojas.)

A: Nontreponemal titers should be obtained just before initiating therapy.

Monitoring with serologic tests (a fourfold decline in the titer is considered an acceptable response).

T: Non-neurosyphilis: Penicillin G benzathine intramuscularly (IM) 2.4 UI (three doses with an interval of 1 week between each) or doxycycline 100 mg bid or ceftriaxone 1 to 2 g IV daily for 14 days. Neurosyphilis: Penicillin G IV 18 to 24 million units/day divided every 4 hours (or continuous infusion) for 10 to 14 days. For allergic patients, alternative agents include, ceftriaxone (2 g q24h) or amoxicillin (3 g) with probenecid (500 mg) orally bid for 14 days or doxycicline 100 mg bid for 21 days.

O: Persons exposed sexually to a partner with syphilis should be evaluated clinically and serologically for infection.

3. *Afebrile/nontoxic, central or peripheral.*

Patients in this classification are much less likely to have a life-threatening diagnosis. Consider drug reactions, pityriasis, scabies, eczema, and psoriasis.

ERYTHEMATOUS RASH

These are characterized by diffuse red skin from capillary congestion, mimicking severe sunburn, and can occur in a variety of inflammatory and infectious conditions

Two points are important to consider and narrow the diagnosis in these patients. Consider whether or not the patient is febrile or toxic and assess the Nikolsky sign (the top layer of the skin slips away from the lower layers when rubbed).

1. *Febrile and positive Nikolsky sign.*

Patients have the potential to develop a life-threatening diagnosis, as well as the risk of losing a large amount of the epidermis, which can lead to dehydration. In this classification, toxic epidermal necrolysis is a differential diagnosis, because mortality can reach up 30% to 35%.

The following pathologies are included in this classification.

STAPHYLOCOCCAL SCALDED SKIN SYNDROME

I: Occurs in children (neonates and infants younger than 1 year), mortality rate is <5%. It rarely occurs in adults and is often associated with an underlying condition. Mortality can be more than 50%.

C: Two presentations: generalized and localized. Localized: Self-limited and wanes within 4 to 5 days. It looks like a bullous impetigo and appears around a wound or umbilicus (neonates). Generalized: Abrupt onset of fever, irritability, lethargy, and nasal or conjunctival secretions.

R: Diffuse, tender erythema, often with bullae and desquamation. Blanching skin erythema, usually beginning on the neck, axillae, and groin, associated with skin tenderness. Mucous membranes are not involved.

A: Skin biopsy is diagnostic and routinely done to distinguish from toxic epidermal necrolysis. Cultures from bullae, blood, urine, eyes, nose, and throat are helpful.

T: General measures: Antiseptic wound dressings and fluid support. Specific therapy: penicillinase-resistant beta-lactams: ceftobiprole 500 mg IV tid; ceftaroline 600 mg IV bid; vancomycin in critically ill patients, with loading dose 25 to 30 mg/kg IV, then 15 to 20 mg/kg IV bid or tid; and daptomycin 4 mg/kg IV every day.

O: Nasal carriage of the organism should be screened in the medical staff and in all caretakers; decolonization with mupirocin nasal ointment 2% bid for 5 days and daily total-body washing with or without chlorhexidine-based soap during 1 week.

2. *Febrile and negative Nikolsky sign.*

TOXIC SHOCK SYNDROME

I: Nasal colonization with *Staphylococcus aureus*, injection drug use, indwelling vascular catheters, use of absorbent tampons, nasal packing, surgical wounds, postpartum infection, and abscesses. Mortality rate with adequate treatment is 5%.
C: Patients are febrile (usually >39° C), toxic appearance, hypotension refractory to fluids, and multiorgan dysfunction.
R: Diffuse erythematous rash on the hands and feet. Desquamation occurs 7 to 10 days of illness.
A: Cultures should be obtained from blood, urine, nasopharynx, or any suspected focus of infection.
T: Removal of the infected materials. Clindamycin 900 mg IV tid and vancomycin in critically ill patients (loading dose 25 to 30 mg/kg IV, then 15 to 20 mg/kg IV every 8 to 12 hours [q8 to 12h]). Fluid and electrolyte management, vasoactive medications, and intensive care unit admission.
O: Avoiding the use of hyper-absorbent tampons and preventing staphylococcal colonization of wounds and mucosa. In nasal carriers, decontamination is suggested.

STREPTOCOCCAL TOXIC SHOCK SYNDROME

I: Most commonly in the setting of pharyngitis from group A streptococcus (GAS). Other portals of entry are the vagina, mucosa, and skin. Mortality rate >30%. During pregnancy is an important cause of maternal and infant mortality.
C: Pain precedes physical findings of infection. At the site of minor trauma, patients develop deep infection such as necrotizing fasciitis or myonecrosis within 24 to 72 hours, often with no visible break in the skin. Multiorgan failure, hypotension, and abdominal pain can develop fast.
R: Coarse, sandpaper-like, erythematous, blanching rash, which ultimately desquamates. This is accompanied by circumoral pallor and strawberry tongue.
A: Thrombocytopenia, coagulopathy, liver dysfunction. Cultures from blood, cerebrospinal, pleural, or peritoneal fluid; tissue biopsy; or surgical wound are indicated.
T: Treatment of septic shock and associated complications, surgical debridement of infection, and antimicrobial therapy. Empiric regimen includes clindamycin 900 mg IV tid plus penicillin G 4 million units IV q4h or clindamycin plus ceftriaxone 2 g IV every day.
O: Life-threatening disease. Routine screening for and prophylaxis against GAS are not recommended for household contacts of index patients.

SCARLET FEVER

I: Nonsuppurative complication of GAS. It is associated with pharyngeal infections or may follow streptococcal infections at other sites.
C: Most common in children 2 to 10 years. High fever and marked systemic toxicity, pharyngitis, headache, vomiting, and abdominal pain. It may complicate with arthritis and jaundice.
R: Diffuse blanchable erythema, numerous small papular elevations, giving a sandpaper texture to skin. It begins on the upper part of the chest and spreads to trunk and extremities. Palms, soles, and usually the face are spared. There is an accentuation of linear erythema in skin folds (Pastia lines). Enanthem characterized by small, red, hemorrhagic spots on palate. Strawberry tongue.
A: Modest eosinophilia early in the course of illness. Antistreptolysin O titer; throat culture, rapid antigen detection tests.

T: Penicillin VK 500 mg bid or amoxicillin 50 mg/kg/day (maximum 1 g) bid. In allergic patients, cephalexin 500 mg PO bid, azithromycin 500 mg PO on day 1 and then 250 mg PO daily on days 2 through 5 or clindamycin 300 mg PO tid for 10 days.
O: Treatment of streptococcal tonsillopharyngitis with antibiotic therapy is important for reducing complications.

3. *Afebrile with Nikolsky sign.*
Toxic epidermal necrolysis could be included in this classification. It is a rare condition (2 cases/1,000,000 population per year) with a mortality rate of 30% to 50%. Involves greater than 30% of the total body surface. In adults, the most frequent cause is drug induced; in children, is frequently associated with Mycoplasma pneumoniae or herpes virus infection.

4. *Afebrile without Nikolsky sign.*
Most of these conditions are noninfectious, such as anaphylaxis, scombroid, alcohol flush, and medications.

Purpuric/Petechial Rash

Petechiae are small (<5 mm) papular or macular nonblanching lesions that are due to extravasation of red blood cells. Lesions > 0.5 cm are called *purpura*. Palpable lesions are the result of either perivascular inflammation (vasculitis) or infection. Nonpalpable lesions usually occur in low-platelet conditions such as idiopathic thrombocytopenic purpura and disseminated intravascular coagulation.

Two characteristics help define the diagnosis: the presence of fever and palpable lesions.

1. *Febrile and palpable.*
A petechial rash plus fever or toxic appearance should be considered a life-threatening condition, because severe infections such as acute meningococcemia are included in this classification. Noninfectious causes should consider Henoch–Schönlein purpura.

ACUTE MENINGOCOCCEMIA

I: Caused by *Neisseria meningitidis*. Outbreaks can occur among groups with confined living conditions (military bases, day care centers, and dormitories). Most common in children, patients with asplenia, or complement deficiency. It is a medical emergency and may be rapidly fatal, with mortality rates between 10% and 25%.
C: Sudden onset of fever, chills, malaise, myalgias, somnolence, weakness, cold extremities, skin pallor, headache, and hypotension. Patients can present with severe, persistent shock; peripheral vasoconstriction; multiorgan failure; and disseminated intravascular coagulation.
R: Initially can be maculopapular, appearing on the wrist and ankles. It becomes palpable petechia in 40% to 80% of patients and spreads to the rest of the body coalescing into purpura.
A: Leukocytosis or leukopenia. Positive buffy coat. Gram stain: negative encapsulated diplococcus. Positive cultures taken from blood, lesions, and cerebrospinal fluid. Severe forms require head CT and/or brain MRI.
T: Early antibiotic treatment with ceftriaxone 1 to 2 g IV bid or cefotaxime 50 to 75 mg/kg q6 to 8h (maximum dose 12 g/day) or penicillin G 4 million U q4h (maximum dose 24 g/day) or meropenem 2 g IV tid for 7 to 14 days. Adjuvant therapy and supportive care should be provided.
O: Prophylaxis is indicated for anyone potentially exposed to respiratory secretions. Recommended drugs are rifampin 600 mg bid for 2 days, ciprofloxacin 500 mg single dose, azithromycin 10 mg/kg (maximum 500 mg) single dose, or ceftriaxone 250 mg, single IM dose.

Meningococcal polysaccharide-conjugate vaccines are recommended for adolescents and others at risk of infection.

DISSEMINATED GONOCOCAL INFECTION

I: Sexually active individuals, some with complement deficiency. Caused by bacteremic dissemination of *Neisseria gonorrhoeae*.
C: It causes urethritis and cervicitis, but also pharyngitis, proctitis, conjunctivitis, tenosynovitis, and polyarthralgias (involve knees, elbows, and more distal joints). Fever and systemic toxicity are common.
R: Rash in 75% of patients; begins as petechial macules, progresses to papules, evolves over 1 to 2 days into hemorrhagic pustules, and later develops a necrotic center. The lesions (usually 5 to 40) are distributed peripherally near joints.
A: Gonococci can be recovered from blood, skin lesions, cervical, or urethral secretions. Synovial fluid contains fewer than 20,000 leucocytes/mm^3 and is sterile. Nucleic acid amplification tests are useful.
T: Ceftriaxone 1 g IV q24h for at least 7 days + azithromycin 1 g PO in a single dose. After improvement it can be changed to an oral cephalosporin (cefixime 400 mg bid) or a fluoroquinolone (levofloxacin 500 mg every day) for 7 to 10 days.
O: Screening of sexually active people in certain settings, such as sexually transmitted disease (STD) clinics. Patients should be tested for other STD infections. Prevention includes proper use of male condoms.

2. Febrile and nonpalpable.
This category includes thrombotic thrombocytopenic purpura (TTP), disseminated intravascular coagulation, purpura fulminans, and enteroviral rash.

ENTEROVIRAL RASH

I: Eighty percent of infections occur in infants, children, and adolescents. *Enterovirus* includes poliovirus, coxsackieviruses, and echoviruses.
C: Incubation period: 3 to 5 days. Symptoms: Pharyngitis, headache, aseptic meningitis, pleurodynia, and myopericarditis.
R: Maculopapular, petechial and purpuric, and urticarial eruptions have been described. Sometimes associated with enanthems.
A: Reverse transcription polymerase chain reaction (RT-PCR) for *Enterovirus* or *Parechovirus* detection, or viral isolation in cell culture.
T: Most infections are self-limited and only require symptomatic and supportive care. For more serious infection, serum IG can be used.
O: Handwashing is important to prevent the spread of infection.

3. Afebrile and palpable lesions.
Patients with palpable petechiae or purpura who are neither febrile nor toxic appearing are more likely to be suffering from one of many causes of perivascular inflammation. Autoimmune vasculitis includes many rheumatologic causes, including lupus erythematosus, rheumatoid arthritis, and systemic vasculitides (e.g., Wegener granulomatosis). Other causes include chronic hepatitis B or C and medications (Fig. 7.6).

4. Afebrile and nonpalpable lesions.
These patients have idiopathic thrombocytopenia purpura (ITP), sometimes associated with a recent viral infection; is more common in children and adolescents.

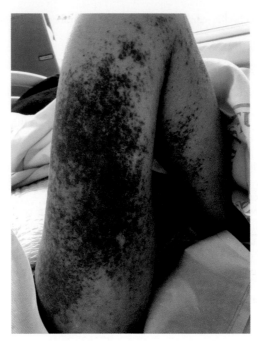

Fig. 7.6   Drug-induced purpuric macules in a patient with cancer. (Courtesy Dr. Elizabeth Salazar-Rojas.)

VESICULOBULLOUS RASHES

Vesiculobullous disorders are characterized by involvement of the dermal–epidermal junction causing fluid-filled lesions. By definition, vesicles are small (<0.5 cm in size), whereas bullae are larger (≥0.5 cm).

It is necessary to first consider if the individual looks toxic, as this may be indicative of a life-threatening diagnosis. Another important point to look at during the examination is if these lesions are diffuse or localized.

In this category, there are also nonfebrile vesiculobullous rashes of medical importance, such as the bullous pemphigoid and the pemphigus vulgaris, both with a diffuse distribution, whereas herpes zoster shows a localized distribution. Although fever is not a defining characteristic, severe forms of these diseases may present with some degree of fever.

1. *Febrile with disseminated lesions.*

VARICELLA (CHICKENPOX)

I: Caused by varicella zoster virus (VZV). More common in children, during winter and spring. With the introduction of the vaccine, its prevalence has decreased. It is transmitted by aerosolized droplets from nasopharyngeal secretions.

C: Incubation period: 14 to 21 days. Usually begins with a prodrome of malaise, low-grade fever, and pharyngitis followed by rash. In adults and immunocompromised patients, severe disease involves the pulmonary system and central nervous system (CNS).

R: Macules, evolving to papules (sometimes umbilicated), pustules, and vesicles that will crust quickly (24 hours or less). All types of lesions can be seen simultaneously. The rash has a centripetal distribution with greater concentration of lesions on the trunk and the fewest lesions on the distal extremities (Fig. 7.7).

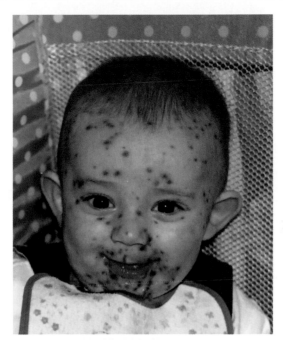

Fig. 7.7 Vesicles and crusts caused by varicella herpes virus in a 5-month-old infant. (Courtesy Dr. Diana Vilar-Compte.)

A: In high-risk patients with clinical data consistent with CNS or lung involvement, CT thorax scan and brain MRI are indicated. Tzanck smear impression (low sensitivity), VZV DNA by PCR, serologic assays, or VZV isolation in tissue culture lines. Confirmation is not required.

T: Symptomatic and supportive care. Good hygiene and topical treatment to relieve itching. In adults, immunocompromised patients, or those with varicella pneumonia or CNS involvement, acyclovir 10 mg/kg tid for 7 days (initiate within 24 hours of symptoms).

O: In the hospital, institute contact and airborne precautions immediately; discharge as soon as possible. Vaccinate susceptible contacts, and consider using IG if close contacts with high risk of severe disease.

2. Febrile with localized lesions distribution.

HAND–FOOT–MOUTH DISEASE

I: Enteroviruses type A cause 90%; the remaining are caused by coxsackievirus. More common in children <7 years; adults can be infected during outbreaks in day cares, summer camps, or within the family. Males are more likely to develop symptoms, to have diffuse infections, and to need medical assistance. The disease is more common during late spring and early summer.

C: Transmission: Oral ingestion of the shed virus from feces, respiratory tract, or via vesicle fluid or oral secretions. Incubation period: 3 to 5 days. The disease is usually mild, with low-grade fever and malaise. In severe cases (1.1%), aseptic meningitis, acute flaccid paralysis, and encephalomyelitis with or without muscle weakness may be present. Sequelae may be present. Adults can be asymptomatic.

R: Maculopapular rash evolving into painful blisters on the hands, soles, and buttocks. Tender ulcerative lesions of the mouth, throat, and tongue. Up to 50% of patients present with desquamation of palms and soles 1 to 3 weeks after the initial presentation (Figs. 7.8 and 7.9).

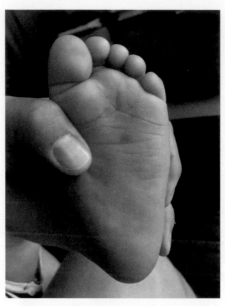

Fig. 7.8 Erythematous bullous lesions on the sole of a 1-year-old child with hand–foot–mouth disease.

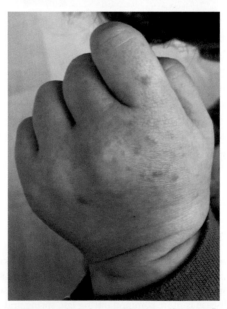

Fig. 7.9 Small vesicles and papules caused in a 2-year-old toddler. (Courtesy Dr. Alexandra Martin and Rafael Franco.)

A: If available, RT-PCR. In patients with high risk of complications, severe illness or deterioration, or during outbreak investigation, *Enterovirus* and coxsackievirus strain identification is highly desirable. Depending on the symptoms and severity of the disease, laboratory studies and CNS imaging.

T: Symptomatic and supportive care. Avoid the use of steroids (increase the risk of CNS disease). IG has been suggested to treat severe infections.

O: Case isolation at home for 10 days. Frequent handwashing plus cleaning and disinfection of high-touch surfaces. When day care center, school classroom, indoor, or recreation facilities are involved in an outbreak, suspension of daily activities is needed plus thoroughly cleaning and disinfection. Use contact and droplet precautions in hospitalized patients.

3. *Nonfebrile with localized lesion distribution.*

HERPES ZOSTER (SHINGLES)

I: Caused by reactivation of latent VZV from the dorsal root ganglia. It can occur at all ages, but it is highest in individuals among the sixth and eight decades.

C: The onset of disease is usually heralded by pain 48 to 72 hours before the onset of skin lesions. VZV may affect the facial nerve, causing Ramsey Hunt syndrome, characterized by pain and vesicles in the external auditory canal with changes in the sense of taste in the anterior two-thirds of the tongue, with ipsilateral facial palsy. Meningo-encephalitis may occur. In the immunocompromised, disease is more severe, with cutaneous dissemination, pneumonitis, meningoencephalitis, or other serious life-threatening complications. Pain associated with acute neuritis and postherpetic neuralgia weeks or months after the skin lesions.

R: Painful, unilateral eruption of vesicular lesions within a dermatome. When branches of the trigeminal nerve are involved, lesions may appear in the face, in the mouth, on the eye, or on the tongue. At the beginning, an erythematous maculopapular rash is seen, rapidly evolving into vesicular lesions. In a normal host, the rash lasts between 7 and 10 days (Figs. 7.10 and 7.11).

A: To confirm the diagnosis, Tzanck smear, immunofluorescence, and the detection of viral DNA from the vesicular fluid are useful.

T: Antivirals are most beneficial if given within the first 72 hours of the onset of symptoms. Valacyclovir 1000 mg PO tid or famciclovir 500 mg PO tid for 7 days. Acyclovir is also effective but less convenient: 800 mg PO 5 times a day for 7 days. In patients with ocular or neurologic or disseminated disease, admit to the hospital and start acyclovir 10 mg/kg day IV (infusion over 1 hour) tid for 7 to 14 days.

Corticosteroids should be considered in older patients within 72 hours of clinical presentation or if new lesions are still appearing; analgesics depending on pain intensity; opioids may be necessary. Local treatment with compresses using cool tap water or solutions help to break the vesicles and remove serum and crust.

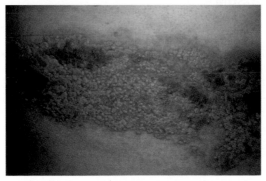

Fig. 7.10 Multiple coalescent vesicles on an erythematous base and necrotic areas caused by herpes zoster virus.

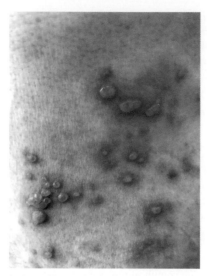

Fig. 7.11   Vesicles grouped into lesions with surrounding erythema in a patient with herpes zoster. (Courtesy Dr. Elizabeth Salazar-Rojas.)

O: Contact precautions. Vaccine available for >50 years old and high-risk groups. Most useful to prevent postherpetic neuralgia. Live-attenuated vaccine is contraindicated in severely immunosuppressed patients.

NODULAR, ULCERS, AND ESCHAR-FORMING RASHES

In this type of rash, erythema nodosum is a common associated eruption with infections and other systemic diseases. Nodules are deep-seated, rounded lesions that can involve the epidermal, dermal, and subcutaneous tissue. These nodules can also be associated with disseminated infection.

   Ulcers and eschar-forming lesions are defects in the skin that extend beyond the upper layer of the dermis with necrotic lesions and crust forming. Two causative agents, *Bacillus anthracis* and *Fransicsella tularensis*, are considered potential bioterror threats.

ERYTHEMA NODOSUM

I: The most frequent causes are infections (antecedent streptococcal infections, 45%, and tuberculosis, 6%), sarcoidosis, inflammatory bowel disease, pregnancy, drugs, and malignancy. Up to 55% are idiopathic. In endemic areas, coccidioidomycosis is a common antecedent. It can also be associated with multiple autoimmune diseases, leukemia, lymphoma, and various drugs.

C: More frequently in women (ratio 5:1). Peak incidence between 15 and 45 years. Prodromal symptoms: fatigue, fever, malaise, arthralgias and arthritis, and symptoms of respiratory tract infection may precede the eruption by several days. Some patients develop pulmonary adenopathy, most commonly seen in sarcoidosis.

R: Painful, red, cutaneous, 1- to 5-cm nodules on the anterior surface of legs, more rarely on the arms. They involve over the days or weeks, leaving some degree of pigmented areas. They may recur in about one-third of cases (see Fig. 7.11).

A: Initial evaluation should include blood cell count, erythrocyte sedimentation rate, purified protein derivative (PPD), chest x-rays, antistreptolysin O titer, and tuberculin skin test. Consider a urine culture, and if the patient has diarrhea, order stool cultures.

T: It is usually self-limiting in 3 to 4 weeks; relapses are frequent. Direct treatment toward symptoms and/or underlying cause of disease. If possible, discontinue the drugs that may be causing the condition. Use nonsteroidal antiinflammatory drugs (NSAIDs) and other supportive measures to relieve pain and inflammation. Prednisone 40 to 60 mg PO per day for a few days if necessary, with a rapid decrease in the dosage.
O: Consult a dermatologist and/or infectious diseases physician. Other specialists may be called, depending on the most probable diagnosis.

CUTANEOUS ANTHRAX

I: Anthrax is a zoonosis, caused by *B. anthracis*, a bacterium that produces spores extremely resistant that primarily affects grazing herbivorous animals. Humans are incidental hosts; most infections are considered an occupational disease. More recently, injectional anthrax has emerged (mainly in Europe), related to heroin contaminated with anthrax spores that are inoculated by IM or subcutaneous injection. Mortality is 20% in those without treatment and 1% with early and appropriate treatment. If lesions are located on the face, neck, or chest, clinical symptoms may be life-threatening.
C: Depending on the route of infection, three primary forms are recognized: cutaneous, pulmonary, and gastrointestinal. Incubation period: 2 to 7 days. Hemorrhagic lymphadenopathy, constitutional symptoms, and even septicemia may accompany the cutaneous lesion.
R: Skin lesions show as a pruritic, enlarging papule evolving into 1- to 3-cm painless ulcer surrounded by vesicles. The vesicles rupture with a discharge of clear fluid, forming a depressed black necrotic lesion (eschar). The eschar resolves in about 10 days, but may take longer. Lesions usually appear on exposed areas (face, neck, arms, and hands). Painful lymphadenitis may be seen.
    Injectional anthrax syndrome: A severe soft tissue infection at the injection site, with cellulitis, abscess, or necrotizing fasciitis. Is often life-threatening. It does not form a black eschar as in cutaneous anthrax.
A: Gram stain and culture isolation, swab extraction tube system, RT-PCR, and immunohistochemical staining of *B. anthracis* with monoclonal antibodies in biopsies are good diagnostic methods. Advise laboratory and pathology personnel about the possible diagnosis, as *Anthrax* is highly infective.
T: Amoxicillin 1 g PO qid or penicillin V 500 mg PO qid or ciprofloxacin 500 mg PO bid or levofloxacin 750 mg every day or doxycycline 100 mg PO bid for 10 days if naturally acquired. Surgical debridement may be needed.
O: An inactivated anthrax vaccine is only recommended for individuals engaged in some laboratory work, in certain remediation efforts, and in military personnel deployed to certain geographies. Consider PEP for health care workers and family members who might have been exposed. Can be a bioterrorism threat, especially the respiratory anthrax; in these cases, contact public health authorities.

TULAREMIA

I: Caused by *F. tularensis*. Occurs worldwide—ticks, hares, rabbits, and rodents are the most important sources of transmission to humans. Hunters, trappers, butchers, agricultural workers, campers, sheep herders, mink farmers, and laboratory workers are at increased risk of acquiring the infection.
C: Myalgias, fatigue, malaise, headache, chills, and fever progress shortly after the infection (3 to 6 days). A third of patients present with cough. Pericarditis, acute respiratory distress syndrome, pneumonia, pleural effusions, sore throat, and skin ulcers may be noted as well. Presentation depends on if the disease is localized to an entry site and its regional lymph nodes (ulceroglandular,

glandular, oculoglandular, and oropharyngeal) or more invasive and generalized forms (typhoidal and pulmonary).

R: Ulcerogandular: Inflamed papule within 24 to 48 hours of infection. The papule ulcerates and becomes pustular, and an ulcer crater with colorless exudate forms. Draining suppuration may be noted in regions of lymphadenopathy. Nodes are painful, with necrosis and even rupture. In children, posterior auricular or cervical nodes are commonly affected; in adults, the femoral and inguinal ones.

A: Diagnosis is made with serologic testing. In some settings, PCR is available.
Culture is the gold standard, but aspiration of the affected lymph nodes increases the risk of infections to health care workers.

T: For mild disease: Ciprofloxacin 400 mg IV or 750 mg PO bid or doxycycline 100 mg PO bid for 14 to 21 days. For pregancy, treatment is uncertain, but streptomycin or chlomphenicol 15 mg/kg qid for at least 14 days has been suggested.

O: Advise all health care personnel, especially those handling samples. No barrier precautions are needed. Alert the public health authorities if there is a high suspicion of it being used as a bioterrorism agent.

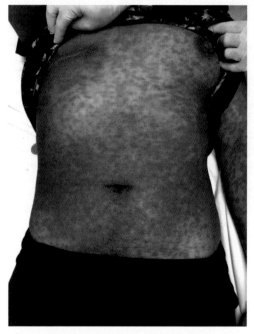

Fig. 7.12 Erythematous rash in a patient with metastatic breast cancer with Stevens–Johnson syndrome caused by diphenylhydantoin. (Courtesy Dr. Elizabeth Salazar-Rojas.)

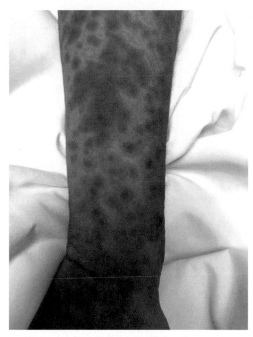

Fig. 7.13 Erythematous rash caused by erythema multiforme. (Courtesy Dr. Elizabeth Salazar-Rojas.)

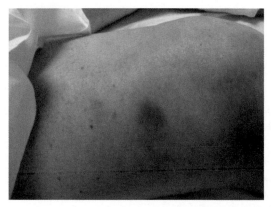

Fig. 7.14 Painful, erythematous, 1-cm nodule on the leg of a patient with Sweet syndrome. (Courtesy Dr. Stefanie Arroyo.)

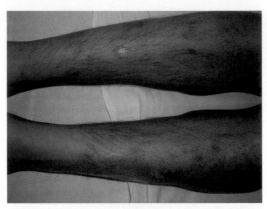

Fig. 7.15 Multiple erythematous, painful nodules on the anterior surface of the inferior extremities. Erythema nodosum. (Courtesy Dr. Teresa Vega.)

Suggested Reading

Blake T, Manahan M, Rodinsk K. Erythema nodosum. A review of an uncommon panniculitis. *Dermatol Online J.* 2014;20(4):22376.
Bolgiano EB, Sexton J. Tickborne illnesses (chapter 126). In: Wallas R, Hockberger R, Gausche-Hill M, eds. *Rosen's Emergency Medicine*. Philadelphia, PA: Elsevier; 2018:1657–1681.
Chen LH, Wilson ME. Dengue and chikungunya in travelers. *Curr Opin Infect Dis.* 2010;23:438–444.
Cohen JI. Herpes zoster. *N Engl J Med.* 2013;369:255–263.
Esposito S, Principi N. Hand, foot and mouth disease: current knowledge on clinical manifestations, epidemiology, aetiology and prevention. *Eur J Clin Microbiol Infect Dis.* 2018;37:391–398.
Korzeniewski K, Juszczak D, Jerzemowski J. Skin lesions in returning travellers. *Int Marit Health.* 2015;66:173–180.
Lamb LEM, Sriskandan S, Tan LKK. Bromine, bear-claw scratch fasciotomies, and the eagle effect: management of group a streptococcal necrotizing fasciitis and its association with trauma. *Lancet Infect Dis.* 2015;15:109–121.
Napolitano L. Severe soft tissue infections. *Infect Dis Clin N Am.* 2009;23:571–591.
Parola P, Paddock CD, Socolovschi C, et al. Update on tick-borne rickettsioses around the world: a geographic approach. *Clin Microbiol Rev.* 2013;26:657–702.
Patterson JW, Brown PC, Broecker AH. Infection-induced panniculitis. *J Cutan Patho.* 1989;16:183–193.
Porter A, Goldfarb J. Measles: a dangerous vaccine-preventable disease returns. *Cleve Clin J Med.* 2019;86(6):393–398.
Pujalte GGA, Marberry S, Libertin C. Tick-borne illnesses in the United States. *Prim Care Office Pract.* 2018;45:379–391.
Santistevan J, Long B, Koyfman A. Rash decisions: an approach to dangerous rashes based on morphology. *J Emerg Med.* 2017;52:457–471.
Sharma H, Yates J, Smith P. Fever and rash. *Medicine.* 2018;46(1):38–43.
Stevens DL, Bisno AL, Chambers HF, et al. Infectious diseases society of america. Practice guidelines for the diagnosis and management of skin and soft tissue infections: 2014 update by the infectious diseases society of america. *Clin Infect Dis.* 2014;59:e10–e52.
Weber DJ, Cohen MS, Rutala WA. The acute ill patients with fever and rash. In: Bennet JE, Dolin R, MJ Blaser MJ, eds. *Principles and Practice of Infectious Diseases*. 8th ed. Philadelphia, PA: Elsevier Saunders; 2015:732–747.
www.cdc.gov (Measles home). Last accessed: July 3, 2019.
Zasada AA. Injectional anthrax in humans: a new face of the old disease. *Adv Clin Exp Med.* 2018;27:553–558.

CHAPTER 8

Ear, Nose, Throat, and Neck Infections

John C. O'Horo ■ Kelly Cawcutt

CHAPTER OUTLINE

Pathogens	**Pharyngitis**
Diagnostic Testing	**Epiglottitis, Croup, and Laryngitis**
Otitis Externa	**Deep Neck Infections**
Otitis Media	**Lymphadenopathy and Lymphadenitis**
Rhinosinusitis	

Infections of the ear, nose, and throat (ENT) run the gamut from annoying but relatively harmless otitis externa to life-threatening infections of the airway. Despite the broad array of syndromes, most of these share a common set of pathogens and similar principles of evaluation and treatment. This chapter will discuss these pathogens and diagnostic tests before discussing anatomically distinct syndromes and specific treatments.

Pathogens

The anatomic continuity of the ENT with the outside environment lends it to extensive colonization with a variety of organisms. Inherently, colonization is a nonpathogenic state; however, these organisms may still evolve into an infection, thus making diagnosis challenging. The most common causes of ear and nose infections is *Streptococcus pneumoniae*, followed by *Haemophilus influenzae* and *Moraxella catarrhalis*. *Staphylococcus aureus* is a common colonizer of the nares but can also cause infections in this area. Group A streptococcus is also found throughout the ENT, although significant disease with this pathogen has become less common in the era of antibiotics.

Viruses can also frequently cause ENT infections, particularly respiratory syncytial virus (RSV), rhinovirus, parainfluenza, adenovirus, coronavirus, herpes viruses (herpes simplex viruses [HSV] 1 and 2, varicella zoster virus [VZV]), and influenza. However, most of these viruses do not cause pure ENT disease but involve the ENT as part of a larger syndrome (e.g., RSV and influenza cause significant lower respiratory tract infections).

Fungal organisms are rare, but can cause critical illness in the correct host. Mucormycosis of the sinuses in immunocompromised (including diabetic) patients is a surgical emergency because it is angioinvasive and has the potential to spread quickly. Aspergillosis can also cause fungal sinus infections whereby fungal "balls" obstruct the sinus outlets. This can occur even more quickly with mucormycosis. Endemic fungi, such as histoplasmosis, blastomycosis, and coccidiomycosis, can also cause infections of the sinuses, but this typically occurs as part of a more systemic syndrome, where the ENT symptoms are secondary considerations.

TABLE 8.1 ■ Common Causes of Bacterial ENT Infections

Organism	Syndrome(s)	Testing	Comments
S. pneumoniae	Otitis, rhinosinusitis	Culture Urine antigen test (disseminated/ systemic disease only)	Most common bacterial cause of ENT infections
H. influenzae	Otitis, sinusitis, pharyngitis epiglottitis	Culture	Less frequent cause of epiglottis since HiB vaccination became common
M. catarrhalis	Otitis, rhinosinusitis, pharyngitis	Culture	More common in children than adults
Group A streptococci	Pharyngitis, necrotizing fasciitis of the head and neck	Culture, rapid antigen test	Left untreated, has significant immunologic sequelae (rheumatic fever/heart disease, post-streptococcal glomerulonephritis
S. aureus	Otitis externa, otitis media, rhinosinusitis, pharyngitis, deep tissue infections	Culture, PCR	Can cause virtually any infection, but typically is either health care associated or related to antecedent trauma
Pseudomonas spp. (and other resistant Gram-negative organisms)	Otitis externa, otitis media, sinusitis, pharyngitis	Culture	Most often seen with health care–associated infection Some increased risk in diabetics
Fusarium spp.	Pharyngitis, Lemierre disease	Culture	
N. gonorrhoeae	Pharyngitis	Culture, PCR	

ENT, Ear, nose, and throat; *HiB, Haeomophilus influenzae* B; *PCR*, polymerase chain reaction.

Diagnostic Testing

Given that similar pathogens infect all anatomic parts of the ENT tract, diagnostic laboratory-based testing is uniform, regardless of the specific anatomy involved. A list of pathogens, syndromes, and recommended diagnostic tests is found in Table 8.1.

Culture-based testing is useful, particularly for bacteria and fungi, but the clinical significance of the results must be interpreted in the context of possible chronic colonization. Rapid diagnostic tests, such as polymerase chain reaction (PCR) testing, are valuable for detecting viruses because viral cultures are laborious and have poor sensitivity and specificity. Additionally, pathology from biopsy specimens may identify the class of pathogen by morphologic features, which suggest identification of the specific organism. Of note, culture remains the primary method for assessing antimicrobial susceptibilities (Tables 8.2 and 8.3).

Otitis Externa

Otitis externa is an infection of the outer ear canal. Commonly called *swimmer's ear*, this is associated with *Pseudomonas* spp. and *S. aureus*, but may be polymicrobial. Typically, otitis externa causes significant pain, especially with manipulation of the ear, including movement of the auricle. Most cases are mild and can be treated topically with antimicrobial-based otic ear drop solutions. However, in immunocompromised hosts, otitis externa can cause significant disease. In the elderly, diabetics, and those with a compromised immune system, the disease can be invasive and evolve

TABLE 8.2 ■ Common Causes of Viral ENT Infections

Organism	Syndrome(s)	Testing	Comments
Rhinovirus	Acute otitis media, rhinosinusitis, pharyngitis	PCR (rarely needed)	Treatment is supportive, and disease is largely self-limiting
Enterovirus spp.	Acute otitis media, rhinosinusitis, pharyngitis	PCR (rarely needed)	Treatment is supportive, and disease is largely self-limiting
Coronavirus	Acute otitis media, rhinosinusitis, pharyngitis	PCR (rarely needed)	Treatment is supportive, and disease is largely self-limiting
Adenovirus	Acute otitis media, rhinosinusitis, pharyngitis	PCR (rarely needed)	Treatment is supportive, and disease is largely self-limiting
Parainfluenza	Acute otitis media, rhinosinusitis, pharyngitis, laryngotracheitis (croup)	PCR (rarely needed)	Treatment is supportive, and disease is largely self-limiting
Influenza	Acute otitis media, rhinosinusitis, pharyngitis	PCR	
RSV	Acute otitis media, rhinosinusitis, pharyngitis	PCR	
HSV	Pharyngitis, skin and soft tissue infection	PCR	
VZV	Ramsay Hunt syndrome (otitis mimic), pharyngitis, skin and soft tissue infection	PCR	

ENT, Ear, nose, and throat; HSV, herpes simplex virus; PCR, polymerase chain reaction; RSV, respiratory syncytial virus; VZV, varicella zoster virus.

TABLE 8.3 ■ Common Causes of Fungal of ENT Infections

Organism	Syndrome(s)	Testing	Comments
Mucorales spp. (Rhizopus, Rhizomucor, Mucor, Lichtheimia, Cunninghamella)	Mucormycosis; invasive sinus infection	Imaging, pathology	Mucormycosis is a surgical emergency. Usually seen in patients with hematologic malignancy, but also associated with other immunosuppression such as diabetic ketoacidosis.
Aspergillus spp.	Chronic sinusitis	Imaging, culture	May require treatment as an adjunct to surgical/mechanical drainage approaches.
Endemic fungi (histoplasmosis, blastomyces, coccidiomycosis, paracoccidioidomycosis)	Sinusitis, laryngitis, deep tissue infections	Pathology, culture, urine antigen testing PCR	Much less common as etiologies of isolated ENT infections.

ENT, Ear, nose, and throat; PCR, polymerase chain reaction.

to a skull-base osteomyelitis and even meningitis, resulting in a higher morbidity and mortality. This manifestation requires systemic antibiotics and optimization of glucose control in diabetics. Although surgical consultation should be obtained, aggressive debridement is rarely indicated.

Herpes zoster infection of the ear canal can be mistaken for otitis externa. Tinnitus, vesicular lesions in the ear, and facial paralysis are all hints that a patient may have HSV causing Ramsay

Hunt syndrome instead of otitis externa, which would require antiviral medication for the zoster infection.

Otitis Media

Acute otitis media (AOM) is typically contracted when an infection in the sinus moves into the middle ear space via the eustachian tube, often while blowing the nose. As such, the pathogens causing rhinosinusitis and AOM are identical. AOM is diagnosed by identifying fluid behind the ear on otoscopic examination, which is associated with local signs of inflammation such as erythema or even spontaneous eardrum rupture and drainage.

Similar to rhinosinusitis discussed later, most cases of otitis media are viral, and thus no specific antimicrobial therapy is usually indicated. Symptom-based treatments (decongestants, antihistamines, and analgesics) may help but do not decrease the duration of symptoms. If a bacterial infection is suspected (usually because the illness is not improving after 3 to 5 days), empiric antimicrobial treatment should target *S. pneumoniae* and *H. influenzae,* which are the most common bacterial causes. A combination β-lactam–β-lactamase inhibitor (such as amoxicillin/clavulanate) or a macrolide antibiotic (such as azithromycin) would be appropriate empiric therapy. Fluoroquinolones that cover respiratory pathogens (levofloxacin and moxifloxacin) are also effective, but are typically reserved for refractory infections. The recommended duration of therapy is 10 days.

Rhinosinusitis

Rhinitis and sinusitis often present in combination as rhinosinusitis. Acutely, this typically manifests as the "common cold," where rhinovirus, parainfluenza virus, or influenza virus is introduced into the paranasal sinuses, which is otherwise sterile. In warm moist sinuses, the viruses replicate and cause thickened mucus and impaired ciliary clearance associated with common cold symptoms. Aside from influenza, where antivirals such as oseltamivir can be given, there are no targeted therapies for other causes of viral rhinosinusitis. Bacterial rhinosinusitis lasts longer (often >10 days) and can be associated with a "double worsening," where there is improvement followed by decline over the course of the illness. For this reason, antibacterial therapy is usually withheld unless the patient has had symptoms for over a week without improvement.

In immunocompromised hosts, including poorly controlled diabetics, invasive fungal sinusitis is a clinically significant entity. These fungal infections typically present as fever, facial pain, and possibly associated nerve palsy. Emergent surgical evaluation and debridement are paramount to an optimal patient outcome.

Other bacteria and nonmucorales fungi, such as *Aspergillus* spp., can also cause chronic sinusitis. Chronic sinusitis is managed primarily through surgical approaches to improve mechanical drainage. Adjunctive antifungals and antibiotics may be indicated as part of a comprehensive approach, but are rarely curative. Topical antibiotic rinses may have a role in treatment, particularly perioperatively, but the evidence for selecting and using specific regimens is lacking.

Pharyngitis

Acute pharyngitis is one of the most common causes of primary care visits in the United States annually. Unfortunately, like rhinitis, most of the time these are due to viral infections and only require symptomatic treatment. Viral causes of pharyngitis may include infectious mononucleosis secondary to Epstein–Barr virus (EBV), cytomegalovirus (CMV), acute human immunodeficiency virus (HIV) infection, and influenza, among other viruses. Discernment between viral and bacterial pharyngitis relies on history of additional viral symptoms, physical examination assessing lymphadenopathy, appearance of the oropharynx, and rapid diagnostics such as a heterophile antibody test for EBV. It is critical to determine whether the symptoms are due to infectious mononucleosis, given the risk of splenic enlargement and possible rupture with this syndrome. The primary bacterial cause of pharyngitis is group A streptococcal infection, which can be associated with glomerulonephritis, acute rheumatic fever, and rheumatic heart disease if not promptly treated with antimicrobials. Since antimicrobials have become more readily available, these complications are increasingly rare, but prompt diagnosis, usually based on a rapid antigen test, is critical to prevent these serious ramifications. Penicillin is the treatment of choice for group A streptococcal infections, including pharyngitis. *Neisseria gonorrhoeae*, group C streptococci, and some anaerobic bacteria, may also cause bacterial pharyngitis.

Fusobacterium spp., particularly *Fusobacterium necrophorum*, can cause pharyngitis and potentially progress to Lemierre disease. In this illness, the bacteria infect the deep pharyngeal structures, causing a peritonsillar abscess and infection of the lateral pharyngeal spaces. Once *Fusobacterium* has invaded these spaces, it can infect the carotid artery and internal jugular vein, resulting in septic thrombophlebitis, most often of the internal jugular vein. Treatment is an antimicrobial with anaerobic activity, such as clindamycin or ampicillin/sulbactam, coupled with surgical drainage of any infected structures.

Another rare complication of pharyngitis is peritonsillar cellulitis, which can progress to peritonsillar abscess. Peritonsillar cellulitis occurs when a phlegmon develops between the palatine tonsil and pharyngeal muscles without a discrete pus collection. In a peritonsillar abscess, pus is present in this space. Although these typically start as pharyngitis, the abscesses tend to be polymicrobial with oral flora. Symptoms include peritonsillar swelling (often with deviation of the uvula), trismus, and voice changes. If abscess is suspected, aspiration or incision to evacuate the collection is recommended. If only cellulitis is suspected, intravenous (IV) antimicrobials alone are sufficient. Typical empiric regimens are either ampicillin/sulbactam or clindamycin, with or without vancomycin, depending on the patient's risk for methicillin-resistant *S. aureus* (MRSA) colonization.

Epiglottitis, Croup, and Laryngitis

Epiglottitis is an acute infection of the epiglottis, which can cause inflammation resulting in airway compromise if not treated. The *H. influenzae* B vaccine (B refers to the serotype of bacteria covered by the vaccine) has drastically reduced this entity, though cases still occur in the nonimmune or with *H. influenzae* serotypes not covered by the vaccine. On a lateral x-ray of the neck, edema of the epiglottis can be identified by the "thumbprint sign," indicating epiglottitis is present (Fig. 8.1).

The most important first step of management is to ensure that the airway is secure. Delayed airway security can lead to obstruction; evaluation with an advanced airway expert is highly recommended. Other important steps in the evaluation and treatment include obtaining blood cultures (bacteremia is highly prevalent in epiglottitis) and starting empiric antimicrobial therapy with a β-lactam/β-lactamase inhibitor or third-generation cephalosporin. Household contacts that are unvaccinated may need to be evaluated for prophylaxis with rifampin.

Croup (laryngotracheitis) is associated with subglottic inflammation causing a characteristic inspiratory stridor and a "seal bark" cough. Despite the stridor, most patients can be managed conservatively, because respiratory failure is rare. Nonetheless, a toxic-appearing patient, particularly those with increased work of breathing, may require hospital admission and even ventilatory support. Dexamethasone and nebulized epinephrine can help reduce airway inflammation and symptoms. Antibiotics do not have a role in the management of laryngotracheitis, as the underlying etiology of croup is a viral infection, most commonly parainfluenza virus.

Laryngitis is a common sequelae of infection of the entire respiratory system, particularly viral infections, though noninfectious causes of laryngeal inflammation also exist. Chronic laryngitis

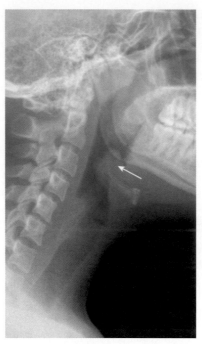

Fig. 8.1 Thumbprint sign in the epiglottitis. (From Nadgir RN, Barest GD, Sakai O, Mian AZ. Traumatic and nontraumatic emergencies of the brain, head, and neck. In JA Soto, BC Lucey, eds. *Emergency Radiology: The Requisites.* 2nd ed. Philadelphia, PA: Elsevier 2017: Fig. 1-64.)

can rarely be caused by fungal infections, but this is typically a manifestation of larger systemic disease rather than an isolated finding. Tuberculosis (TB) is also a rare cause of laryngitis, yet notable because of the higher risk of transmission for health care workers. TB laryngitis may also mimic laryngeal cancer due to its appearance. Typically, this is associated with pulmonary disease, but can occur in isolation. Fortunately, this is rare in the modern era.

Deep Neck Infections

Infections of the neck structures usually originate from an oropharyngeal source. Given the multitude of critical vascular and neurologic structures in the neck, deep space infections are often life-threatening if not promptly treated. Three such examples (Lemierre syndrome, peritonsillar cellulitis, and peritonsillar abscess) are discussed under "Pharyngitis" earlier. Another serious deep neck infection occurs in the submandibular space as a result of an infected tooth, known as *Ludwig angina*. Infection in this space can spread into the hypopharynx rapidly, causing increase in the size of the tongue, and can further spread into the parapharyngeal space. The characteristic appearance of Ludwig angina is a "woody induration" of the submental space, an inability to close the mouth due to the swollen tongue, and absent lymphadenopathy. This is typically associated with oral anaerobes, such as *Peptostreptococcus* and *Bacteroides* spp., but can involve *S. aureus* and *Fusobacterium* species. The first priority of treatment is to secure the airway. Once this is accomplished, patients require broad-spectrum antibiotics effective against oral anaerobes, Gram-negative organisms, and potentially MRSA coverage if the patient has risk factors for MRSA colonization. Surgery may be needed, but often is delayed, as the abscesses have not yet organized early in the course of illness.

All deep neck space infections require prompt evaluation for airway stability and evaluation with a surgical specialist. Empiric antibiotics should cover oral flora until culture data can guide therapy.

Lymphadenopathy and Lymphadenitis

Lymphadenopathy is often a sign of systemic infection rather than an isolated infection of the head and neck, but when isolated to the cervical chain, there are some specific ENT infections to consider. Aside from any of the infection syndromes mentioned earlier, isolated cervical adenopathy can be seen with viral infections, various bacterial infections, cervicofacial actinomycosis, mycobacterial infection, and fungal infections, as well as a bevy of noninfectious etiologies, particularly malignancies.

The most common viral infection associated with lymphadenopathy is mononucleosis, caused by both EBV and CMV (also mentioned earlier under "Pharyngitis"). Both can cause an influenza-like illness with malaise and prominent lymphadenopathy, and in immune-competent hosts, neither requires directed treatment. In immunocompromised hosts, targeted treatment can be considered for CMV.

Cervicofacial actinomycosis is manifested by abscesses, sinus tracts, and fibrosis. It is usually found during an evaluation of malignancy, as it can mimic several malignancies of the head, neck, and chest, given that it is frequently subacute and masslike in nature. Treatment may require surgical excision of any masses based on related tissue destruction, and antimicrobial therapy with a β-lactam/β-lactamase inhibitor is often initiated, with transition to a β-lactam–only antibiotic for several months to complete the course of treatment.

Bartonella henselae is the bacteria that causes cat scratch fever. This pathogen can cause auricular, cervical, and axillary adenitis resulting from exposure to infected cat saliva as a result of scratches, bites, and even potentially flea exposure. Parinaud oculoglandular syndrome due to *Bartonella* presents with tender lymphadenopathy in the preauricular, submandibular, and/or cervical lymph nodes with concurrent unilateral infection of the eye. Diagnosis is generally made via serology and pathology. Treatment for *B. henselae* infections varies from self-limited adenopathy that resolves over a few weeks to months; to monotherapy with azithromycin, doxycycline, or rifampin for simple lymphadenitis; to multiantibiotic therapy for disseminated disease.

Parinaud oculoglandular syndrome can also be caused by *Francisella tularensis*, the etiologic agent responsible for tularemia. This is a zoonotic agent that infects >100 species of both vertebrates and invertebrates, making identifying a specific risk factor difficult in many cases. Tularemia is endemic in many parts of the United States, but particularly within the southern Midwest regions. Tularemia can present with a multitude of different findings, but often presents with tender lymphadenitis that may evolve to ulceration, eschar, or suppuration. Pharyngeal tularemia may also present as severe pharyngitis with adenopathy not responding to empiric penicillin therapy for presumed group A streptococcal infection. The primary treatment for tularemia is with aminoglycoside therapy (streptomycin, gentamicin), tetracyclines, and fluoroquinolones. Use of multidrug therapy and the duration are dependent on the severity and dissemination of infection. In some instances, localized, simple infections may be treated with tetracycline therapy alone.

Mycobacterial infections can cause matted or fluctuant enlargement of lymph nodes, as seen in tuberculous lymphadenitis or scrofula. This likely occurs due to primary infection of the tonsils and adenoids. TB adenitis is a leading cause of peripheral lymphadenopathy in resource-limited settings where TB is highly prevalent. Diagnosis of *Mycobacteria* lymphadenitis is made based on culture and biopsy. All patients with suspected *Mycobacterial* lymphadenitis should have an HIV test and chest imaging to assess for complicated infections. Treatment is dictated by the specific *Mycobacteria* isolated and is often several months in duration. Occasionally, isolated adenitis can be surgically excised and resolved.

Suggested Reading

Chow AW, Benninger MS, Brook I, File JL. IDSA Clinical practice guideline for acute bacterial rhinosinusitis in children and adults. *Clin Infect Dis*. 2012;54(8):e72–e112.

Rosenfeld RM, Piccirillo JF, Chandrasekhar SS, et al. Clinical practice guideline (update): adult sinusitis. *Discourse Soc*. 2015;152(suppl 2):115–132.

Rosenfeld RM, Shin JJ, Schwartz SR. Clinical practice guideline: otitis media with effusion (update). *Otolaryngol Head Neck Surg*. 2016;154(suppl 1):S1–S41.

CHAPTER 9

Lower Respiratory Tract Infections

John C. O'Horo ■ Kelly Cawcutt

Lower respiratory tract infections (LRTIs) are among the most frequently encountered and difficult to diagnose infectious syndromes. Symptoms of most LRTIs overlap with other clinical conditions, such as congestive heart failure and obstructive lung disease, such asthma and chronic obstructive pulmonary disease (COPD). Diagnostic tests are not specific to LRTIs, and even invasive studies have a low yield in terms of confirming the diagnosis. This means that a thorough understanding of the epidemiology, clinical presentation, and patient factors is critical to providing care for those suffering from respiratory tract infections.

Broadly speaking, LRTIs can be divided into different categories based on patient exposures and characteristics. The most common of these would be community-acquired pneumonia (CAP) followed by health care–associated pneumonia (HAP). Additionally, there are a subset of patients and risk factors that merit special consideration. These pertain to endemic illnesses and respiratory tract infections in immunocompromised hosts. This chapter will discuss each of these groups.

Community-Acquired Pneumonia

Pneumonia, and CAP in particular, is a leading cause of death in the United States, particularly in the elderly. This is in part due to the nonspecific presentation and lack of a practical diagnostic gold standard to confirm CAP; therefore the diagnosis frequently relies upon symptom assessment and clinical gestalt. Several critical decisions must be made early in the course of CAP: first, whether CAP is present; second, if the patient has risk factors for multidrug-resistant organisms (MDROs); third, which clinical setting (outpatient, inpatient, or intensive care unit [ICU]) is appropriate for management; and fourth, which antimicrobial agents and what duration of therapy are most appropriate. The Infectious Disease Society of America and the American Thoracic Society have issued joint guidelines on the management and diagnosis of CAP, which integrate evidence-based approaches to these dilemmas and have been proven to reduce mortality.

Diagnosis is based on respiratory and infectious symptoms such as cough, fever, and malaise associated with radiographic infiltrate suggestive of pneumonia. Although it is possible for a chest radiograph to be clear in pneumonia, this is highly unusual, and typically further imaging (e.g., computed tomography) is not required to establish a clinically significant pneumonia.

TABLE 9.1 ■ Evaluation for Community-Acquired Pneumonia

Setting	Blood Culture	Sputum Culture	Urine Testing	Other Testing
ICU admission	X	X	*Legionella* and pneumococcal antigens	Multiplex PCR
Failure of outpatient treatment		X	*Legionella* and pneumococcal antigens	Multiplex PCR
Asplenia or leukopenia	X	X	Pneumococcal antigen	Multiplex PCR Consider bronchoscopy
Alcohol abuse	X	X	*Legionella* and pneumococcal antigens	Multiplex PCR
Recent travel			*Legionella* antigen	
Pleural effusion	X	X	*Legionella* and pneumococcal antigen	Multiplex PCR, thoracentesis
Cavitary disease	X	X	None	Fungal and mycobacterial blood cultures, consider bronchoscopy

ICU, Intensive care unit; *PCR,* polymerase chain reaction.

Other testing can support the diagnosis or help with risk stratification, but normal results do not rule out pneumonia. For example, sputum microbiology, although helpful if positive, is negative in greater than half of patients with pneumonia. Renal function, leukocyte count, and hematocrit are all useful in risk stratification schemes, such as the Pneumonia Severity Index, but do little for establishing or refuting a diagnosis. Novel biomarkers, such as procalcitonin, have shown promise in study settings, but practical implementation trials to date have shown no known diagnostic benefit, and biomarkers are currently not part of any guideline-driven CAP treatment protocols.

The next decision is where to place the patient for clinical management; the outpatient setting is appropriate for the mildly to moderately ill, the inpatient setting is needed for the moderately to severely ill, and the intensive care setting for the severely ill. Tools like the Pneumonia Severity Index (a complex score typically requiring a calculator to use, but reasonably accurate) or the CURB-65 (a simple, but less accurate, score) can be used to assist such risk stratification, but ultimately, this is a clinical decision based on the patient's appearance, baseline level of health, and risk for progression of disease.

Once the patient's risk factors are categorized and a working diagnosis of pneumonia is established, the next step is to obtain additional diagnostic tests based on the most likely etiologies and risk factors for the patient. This is shown in Table 9.1.

Once diagnostics are underway, appropriate empiric treatment should be initiated based on the patient's clinical situation. Empiric therapy is targeted at common organisms, knowing that the most commonly isolated pathogen in CAP is *Streptococcus pneumoniae*, with other typical organisms, including *Haemophilus influenzae, Moraxella catarrhalis,* and atypical organisms such as *Legionella* spp. and *Mycoplasma pneumoniae*. Viral causes of illness, such as influenza and parainfluenza, are also common, but given the propensity for bacterial superinfections to occur in the critically ill, antibacterial therapy is often given when empirically treating a severe viral pneumonia. Of note, *H. influenzae* is thus named because of being mistakenly attributed as the cause

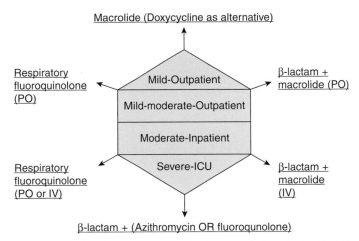

Fig. 9.1 Empiric treatment options for community-acquired pneumonia. In patients with defined risk factors or pathogens, further treatment may be indicated. *ICU,* intensive care unit; *IV,* Intravenous; *PO,* by mouth.

of influenza in the 1890s due to this organism frequently being isolated from influenza patients during a pandemic.

Conversely, it should be noted that viruses can mimic bacterial pneumonia and, particularly during influenza season, testing for influenza and other viral pathogens should be performed in hospitalized patients, both for accurate diagnosis of viral, bacterial, or coinfections causing pneumonia and in order to initiate infection prevention strategies to limit the risk of nosocomial spread of viral infections.

CAP patients may be at risk for infections with MDROs in certain settings. Patients who were recently hospitalized, on antibiotics, or chronically ill with immune or pulmonary disease or chronic illness may lead to colonization with organisms such as *Pseudomonas aeruginosa*, notorious for developing resistance to first-line antimicrobial agents.

For common organisms (not the potential MDROs), empiric treatment is targeted at these organisms. For mild cases, a macrolide antibiotic or, as an alternative, doxycycline may be appropriate. As patients become more severely ill, options diverge to either be fluoroquinolone based or a combination of a β-lactam and macrolide, as this provides common and atypical bacteria coverage, and dual therapy carries potential morbidity and mortality benefits for those with severe *S. pneumoniae* pneumonia. In the ICU setting, a combination of a β-lactam (or cephalosporin) plus a macrolide or fluoroquinolone antibiotic is appropriate empiric coverage (Fig. 9.1). In patient at risk for MDRO, coverage for specific organisms (methicillin-resistant *Staphylococcus aureus* [MRSA], resistant *Pseudomonas*, etc.) may be indicated.

Generally speaking, factors that increase the suspicion for MRSA include Gram-positive cocci on the sputum Gram stain, known intravenous (IV) drug abuse, recent influenza infection, prior recent antimicrobial exposure, or if patient is on dialysis. In these situations, vancomycin or linezolid may need to be added to the regimen for empiric MRSA coverage. Of note, daptomycin should not be used for pulmonary infections because it is inactivated by surfactant and therefore cannot adequately penetrate the lungs to treat pneumonia.

Viral causes of CAP are common, with influenza being the most concerning. Some strains of influenza can be treated with antiviral medications such as oseltamivir, but meta-analytic reports have not consistently shown a benefit with this treatment, particularly if started >48 hours after symptom onset. Nonetheless, antiviral treatment remains part of most practitioners' approach to suspected or confirmed influenza.

A final consideration for CAP is aspiration pneumonia; in patients with known dysphagia or considered at risk for aspiration, the organisms involved may include more oral anaerobes than those typically micro-aspirated in CAP. In such a situation, it is reasonable to add anaerobic coverage such as amoxicillin–clavulanate or clindamycin to the empiric coverage. This is controversial, as much of the radiographic and clinical presentation of aspiration may be due to chemical pneumonitis from stomach contents, as opposed to true infection, and thus the need for any antimicrobial therapy is a clinical judgement call.

Duration of antimicrobial therapy for any of the described CAP infections is typically 5 to 7 days, depending on clinical improvement. Often, patients can be de-escalated or have antimicrobials stopped altogether if a single etiologic agent is identified and can be targeted or a better alternative diagnosis becomes evident.

Health Care–Associated Pneumonia and Ventilator-Associated Pneumonia

HAP and ventilator-associated pneumonia (VAP) are clinically differentiated from CAP based on the risk factors noted within their names. A pneumonia is considered "health care associated" if symptom onset is ≥48 hours after hospital admission, and VAP is similarly defined by onset ≥48 hours after intubation (noting that there is a difference between clinical definitions and the reported infection control definitions used). Similar to other pneumonias, the pathogenesis of HAP is thought to be due to micro-aspiration of oropharyngeal flora. However, due to the more vulnerable population seen in the hospital, their risk for aspiration is presumed to be higher, and their oral flora is anticipated to change to reflect the higher proportion of MDROs in the hospital setting relatively quickly. Thus a patient is considered at risk for HAP after being in the hospital after 48 hours, though the longer a patient is hospitalized, the greater their risk for MDRO becomes.

Among the hospital flora, the most common Gram-negative organisms of concern are *Escherichia coli, Klebsiella pneumoniae, Enterobacter* spp., *Pseudomonas,* and *Acinetobacter.* The main Gram-positive bacteria of concern is MRSA. The risk factors for MDRO in this population are prolonged hospitalization (>4 days), recent use of (>4 days) IV antimicrobials (within the last 90 days), presence of acute respiratory distress syndrome (ARDS) or shock, need for renal replacement therapy, or a high prevalence of MDROs in the community. For the purposes of risk stratification, a high prevalence is considered 10% to 20% of *S. aureus* isolates being MRSA or 10% of Gram-negative rods demonstrating multidrug resistance. Many institutions now internally report "antibiograms," which list the rates of bacterial resistance to make clinicians aware of the prevalence of antimicrobial resistance and help guide empiric antimicrobial drug choices. If local resistance is unknown, it should be considered high until proven otherwise.

Viral and fungal causes of HAP and VAP are less common, though influenza can cause both HAP and VAP if infection control adherence is suboptimal. Cytomegalovirus (CMV) and Epstein–Barr virus (EBV) are rare causes of HAP or VAP and more commonly represent reactivation of the virus due to severe illness and thus do not represent invasive disease or require antiviral therapy. Another common point of confusion in this population is whether *Candida* species noted on Gram stain or bronchoalveolar lavage are pathogens. Once again, pneumonia caused by *Candida* species is rare and most often represents colonization of the airway with this organism, not invasive pathogenic infection. It has been questioned whether *Candida* pneumonia exists as a clinical entity at all, but if it does occur, it is only in the most severely immune compromised hosts.

The clinical diagnosis of HAP/VAP, similar to CAP, is primarily clinical. Infiltrates are usually seen on chest radiography, but other signs of infection such as fever, purulent sputum, hypoxia, and leukocytosis are not as consistent and require interpretation in each individual case. Sputum cultures have low sensitivity in HAP, but negative sputum is considerably more useful for ruling out VAP, likely reflecting the ease of obtaining a higher-quality specimen than can be obtained via an endotracheal tube. Molecular tests can be used, such as multiplex polymerase chain reaction (PCR), but these should be considered for de-escalation purposes based on identification of an etiologic agent, not as the basis for withholding or administering antibiotics.

In patients without MDRO risk factors, piperacillin–tazobactam, cefepime, or levofloxacin are appropriate empiric regimens. If an MDRO is suspected, empiric coverage options include piperacillin–tazobactam, cefepime, ceftazidime, imipenem, meropenem, or aztreonam for Gram-negative coverage. Double coverage for *Pseudomonas aeruginosa* can be used for high-risk patients by adding an aminoglycoside for additional coverage for highly resistant organisms. Further use of double antimicrobial coverage should depend on local "antibiogram" data. The need for empiric coverage of Gram-positive MDROs is identical to that of CAP. As noted earlier, in patients at risk for MDRO pneumonia, vancomycin or linezolid are appropriate first-line choices for MRSA coverage.

Duration of therapy is typically 7 days for HAP and VAP. Longer regimens used to be used for select organisms such as *Acinetobacter* and *Pseudomonas*, but in the most recent guidelines, the recommended duration was shortened to only 14 days. De-escalation should occur when susceptibility and culture results are available, or 48 hours after cultures are obtained if there is no growth. Typical antimicrobial de-escalation removes MDRO coverage in the absence of a demonstrated MDRO at that time and sets a definitive end date for the treatment program.

Biomarkers play a limited role in HAP and VAP. Procalcitonin, probably the most studied of these, is not recommended to use as a basis for initiating or withholding treatment. Current guidelines advise considering serial procalcitonins for de-escalation for patients beyond the 7-day treatment time frame; thus in most cases, procalcitonin should not affect therapy. Other biomarkers have less data to advise their proper use.

SPECIAL CONSIDERATIONS

Fungi in Immune Competent Hosts

In some areas, endemic fungal infections can be broadly considered within the diagnosis of CAP. Histoplasmosis is endemic in the Mississippi River Valley, blastomycosis in the Ohio River Valley, and coccidiomycosis in the American Southwest. In each of these regions, a pneumonia-like presentation is a common manifestation of early illness and should be considered in the differential diagnosis for CAP.

Other fungi are generally of little significance in CAP. The presence of yeast or *Candida* spp. on sputum cultures almost always represents an oropharyngeal contaminant. Likewise, *Aspergillus* spp. are usually not clinically relevant unless present in a severely immunocompromised host. *Cryptococcus* rarely causes infection in immunocompetent hosts, but can cause a pneumonia presentation and should not be dismissed without consideration as a pathogen.

Immunocompromised Hosts

Even among immunocompromised hosts, common organisms predominate. *S. pneumoniae* and influenza remain the leading causes of bacterial and viral pneumonia, respectively. However, a number of other potential pathogens should be considered.

Pneumocystis jirovici pneumonia (PCP) classically occurs in people living with HIV, but can be seen in any individual with compromised cellular immunity. High-dose steroids and certain chemotherapeutic regimens merit prophylaxis with trimethoprim–sulfamethoxazole, dapsone, or pentamidine to prevent this infection. Presumed diagnosis is often made based on the host, chest imaging, and possible laboratory findings. However, definite diagnosis is made with a special smear/stain or with a PCR test on sputum or bronchoalveolar lavage. The drug of choice for PCP treatment remains trimethoprim–sulfamethoxazole and consideration of adjunctive steroids based on the severity of associated hypoxia.

CMV can also cause pneumonitis in a host with impaired cellular immunity. Diagnosis can be challenging, as CMV can be shed during times of inflammation without indicating a true invasive infection. Symptoms are fairly nonspecific, but can include nonproductive cough; decrease in pulmonary function; and patchy, diffuse infiltrates. CMV is similar in presentation to transplant rejection (in a transplanted allograft), and a biopsy may be required to differentiate between invasive CMV disease, allograft rejection, or just colonization. Treatment is affected by a number of factors, including the predisposing immune-compromising condition (transplant, chemotherapy, etc.), prior treatments, and prophylaxis, as well as other medications such as immunosuppressant agents in use. Treatment decisions for CMV are best done in concert with an infectious diseases specialist.

Varicella zoster virus (VZV) and herpes simplex virus (HSV) likewise can cause clinically insignificant shedding or cause an invasive viral pneumonitis and are also difficult to differentiate. Directed antiviral therapy is available, but typically pulmonary involvement indicates a life-threatening disseminated disease, which requires aggressive treatment and further evaluation of overall health status.

Invasive pulmonary aspergillosis can be another cause of pneumonia in the high-risk patient. Diagnosis is associated with characteristic imaging (the "halo sign") and immune compromise (particularly from hematologic malignancies and associated treatments, or other causes of neutropenia). Diagnostic tests like galactomannan can be helpful, but false positives are common. Azole therapy, specifically voriconazole, is frequently the first line for treatment, but the comorbidities of this population can make effective treatment challenging.

Mucormycosis can also be a cause of pneumonia for the severely immune compromised hosts, in which it can develop and spread rapidly. Pulmonary mucormycosis often presents as a mass-like lesion; thus surgical debridement may be needed, but often the fungus spreads too quickly to make lobectomy practical. IV amphotericin B is the backbone of primary treatment for mucormycosis, with potential use of newer azoles as step-down therapy after clinical improvement.

Toxoplasma pneumonia is rare and typically results from reactivation of latent infection. Typical presentation is a reticulonodular infiltrate, fever, and cough. Clinically, this appears similar to PCP pneumonia and has substantial overlap in patient risk factors. Sulfadiazine and pyrimethamine are first-line therapy.

Cryptococcal pneumonia in immunocompromised hosts can vary from a solitary pulmonary nodule to influenza-like illness with or without ARDS. HIV is a significant risk factor for developing cryptococcal pneumonia and is associated with substantially increased severity of disease. Cryptococcal antigens have a low false-positive rate, but a negative result does not rule out disease. Treatment is dependent on the extent of disease (e.g., if meningitis is present, treatment as cryptococcal meningitis is appropriate). However, if the disease is isolated and nonsevere, azole monotherapy may be adequate.

Other Unusual Pathogens

When discussing agents of bioterrorism, several of the high-risk agents primarily transmit as a respiratory infection. Being alert for unusual symptoms or syndromes, particularly if a cluster of patients is presenting, occurring outside of expected areas and populations is the best defense against bioterrorism and the best chance for early identification. This chapter will discuss two inhalational pathogens: hantavirus and anthrax.

An unusual cause of pneumonia-like presentation worth noting is hantavirus cardiopulmonary syndrome. Hantavirus family diseases (including Sin nombre, Laguna Negra, Andes virus, and more than a dozen others) are associated with inhaling the pathogen from infected rodent urine, resulting in infection and development of ARDS-like presentation. Treatment is primarily supportive, with a potential role for extracorporeal membrane oxygenation (ECMO). Ribavirin, although active against some strains in vitro, failed to show any survival benefit in vivo.

Anthrax infection can present as many different syndromes, but when acquired through inhalation, can develop into a pneumonia and influenza-like illness over the course of a week, followed by a fulminant phase where treatment rarely succeeds. In the absence of meningitis, ciprofloxacin plus clindamycin is the initial therapy of choice. Antitoxins are also available via the US Strategic Stockpile and can be obtained via the Centers for Disease Control and Prevention in the situation of a suspected or confirmed anthrax case.

Suggested Reading

Bernstein JM. Treatment of community-acquired pneumonia: IDSA guidelines. *Chest*. 1999;115(suppl 3):9S–13S.

Kalil AC, et al. Management of adults with hospital-acquired and ventilator-associated pneumonia: 2016 clinical practice guidelines by the infectious diseases society of america and the american thoracic society. *Clin Infect Dis*. 2016;3(5):e61–e111.

CHAPTER 10

Select Gastrointestinal and Hepatobiliary Infections

Robert Orenstein

Esophagitis

Esophagitis is an inflammatory mucosal injury disorder that may be caused by infectious agents and local irritants. The inflammation may present with substernal pain, odynophagia, and occasionally dysphagia. The risk factors for esophageal inflammatory disorders may be iatrogenic (i.e., pill esophagitis, chemical injuries) or disease related. Infectious esophagitis often presents with odynophagia in the setting of immunosuppression, recent antibiotics, corticosteroids, or neutropenia. Most infectious esophagitis is viral or due to *Candida*.

- Microbiology: Most commonly viral—herpes simplex virus (HSV) but can be due to cytomegalovirus (CMV) or fungal *(Candida)*
  - HSV—seen in immune compromised host (ICH); endoscopically ulcers, vesicles
  - *Candida* spp.—usually with oral thrush; one-third without—endoscopically, white plaques, hyphae on biopsy
- Diagnostics: Endoscopic examination, histology (HSV—multinucleated giant cells; CMV—"owl's eye," *Candida*—hyphae), bacterial or fungal cultures or polymerase chain reaction (PCR) (HSV, CMV)
- Treatment: *Candida*—fluconazole 200 mg/day for 14 days; HSV—acyclovir 5 mg/kg intravenous (IV) q8h for 14 to 21 days; CMV—ganciclovir 5 mg/kg IV q12h for 14 to 21 days

Gastritis/Duodenitis

Gastritis and duodenitis are mucosal inflammatory disorders of the stomach and duodenum, most often due to *Helicobacter pylori*. Patients commonly present with epigastric pain, nausea, and vomiting without fever.

- Microbiology: *H. pylori*—a urease-producing, curved, Gram-negative rod
  - Less common causes—Immunocompromised hosts—CMV
  - Granulomatous gastritis—syphilis, tuberculosis (TB), nontuberculous mycobacteria (NTM), Whipple disease, cryptococcus, anisakiasis, schistosomiasis
- Chronic gastritis is common—usually asymptomatic
- Symptomatic peptic ulcer disease (95% of duodenal ulcer and 70% gastric ulcer cases are associated with *H. pylori*), gastric cancer, or mucosa-associated lymphoid tissue (MALT) lymphoma; idiopathic thrombocytopenic purpura (ITP) rarely
- Diagnosis: Upper endoscopy when warning symptoms—biopsies, histopathology; urease (Campylobacter-like organism [CLO]) test on gastric tissue samples for *H. pylori*; urea breath test for *H. pylori*; fecal antigen test for *H. pylori* (both for diagnosis and eradication tests)
  - *H. pylori* serology is not useful for identifying active infection
  - Testing should be done off proton pump inhibitors (PPIs) or H_2 receptor blockers (H_2Bs) for 2 weeks; off antibiotics for 4 weeks
- Treatment: Assess risk for resistance to macrolides: prior exposure, high local resistance >15%
  - If no macrolide risk—triple therapy with macrolide: clarithromycin/amoxicillin/PPI
  - If penicillin allergy—clarithromycin-based triple therapy with metronidazole consists of clarithromycin, metronidazole, and a PPI
  - If resistance: bismuth quadruple therapy—bismuth, metronidazole, tetracycline, and a PPI
  - Treatment should be 14 days
- For recurrent or refractory disease—obtain cultures and sensitivity; refer for infectious diseases (ID) consultation.
- Test for cure at 6 to 8 weeks with stool antigen or urease breath test.

Infectious Diarrhea

Due to the numerous causes of both infectious and noninfectious diarrhea, development of a stepwise approach is critical to management. A simple six-step approach asks the following questions:
1. Is it diarrhea?
2. Is it acute, persistent, or chronic?
3. Who is the host?
4. What are the exposures?
5. What is the severity?
6. Is it inflammatory, noninflammatory, or invasive?

The first step is defining diarrhea—at least three loose stools a day. Use the Bristol Stool Scale (types 6 and 7).

Not all loose stool is diarrhea—fecal incontinence often mimics diarrhea.

Step 2: What is the duration?
- Acute—acute gastroenteritis; lasts <14 days
- Persistent diarrhea—lasts 14 to 30 days
- Chronic diarrhea—lasts more than 30 days, rarely infectious

Step 3: Who is the host?
- Healthy person
- Returning traveler

- Individual with food-borne illness
- Individual with health care or institutional exposures
- Pregnant woman
- Elderly
- Immunocompromised
  - HIV, transplant, hematologic malignancy, medications, asplenia, immune globulin deficient

Step 4: Determine the exposure risks.
- Food and water ingestion
- Water exposures/outdoor exposures
- Daycare/institutional settings
- Pools
- Livestock/pets
- Sexual practices
- Health care exposures

Step 5: What is the severity?
- Uncomplicated watery diarrhea
- Invasive disease
- Dysentery (bloody stools)
- Severe volume-depleting diarrhea

Step 6: Is the diarrhea inflammatory, invasive, or noninflammatory?

Inflammatory diarrhea may be associated with small-volume, mucoid or bloody stools, tenesmus, cramps, and fever—usually involves the colon.

Invasive diarrhea may be associated with fever and periumbilical or right-lower-quadrant abdominal pain. Usually due to *Salmonella, Campylobacter, Yersinia,* or enteroinvasive *Escherichia coli* or *Entamoeba histolytica.*

Noninflammatory diarrhea may be associated with watery, large volume without fever. May be toxin mediated or directly related to the microorganism. These are often viral, parasitic, or toxigenic bacteria.

Tables 10.1 and 10.2 provide epidemiologic links and clinical clues to the etiologic diagnosis of infectious diarrhea. The algorithms illustrated in Figs. 10.1 to 10.3 illustrate approaches to diagnosis and management.

CLOSTRIDOIDES DIFFICILE INFECTION

C. difficile has become an increasingly common cause of both community-onset and health care–associated diarrhea. Its spectrum of illness can range from mild self-limiting diarrhea to severe colitis, sepsis, and death. Community-onset *C. difficile infection* (CDI) tends to occur in younger persons with less antibiotic exposure versus health care–associated infections. Antibiotics are the major risk factor for CDI, especially second- and third-generation cephalosporins and fluoroquinolones. Clindamycin and antianaerobic penicillins have the greatest risk.

- Diagnosis is made by testing of diarrheal (Bristol 5 to 7) stools when there are >3 loose stools/24 hours in the appropriate epidemiologic circumstances.
- Current guidelines recommend a two-step *C. difficile* glutamate dehydrogenase antigen plus *C. difficile* toxin A and B enzyme immunoassay test or a molecular test using polymerase chain reaction (PCR) to the toxin B gene.
  - Repeat testing is not recommended if the initial test is negative.
  - Three to five percent of healthy adults are colonized with C. *difficile.*
  - Twenty to fifty percent of hospitalized or long-term care patients may be colonized.
  - Testing for cure is not indicated, as the test may remain positive despite clinical resolution.
- Treatment of CDI is currently stratified by severity and the initial versus recurrent episodes.

TABLE 10.1 ■ Epidemiologic Considerations in Infectious Diarrhea: Who Is the Host?

Host Factors	Potential Infectious Agents/Associations
Immune status	*Salmonella, Yersinia, Giardia (IgA deficiency)*
Hypogammaglobulinemia	*Salmonella, Mycobacterium avium complex, Listeria,*
Cell-mediated immune deficiencies	CMV, Adenovirus, *Cryptosporidia, Cystoisospora, Cyclospora*
Antimicrobial treatments	*C. difficile* infection
International travel	*E. coli* (mostly ETEC), *Campylobacter, Salmonella, Shigella, Vibrio cholera, E. histolytica* (prolonged diarrhea—*Giardia, Blastocystis, Cyclospora, Cystoisospora, Cryptosporidia*)
Food and water exposures	Norovirus (work parties, cruise ships), *Salmonella, C. perfringens, B. cereus, S. aureus* (picnics, food poisoning), *Campylobacter*, ETEC, STEC (undercooked burgers, cider, veggies), *Listeria* (soft cheeses, cantaloupes), *Shigella, Cyclospora* (raspberries), *Cryptosporidia* (pools)
	Yersinia (pork), *Campylobacter* (poultry), *Trichinella* (pork, bear, jerky),
	C. perfringens (beef, poultry),
	B. cereus (old pasta)
	Brucella (goat cheese, milk)
Institutionalization—child care, long-term care	Norovirus, rotavirus, *C. difficile, Shigella*
Health care exposure—hospitals, nursing facilities	*C. difficile*, Norovirus
Sexual practices	HSV, *Chlamydia, N. gonorrhea, Salmonella, Shigella, Campylobacter, E. histolytica, Cryptosporidia*
Adults vs. children	Rotavirus, *E. coli*—children

CMV, Cytomegalovirus; *ETEC,* enterotoxigenic *E. coli; HSV,* herpes simplex virus; *IgA,* immunoglobulin A; *STEC,* Shiga toxin *E. coli.*

TABLE 10.2 ■ Clinical Considerations in Infectious Diarrhea

Clinical Clues	Infectious Agents
Acute-onset nausea and vomiting <24 hr	Toxin-mediated—*S. aureus, B. cereus*
Acute-onset nausea and vomiting lasts >24 hr Watery diarrhea for several days	Norovirus
Grossly bloody stool, severe abdominal pain (dysentery)	*Shigella*, STEC, *Salmonella, Campylobacter, Yersinia enterocolitica*
Abdominal pain	*C. difficile, Salmonella, Shigella*, STEC, *Campylobacter jejuni, Y. enterocolitica*
Persistent abdominal pain, fever Mimics of appendicitis	*Y. enterocolitica*, pseudotuberculosis *Salmonella typhi* or *paratyphi, Campylobacter*
Persistent diarrhea >14 days	*Giardia lamblia, Cryptosporidia, Cyclospora, Cystoisospora, E. histolytica*

STEC, Shiga toxin *E. coli.*

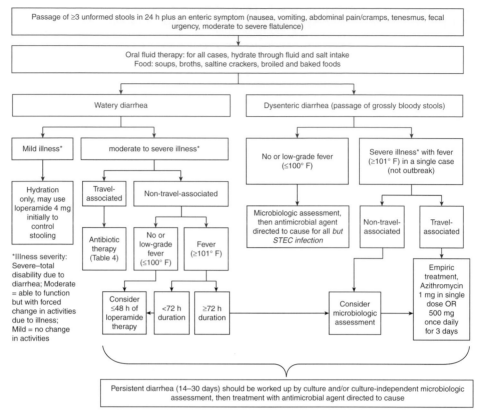

Fig. 10.1   Approach to empirical therapy and management of the adult with acute diarrhea. (From Riddle MS, DuPont HL, Connor BA. ACG Clinical Guideline: Diagnosis, treatment and prevention of acute diarrheal infections in adults. *Am J Gastroenterol.* 2016;111:602–622.)

- First episode, nonsevere—treat with oral vancomycin 125 mg four times a day (QID) for 10 to 14 days or fidaxomicin 200 mg twice a day (BID) for 10 days
  - Recurrence occurs in 20% to 30% after the first episode
- Fulminant CDI initial—vancomycin 500 mg QID oral or via nasogastric (NG) tube. If ileus, rectal vancomycin 500 mg QID as retention enema, plus IV metronidazole 500 mg three times a day (TID) for 10 days.
- Second episode—treat with fidaxomicin 200 mg BID for 10 days if prior vancomycin or if prior fidaxomicin use, vancomycin 125 mg QID for 10 to 14 days followed by BID for 7 days, daily for 7 days, then every 2 to 3 days for 2 to 8 weeks.
- Third or more episode—vancomycin pulse and taper or vancomycin 125 mg QID for 10 days followed by rifaximin 400 mg TID for 20 days or fecal microbiota transplant (investigational)
- Bezlotuxumab (monoclonal antibody against the *C. difficile* toxin B) may be administered in a first episode or beyond in high-risk patients for recurrence.

Acute Appendicitis

Acute appendicitis is thought to result from luminal obstruction of the appendix by a fecalith, leading to distension, bacterial overgrowth, and increased intraluminal pressure followed by

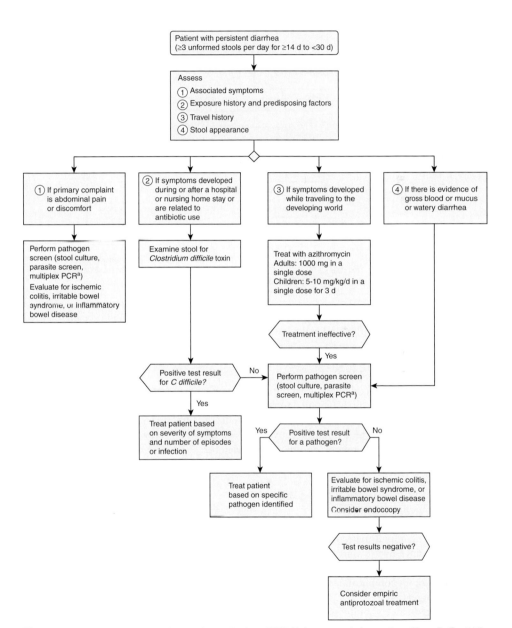

Fig. 10.2   Approach to the adult with persistent diarrhea. *PCR,* Polymerase chain reaction. (From DuPont HL. Persistent diarrhea: A clinical review. *JAMA.* 2016;315:2712–2723.)

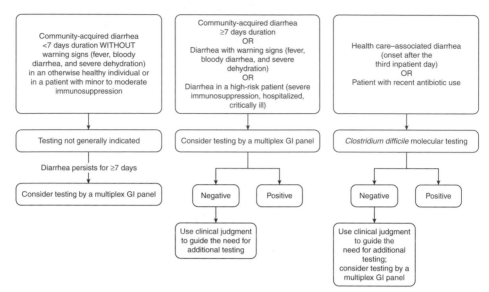

Fig. 10.3 Testing algorithm for infectious diarrhea in immunocompromised hosts. *GI,* Gastrointestinal. (From Liesman RM, Binnicker MJ. The role of multiplex molecular panels for the diagnosis of gastrointestinal infections in immunocompromised patients. *Curr Opin Infect Dis.* 2016;29[4]:359–365, Figure 1.)

gangrene. Patients with acute appendicitis may present with bloating, periumbilical pain followed by anorexia, nausea/vomiting and right-lower-quadrant abdominal pain, fever, and an elevated white blood cell (WBC) count (seen in less than one-third of patients).

- Clinical risk scoring systems for appendicitis include the Alvarado score and Appendicitis Inflammatory Risk (AIR) (Table 10.3).
- Classical signs—Tenderness at McBurney point, psoas sign (retrocecal), obturator sign
- Helical multislice spiral computed tomography (CT) scan is preferred diagnostic test
  - Enlarged >6 cm, thickened wall of the appendix, fecalith, periappendiceal stranding
- Microbiology—Enteric Gram-negatives—*E. coli, Klebsiella, Enterobacter, Proteus* spp.
  - Late prolonged symptoms and rupture—anaerobes, *Pseudomonas aeruginosa*
- Mimics—*Yersinia* enterocolitica, *Campylobacter jejuni, Salmonella,* Crohn disease, gynecologic disease/pregnancy
- Treatment—Two approaches:
  - Antibiotics first and observe
    - Ampicillin–sulbactam 3 g IV q6h, piperacillin–tazobactam 3.375 g IV q6h, ceftriaxone 1g q24h plus metronidazole 500 mg q6–8h for 7 to 10 days if no surgery
    - Twenty-five to thirty percent of patients treated with antibiotics first will eventually need appendectomy
    - Risk for complications (peritonitis, abscess, wound infection) no different with delayed surgery
    - Predictors of antibiotic failure or recurrence: appendicolith seen on imaging
    - Predictors of success with antibiotics-first approach: C-reactive protein (CRP) <60, WBC <12,000, age <60
  - Surgical treatment—laparoscopic or open appendectomy
    - Recent advances in endoscopic retrograde appendicitis therapy with irrigation, appendicolith removal, and stent placement
- Postappendectomy antibiotics

TABLE 10.3 ■ Clinical Risk Scoring Systems for Suspected Acute Appendicitis

Alvarado Score

Clinical Feature	Score
Anorexia	1
Nausea or vomiting	1
Pain migration to right lower quadrant (RLQ)	1
RLQ pain	2
Rebound tenderness	1
Temperature > 37.5° C	1
White blood cell (WBC) count with left shift	1
WBC > 10,000	2
Total	10

Appendicitis Inflammatory Risk Score (AIR)

Clinical Feature	Score
Vomiting	1
RLQ pain	1
Mild rebound tenderness	1
Moderate rebound tenderness	2
Severe rebound tenderness	3
Temperature > 38.5° C	1
Polymorphonuclear (PMN) 70%–84%	1
PMN > 85%	2
WBC 10,000–14,999	1
WBC > 15,000	2
C-reactive protein (CRP) 10–49	1
CRP > 50	2
Total maximum points	12

Appendicitis Risk	Alvarado	AIR
Low	1–4	1–4
Moderate	5–6	5–8
High	7–10	9–12

- Simple appendicitis—not needed postoperatively
- Complicated, perforated appendicitis—3 days if clinically improving

Diverticulitis

Diverticulitis is a common gastrointestinal (GI) inflammatory disorder that occurs in 1% to 5% of those with diverticulosis; 20% of those have recurrent disease within 10 years. Recent theories suggest that prolonged fecal stasis may alter the colonic microbiome leading to an increased ratio of *Firmicutes/Bacteroidetes* and increased *Proteobacteria* resulting in a chronic inflammatory state.

These patients often present with acute or subacute left-lower-quadrant abdominal pain, malaise, fever, elevated WBC, and CRP. A CT scan abdomen with IV and oral contrast is the preferred diagnostic test for diverticulitis.

- Microbiology—colonic flora, principally enteric Gram-negatives, anaerobes, and aerobic and anaerobic streptococci.

TABLE 10.4 ■ Modified Hinchey Classifications for Diverticulitis

Modified Hinchey Stage	Definition	Clinical Classification
0	Clinically mild diverticulitis Diverticula with wall thickening on CT	Uncomplicated
Ia	Colonic wall thickening with Inflammation in pericolonic fat (phlegmon)	Uncomplicated
IIb	Pericolonic or mesenteric abscess proximal to the inflamed tic (diverticular abscess)	Complicated
II	Distant intraabdominal abscess	Complicated
III	Purulent peritonitis	Complicated
IV	Feculent peritonitis	Complicated

CT, Computed tomography.

- May be uncomplicated or complicated—12% of cases; modified Hinchey criteria may help (Table 10.4)
  - Complications—abscess, peritonitis, obstruction, or fistulae; sepsis
- Treatment:
  - Uncomplicated inflammatory disease—may not require antibiotics; supportive management with pain medicines, IV fluids, nothing by mouth (NPO)
    - Probiotics, rifaximin, mesalamine, and nut avoidance of no value to prevent recurrence
    - High-fiber diet and avoidance of nonsteroidal antiinflammatory drugs (NSAIDs) may be helpful in prevention
  - Complicating factors: severe disease, sepsis, immunosuppression, multiple comorbidities—may benefit from antibiotics
    - Four to seven days of antibiotics if source controlled—mild disease
    - Amoxicillin/clavulanate 875/125 mg q12h or if penicillin allergy
    - Ciprofloxacin 750 mg q12h plus metronidazole 500 mg q8h
    - Trimethoprim–sulfamethoxazole (TMP-SMX) 160/800 mg q12h plus metronidazole 500 mg q8h
- Inpatient admission—failure of outpatient treatment for 48 to 72 hours; complicated disease, inability to take oral medicines, complicated morbidities
- Inpatient—mild to moderate disease
  - Ertapenem 1g daily
  - Moxifloxacin 400 mg IV daily
  - Ceftriaxone 1g q 2h IV plus metronidazole 500 mg IV q8h
  - Levofloxacin 750 mg IV plus metronidazole 500 mg IV q8h
- Complicated diverticulitis: IV antibiotics, IV fluids, and NPO
  - Meropenem 1 g IV q8h
  - Piperacillin–tazobactam 3.375 g q6h IV
  - Cefepime 2 g IV q8h plus metronidazole 500 mg IV q8h
  - Levofloxacin 750 mg IV q24h plus metronidazole 500 mg IV q8h
- Diverticular abscesses
  - Abscess < 3 cm—antibiotics and bowel rest
  - Abscess > 3 cm—antibiotics and drainage by CT
  - Indications for surgery: Failure of medical management, persistent sepsis, peritonitis
  - In perforated diverticulitis, surgical resection is preferred over laparoscopic lavage
    - Colonoscopy recommended 6 to 8 weeks after recovery

Typhlitis

Typhlitis is an inflammation of the cecum seen in neutropenic hosts, especially those with leukemia, and is also known as *neutropenic enterocolitis*. The typical clinical features are fever, neutropenia, right-lower-quadrant abdominal pain, and mucositis occurring at around 7 to 10 days of neutropenia.
- Diagnosis: CT scan showing inflammation, thickening, or fluid-filled cecum
- Treatment: NPO, broad-spectrum antibiotics with coverage of *Pseudomonas*, enteric Gram-negative rods and anaerobes:
    - Meropenem, imipenem, doripenem, and cefepime plus metronidazole

Proctitis

Proctitis is an inflammatory disorder of the rectum, which presents with rectal pain, pressure, and tenesmus. Common clinical features are acute rectal pain, mucus discharge, diarrhea, and urgency. Though this can occur in heterosexuals, this should be considered in men who have sex with men (MSM).
- Microbiology: common sexual transmitted diseases—herpes simplex, *Chlamydia*, gonorrhea
- Diagnostic tests:
    - Anoscopy, rectal swabs for gonoococcus and *Chlamydia trachomatis*, HSV, PCR
    - Serology for syphilis
    - Stool studies for enteric pathogens and *C. difficile*
    - In MSM, anal pap and HIV testing is indicated
- Treatment:
    - Bacterial—ceftriaxone 250 mg intramuscular (IM) and doxycycline 100 mg BID for 7 days
    - HSV—valacyclovir 1g BID, famciclovir 500 mg BID, or acyclovir 400 mg TID for 7 to 10 days
    - If mucosal ulcers and suspect lymphogranuloma venereum (LGV), treat with 21 days of doxycycline.

Biliary Tract Infections
CHOLECYSTITIS

Cholecystitis is an inflammatory disorder of the gallbladder that can be caused by obstruction from a stone or in the setting of chronic illness. Calculus cholecystitis is inflammation of the gallbladder usually caused by an obstructing gallstone in the cystic duct—it is not infectious. However, delays in surgery may cause stasis and can lead to infection; thus antibiotics are given in delayed surgery or prolonged observation or complicated cholecystitis.
- Microbiology: Enteric Gram-negative bacteria—*E. coli*, *Klebsiella*, and anaerobes such as *Bacteroides fragilis.*
    - Increasing concern for extended-spectrum β-lactamases and other resistant enteric organisms may alter initial therapy.
- Acalculus cholecystitis seen in critically ill secondary to gallbladder ischemia
- Clinical features: Acute-onset right-upper-quadrant (RUQ) abdominal pain after eating. Nausea, vomiting, fever, elevated WBC, alkaline phosphatase.
- Examination may reveal Murphy sign—palpation of the RUQ elicits a gasp
- Diagnostics tests: Ultrasound with stone, gallbladder thickening >5 mm, pericholecystic fluid, Murphy sign
    - Hepatobiliary iminodiacetic acid (HIDA) scan—absent filling of the gallbladder within 1 hour

- Treatment of uncomplicated cholecystitis:
  - Supportive care, hydration, and rarely antibiotics if evident complications
  - Stop antibiotics within 24 hours after cholecystectomy—no difference in outcomes when stopped postoperatively versus 5 days after procedure
- Definitive treatment is gallbladder removal within 72 hours—decreases length of stay and antibiotic use, but no impact on late complications versus delayed surgery
- Complicated cholecystitis and sepsis
  - Antibiotic therapy to cover enteric Gram-negative rods and *Bacteroides*
    - Piperacillin—tazobactam
    - Ampicillin—sulbactam
    - Cefepime or ceftriaxone and metronidazole
    - Meropenem—health care associated or multiresistant
- Percutaneous cholecystostomy tube plus antibiotics may be indicated in severely ill who are poor operative candidates

ACUTE CHOLANGITIS

Obstruction of the biliary tract can lead to infection of the bile ducts due to stones, tumors, or fibrosis.

Patients with acute cholangitis often present with fever, RUQ pain, and jaundice, known as *Charcot triad*; this is often in association with elevated transaminases and alkaline phosphatase.

- Microbiology: Enteric Gram-negative rods and enterococci, anaerobes
- Diagnostic tests: Ultrasound looking for obstruction, endoscopic ultrasound (EUS) for <10 mm, magnetic resonance cholangiopancreatography (MRCP) for stones >6 mm, endoscopic retrograde cholangiopancreatography (ERCP) for treatment and diagnostics
- Treatment: Source control—relief of obstruction
  - Piperacillin–tazobactam, ampicillin–sulbactam, levofloxacin, or moxifloxacin
  - For Gram-negatives, treat with antibiotics for 4 to 7 days once source controlled
  - If Gram-positive bacteremia present, treat for at least 14 days

LIVER ABSCESS

Hepatic abscesses may occur via hematogenous, portal, or local spread from the biliary tract. Travel history and food history may indicate amebic liver abscess. Identifying the organisms may lead to the source and vice versa. Patients with liver abscesses often present with undifferentiated fever, chills, night sweats, and/or an elevated WBC.

- Microbiology: Gram-negative enteric bacteria (*Klebsiella, E. coli*) or alpha-hemolytic streptococci—especially *S. milleri* group—depending on the originating site
- Diagnosis: CT scan of the abdomen
- Treatment: CT-guided aspiration and drainage; culture-directed antimicrobials for a minimum of 2 weeks of IV followed by 4 to 6 weeks oral
- Amebic abscess – check serology for *E. histolytica*, single large right lobe—treat with metronidazole 750 mg q8h for 10 days then intraluminal agent—paromomycin 500 mg q8h for 7 days

PYLEPHLEBITIS

Pylephlebitis is an uncommonly seen suppurative thrombophlebitis of the portal vein. It can occur secondary to diverticulitis or appendicitis, or in contiguous biliary infections.

- Microbiology: Polymicrobial—usually *B. fragilis* and enteric Gram-negative rods (*E. coli, Klebsiella*), streptococci

- Clinical features—abdominal pain, persistent fever on antibiotics, leukocytosis, elevated alkaline phosphatase, and positive blood cultures
- Diagnostic tests: CT scan with contrast, blood cultures—which often are persistently positive due to the endovascular infection
- Treatment: Antibiotics—ceftriaxone 2g/day, levofloxacin 500 mg/day, or ciprofloxacin 400 mg q12h IV plus metronidazole 500 mg q8h; piperacillin–tazobactam 4.5 g q6h, meropenem 1 g q8h—IV until response and then 2 to 3 weeks, then continue total treatment at least 4 to 6 weeks; anticoagulant therapy is debatable

INFECTED PANCREATIC NECROSIS

Infected pancreatic necrosis may develop in up to one-third of patients with pancreatic necrosis. Clues to this diagnosis are persistent fever, leukocytosis, abdominal pain, and sepsis 7 to 10 days after an episode of acute pancreatitis.

- Diagnosis—CT scan of the abdomen showing gas in peripancreatic space and necrosis
  - CT-guided aspiration of necrosis
- Microbiology—Usually Gram-negative rods such as *E. coli*, *Klebsiella*, *Pseudomonas*, and *Enterococcus*
- Treatment—Antimicrobial therapy with carbapenems, a fluoroquinolone, or cefepime plus metronidazole continued for at least 4 weeks
  - Debridement/necrosectomy for antimicrobial failure
  - Culture-directed antibiotics/antifungals if cultures negative, no antimicrobials

PANCREATIC ABSCESS

Another uncommon complication of pancreatitis is the development of an abscess. This typically occurs 5 to 6 weeks after a bout of pancreatitis.

- Diagnosis is by abdominal CT scan.
- Treatment typically entails percutaneous drainage with culture-directed antimicrobial therapy.

INTRAABDOMINAL ABSCESSES

Abscesses may occur anywhere in the abdominal or pelvic cavity, most often due to a leak or perforation of an abdominal viscus. Typically these infections are polymicrobial and often include enteric Gram-negatives, streptococci, and anaerobes.

- Clinical features may include abdominal pain, fever, and leukocytosis.
- Diagnosis: CT scan abdomen and pelvis.
- Treatment: aspiration, drainage, and culture-directed antimicrobials.
- In cases where there is fistula formation, long-term antimicrobial treatment is typically not recommended.
- In cases of drained perirectal abscesses, a short 5- to 10-day course of antibiotics is recommended to reduce the risk of fistula.

SPLENIC ABSCESS

Splenic abscesses can be seen in infective endocarditis, hemoglobinopathies, and rarely other bacteremic infections. A clinical diagnosis is challenging, and imaging is essential. Some patients will present with persistent fever, leukocytosis, and left-upper-quadrant pain.

- Microbiology: depends on the bacteremic source—enteric Gram-negatives are most common, including *E. coli* and *Salmonella*.

- Diagnostics: CT scan abdomen
- Treatment: <3 cm—percutaneous drainage and antibiotics; >3 cm—splenectomy

PERINEPHRIC AND RENAL CORTICAL ABSCESS

Abscesses arising in and around the kidney are rare in the antibiotic era. Cortical abscesses arise from bacteremia or, rarely, from pyelonephritis. These may present with nonspecific features such as fever, chills, nausea, vomiting, flank pain ,or a prolonged fever after treatment of pyelonephritis. These may be staphylococcal or streptococcal with preceding bacteremias.

Most perinephric abscesses originate from a urinary tract source, especially with stones with perforation into the perinephric space.

- Microbiology: *E. coli, Klebsiella, Proteus, Candida* spp.; hematogenous spreads—*Staphylococcus aureus, Candida*
- Diagnosis: CT scan abdomen
- Treatment: Intrarenal—IV antibiotics 4 to 6 weeks; if >5 cm may need drainage
  - Perinephric abscesses—percutaneous or surgical drainage or nephrectomy.

PERITONITIS

Peritonitis is an inflammatory disorder of the peritoneal cavity. It may be primary (formerly called *spontaneous bacterial peritonitis*) due to transmural bacterial migration into ascites or secondary peritonitis due to an intraabdominal source. The clinical clues are fever in a patient with ascites, abdominal pain, and encephalopathy

- Microbiology—Enteric Gram-negative rods (*E. coli, Klebsiella*), streptococci, enterococci
- Hosts—ascites: Cirrhotics, heart failure, renal failure, metastatic cancer, lymphatic disease
- Diagnosis: Paracentesis with cell count, differential, protein, Gram stain/culture
  - Inoculate 10 mL into blood culture bottle at bedside
  - Blood cultures
- Ascitic fluid WBC cell count >1000 or >250 polymorphonuclear (PMN) cells—positive fluid culture
- Treatment: Ceftriaxone 1g/day IV or cefepime 2g IV q8–12h, ciprofloxacin 400 mg IV q12h, or levofloxacin 500 mg by mouth (PO) or IV plus metronidazole 500 mg q8h or moxifloxacin 400 mg/day for 5 days
- Prophylaxis:
  - In those with recurrent disease and low protein ascites (<1 g/dL)—ciprofloxacin 750 mg/week PO or norfloxacin 400 mg/day (norfloxacin is not available in the United States)
  - Those with GI bleeding—7 days of prophylaxis

Secondary peritonitis—due to ruptured viscus with leakage into peritoneum

- Microbiology—polymicrobial
- Treatment: source control/surgery plus broad-spectrum antibiotics
  - Delayed complications such as abscesses or recurrence are not uncommon: 20% to 25% despite antimicrobial therapy
  - Duration of antibiotics after source control:
    - No difference in complications between 4 and 8 days

Suggested Reading

Alvarado A. A practical score for the early diagnosis of acute appendicitis. *Ann Emerg Med.* 1986;15:557–564.
Andersson M, Andersson RE. The appendicitis inflammatory response score: a tool for the diagnosis of acute appendicitis that outperforms the alvarado score. *World J Surg.* 2008;32:1843–1849.

Ansaloni L, Pisano M, Coccolini F, et al. WSES guidelines on acute calculous cholecystitis. *World J Emerg Surg*. 2016;11:25. https://doi.org/10.1186/s13017-016-0082-5.

Chey WD, Leontiadis GI, Howden CW, Moss SF. ACG Clinical guideline: treatment of *Helicobacter pylori* infection. *Am J Gastroenterol*. 2017;112:212–238.

de Castro SM, Ünlü C, Steller EP, van Wagensveld BA, Vrouenraets BC. Evaluation of the appendicitis inflammatory response scores for patients with acute appendicitis. *World J Surg*. 2012;36:1540–1545.

DuPont HL. Acute infectious diarrhea in immunocompetent adults. *N Engl J Med*. 2014;370:1532.

DuPont HL. Persistent diarrhea: a clinical review. *JAMA*. 2016;315:2712–2723.

Feingold D, Steele SR, Lee S, et al. Practice parameters for the treatment of sigmoid diverticulitis. *Dis Colon Rectum*. 2014;57:284–294.

Gomi H, Solomkin JS, Schlossberg D, et al. Tokyo guidelines 2018: antimicrobial therapy for acute cholangitis and cholecystitis. *J Hepatobiliary Pancreat Sci*. 2018;25:3–16.

McDonald LC, Gerding DN, Johnson S, et al. Clinical practice guidelines for *clostridium difficile* infection in adults and children: 2017 update by the Infectious Diseases Society of America (IDSA) and Society for Healthcare Epidemiology of America (SHEA). *Clin Infect Dis*. 2018;66:987–994.

Miura F, Okamato K, Takada T, et al. Tokyo guidelines 2018: initial management of acute biliary infection and flowchart for acute cholangitis. *J Hepatobiliary Pancreat Sci*. 2018;25:31–40.

Riddle MS, DuPont HL, Connor BA. ACG clinical guideline: diagnosis, treatment and prevention of acute diarrheal infections in adults. *Am J Gastroenterol*. 2016;111:602–622. http://gi.org/guideline/diagnosis-treatment-and-prevention-of-acute-diarrheal-infections-in-adults/.

Ross JT, Matthay MA, Harris HW. Secondary peritonitis: principles of diagnosis and intervention. *BMJ*. 2018;361:k1407.

Salminen P, Tuominen R, Paajanen H, et al. Five-year follow-up of antibiotic therapy for uncomplicated acute appendicitis in the APPAC randomized clinical trial. *JAMA*. 2018;320:1259–1265.

Sceats LA, Trickey AW, Morris AM, Kin C, Staudenmayer KL. Nonoperative management of uncomplicated appendicitis among privately insured patients. *JAMA Surg*. 2019;154(2):141–149.

Schiller LR, Pardi DS, Sellin JH. Chronic diarrhea: diagnosis and management. *Clin Gastro Hepatol*. 2017;15:182–193.

Shane AL, Mody RK, Crump JA, et al. Infectious disease society of america clinical practice guidelines for the diagnosis and management of infectious diarrhea. *Clin Infect Dis*. 2017;65:1963–1973.

Stollman N, Smalley W, Hirano I. American gastroenterological association institute guideline on the management of acute diverticulitis. *Gastroenterology*. 2015;149:1944–1949.

Tenner S, Ballie J, DeWitt J, et al. American college of gastroenterology guideline: management of acute pancreatitis. *Am J Gastroenterol*. 2013;108:1400.

Young-Fadok TM. Diverticulitis. *N Engl J Med*. 2018;379:1635–1642.

Urinary Tract Infections

Dimitri M. Drekonja

Introduction

Urinary tract infection (UTI) is one of the most common infectious diseases, both in ambulatory and hospital settings, and is a major cause of antimicrobial use. This is especially relevant in the era of increasing antimicrobial resistance, and in particular, resistance developing in the Gram-negative organisms, which cause most UTI episodes. In many locations, it is increasingly difficult to select an empiric agent for UTI treatment that is reliably active, without major toxicities, and with robust evidence from clinical trials. Additional challenges in treating UTI are recognizing the distinct clinical syndromes included within the broad category of UTI and being aware of key management differences such as drug selection, therapy duration, and route of administration. The spectrum of distinct entities included under the umbrella of "UTI" ranges from simple cystitis, to pyelonephritis, to life-threatening urosepsis, making appropriate treatment of UTI more challenging than often appreciated.

Finally, it is critical to recognize that 30% to 50% of "UTI" episodes are actually asymptomatic bacteriuria mistakenly labeled as UTI and that any antimicrobial therapy given to these patients confers the risk of harm with no benefit. This chapter will focus on practical definitions of the commonly encountered UTI syndromes and highlight important principles of diagnosis and treatment for each entity.

Microbiology

Escherichia coli is the most important organism in the UTI world, but its relative importance fluctuates based on the specific UTI syndrome and the age and sex of the patient. In the case of uncomplicated cystitis in a premenopausal woman, *E. coli* is the causative organism for >90%

of cases, with the remainder accounted for by *Staphylococcus saprophyticus* and a smattering of non–*E. coli* Enterobacteriaceae. Defining clonal strains of *E. coli* and their epidemiology is an ongoing area of research and is clinically relevant in that rapid expansion of specific clones can lead to widespread emergence of clinically relevant phenotypes, such as fluoroquinolone resistance and extended-spectrum β-lactamase production, both of which are important to consider when choosing empiric antimicrobial therapy, especially in a critically ill patient. In postmenopausal women, and especially in elderly men, non–*E. coli* organisms become more common causes of UTI. Although *E. coli* is still the most common organism isolated from the urine of symptomatic patients, in many cases, it is only a plurality, with non–*E. coli* organisms together comprising a majority. The specific organisms are not crucial to commit to memory, but a few general principles should be noted. Gram-negative organisms predominate, including Enterobacteriaceae such as *Klebsiella*, *Enterobacter*, and *Citrobacter*, but others such as *Pseudomonas aeruginosa* are also encountered, especially in patients with recent hospital exposure. Gram-positive organisms are less likely, but enterococci can be isolated from men, and *Staphylococcus aureus* should also be considered in a patient with hospital exposure.

Other than knowing the relative importance of Gram-negative organisms, the most important tools for a provider regarding UTI treatment is knowledge of how to access a current antibiogram and the ability to obtain a urine Gram stain to help guide empiric therapy. The urine Gram stain can be particularly useful in a patient with a prior history of methicillin-resistant *S. aureus* (MRSA) or vancomycin-resistant *Enterococcus* (VRE) colonization; if such a patient presents with symptoms of pyelonephritis, a urine Gram stain showing only Gram-negative bacilli eliminates the need for empiric therapy targeting those previously isolated organisms and can greatly simplify therapy. Consulting a local antibiogram is essential in selecting an optimal empiric therapy for all UTI syndromes, but in particular for high-acuity syndromes such as pyelonephritis and urosepsis. At a facility where resistance to fluoroquinolones among Gram-negative organisms is below 10%, ciprofloxacin for a patient hospitalized with pyelonephritis is reasonable. If the same patient were to present at a facility with fluoroquinolone resistance rates for Gram-negatives exceeding 25%, ciprofloxacin as empiric therapy would be a questionable choice and could lead to harm.

Sex Differences

The epidemiology of UTI differs by sex, with UTI being far more common in premenopausal women relative to similarly aged men. The shorter urethra in women is believed to contribute to the increased risk of UTI, with bacteria having a shorter distance to travel to reach the bladder. Among postmenopausal women and similarly aged men, rates of UTI are comparable, largely due to rising incidence among men. This is attributed to the increasing frequency of prostatic hypertrophy and to the development of other comorbid conditions such as renal calculi, other prostatic diseases such as cancer, diabetes mellitus, chronic kidney disease, and others. This accumulation of conditions negates the protection accorded by the longer male urethra and whatever other factors may account for the lower rate of UTI in younger men relative to their female counterparts.

Sex differences are relevant in both the diagnosis and treatment of UTI. As mentioned previously, the microbiology of UTI in men is varied and unpredictable, such that a urine culture should always be obtained. In women, the microbiology is so predictable that in the absence of high rates of resistance, a urine culture is superfluous for UTI managed in the ambulatory setting. Among hospitalized patients, urine culture is advisable for all patients with a UTI syndrome to ensure active therapy in these acutely ill patients. Treatment differences between men and women include the fact that known or suspected prostatic involvement may influence drug selection (ideally with an agent known to penetrate prostatic tissue) and that treatment duration is generally longer for men than for women.

Classification of Urinary Tract Infections

WHAT IS A URINARY TRACT INFECTION?

In broad terms, a UTI is the presence of bacteria in the urinary tract with corresponding symptoms and signs. Importantly, although much is made about a specific numeric threshold for bacteria in a urine sample that indicates a true UTI, it is critical to note that patients can be symptomatic with relatively low numbers of bacteria in their urine and completely asymptomatic with high-count bacteriuria (generally defined as >100,000 colony-forming units/milliliter [cfu/mL]). In patients who are neurologically intact and without an indwelling catheter, symptoms of UTI can include frequency, urgency, dysuria, flank pain, pelvic discomfort, suprapubic pain, and acute hematuria. Other less specific symptoms can also be present, including fevers, chills, and rigors. Different UTI syndromes typically present with a subset of these symptoms, which will be reviewed in detail later and are summarized in Table 11.1.

Among patients with neurologic deficits such as multiple sclerosis, spinal cord injury (SCI), and stroke, some symptoms of UTI may not be present or may be reported differently. For instance, a patient with an incomplete SCI at the T10 spinal cord level is not likely to report dysuria, but may report malaise or increased spasticity. Similarly, a patient with a chronic indwelling urinary catheter will not report frequency and may not be able to report dysuria. Patients lacking the ability to accurately report symptoms can also be challenging—this includes sedated patients in the intensive care unit and those with cognitive impairments that preclude accurate reporting of symptoms. These special populations need to be evaluated carefully, and sometimes clinicians must decide whether an unusual symptom such as increased muscle spasticity is representative of a UTI or simply a temporal coincidence.

WHAT IS NOT A URINARY TRACT INFECTION?

Bacterial growth in the urine without corresponding symptoms is not a UTI, but instead reflects asymptomatic bacteriuria (ASB). In research settings this has been defined as >100,000 cfu/mL of the same organism isolated in two urine samples obtained at least 1 week apart, but a clinically

TABLE 11.1 ■ Typical Symptoms, Examination Findings, Urinalysis, and Urine Culture Results in Different Urinary Tract Infection Syndromes and Asymptomatic Bacteriuria

UTI Syndrome	Characteristic Symptoms	Typical Findings	Urinalysis	Urine Culture
Cystitis (uncomplicated and complicated)	Dysuria, frequency, urgency	Suprapubic tenderness	Pyuria	Microbial growth
Pyelonephritis	Fever, flank pain, malaise, nausea, vomiting	CVA tenderness	Pyuria	Microbial growth
Urosepsis	Fever, altered mental status	Varied, including hemodynamic instability	Pyuria	Microbial growth
Bacteriuria/pyuria of undetermined clinical significance	Nonurinary symptoms without signs of systemic illness	Often absent or trivial findings	Pyuria	Microbial growth
Asymptomatic bacteriuria	None	None	Pyuria	Microbial growth

CVA, Costovertebral angle tenderness.

more practical definition is any bacterial growth reported on a urine culture obtained from an asymptomatic patient. Despite guidelines from the Infectious Diseases Society of America that recommend no antimicrobial treatment for ASB outside of two specific scenarios (in pregnant women and before urologic surgery), treatment of ASB that is incorrectly labeled as UTI accounts for a substantial portion of UTIs that are treated with antimicrobials. An abnormal urinalysis or urine culture in an asymptomatic patient is not a UTI.

Specific Syndromes

UNCOMPLICATED CYSTITIS

A 24-year-old woman presents with 24 hours of dysuria and frequency. She is afebrile and without abnormal findings on physical examination, including no vaginal discharge. She reports vaginal intercourse two to four times weekly with a single male partner and uses condoms with spermicide for all episodes. She has no history of UTI or sexually transmitted infections.

The concept of "complicated" and "uncomplicated" in the field of UTI generates considerable confusion, in part because there is some disagreement regarding whether certain features suffice to classify an episode as complicated. In this setting, "complicated" refers to factors that increase the risk of UTI, make eradication of the infection more difficult, broaden the spectrum of causative organisms, or increase the risk of UTI recurrence. Factors that most UTI experts agree upon as conferring "complicated" status include renal calculi, presence of a urinary catheter, abnormal urinary tract anatomy, anatomic or physiologic obstruction (e.g., prostatic hypertrophy or neurogenic bladder, respectively), recent instrumentation, and diabetes. Male sex is a factor that is sometimes invoked as a complicating factor, but agreement is not universal. Certain medications for diabetes can confer an increased risk for UTI, most notably the sodium–glucose cotransporter-2 inhibitors, which are widely used.

The patient in the clinical vignette is presenting with a clear case of cystitis, or what is sometimes described as "lower urinary tract infection." Symptoms are directly referable to the site of infection—the urinary bladder. Systemic symptoms such as fevers or rigors are not present, and there is no indication of pyelonephritis (aka *upper urinary tract infection*) such as flank pain or costovertebral tenderness on examination. Because the patient is sexually active, sexually transmitted infections should be considered, but the lack of vaginal discharge and the history of condom use makes this less likely. Use of spermicide has been linked to an increased risk of UTI through alteration in the normal bacterial flora of the vagina. The suggested diagnostic workup includes a urinalysis and possibly a urine culture. Urinalysis findings suggestive of infection include the presence of white blood cells (or a surrogate marker of white blood cells such as leukocyte esterase), nitrates, and bacteria. If the local antibiogram demonstrates low levels or resistance to first-line agents for cystitis, a urine culture is unlikely to add value. However, if resistance to first-line agents exceeds 20%, or if there is a reason to suspect a more resistant organism such as recent antimicrobial use, then a urine culture should be obtained.

Recommended treatment for cystitis includes nitrofurantoin, fosfomycin, and trimethoprim–sulfamethoxazole (Table 11.2). Fluoroquinolones are not recommended for simple cystitis, despite excellent efficacy. This is because cystitis is typically a self-limiting disease, and widespread use of an oral agent with extended Gram-negative activity will limit its utility for more serious infections by increasing selection for fluoroquinolone-resistant strains. Moreover, increasing recognition of the adverse events caused by fluoroquinolones (hypoglycemia and hyperglycemia, tendon pain and rupture, neuropathy, QT prolongation, and increased rate of aortic aneurysms) have further added to the impetus to avoid these drugs for uncomplicated cystitis, and the US Food and Drug Administration specifically states to not use fluoroquinolones for uncomplicated cystitis. Patients with mild symptoms could be offered symptomatic treatment with ibuprofen and increased fluid intake, particularly if there is a

TABLE 11.2 ■ Recommended Antimicrobial Treatment for Different Urinary Tract Infection Syndromes

UTI Syndrome	Antimicrobial Dose, Route, and Duration	Comments
Uncomplicated cystitis	Nitrofurantoin macrocrystals 100 mg PO twice daily for 5 days TMP/SMZ 160/800 mg PO twice daily for 3 days Fosfomycin 3 g PO once	If treating a man as uncomplicated, consider treating for 7 days
Complicated cystitis	Nitrofurantoin macrocrystals 100 mg PO twice daily for 7–14 days TMP/SMZ 160/800 mg PO twice daily for 7–14 days Ciprofloxacin 500 mg PO twice daily for 7–14 days Fosfomycin 3 g PO every 3 days for two to three doses	For most cases, opting for shorter-duration therapy is preferred. Men with slow-to-resolve symptoms may need longer treatment duration. Fosfomycin dosing beyond once daily is poorly studied.
Pyelonephritis and febrile UTI	Ciprofloxacin 500 mg PO twice daily for 7 to 14 days Ceftriaxone 1 g IV once daily Piperacillin/tazobactam 3.375 grams IV q6h Ampicillin 2 grams IV q4h	If fluoroquinolone resistance exceeds 10%–20%, consider initial dose of ceftriaxone Ampicillin monotherapy suitable if *Enterococcus* suspected from urine Gram stain Step-down to oral agent to complete 7–14 days therapy
Urosepsis	Piperacillin/tazobactam 3.375 g IV q6h plus gentamicin 5 mg/kg/day Meropenem 500 mg IV q6h	Adding gentamicin is suggested for areas with high rates of resistance or for critically ill patients Step-down to oral agent to complete 7–14 days therapy, if possible
Bacteriuria/pyuria of undetermined clinical significance	Unknown if treatment needed	If opting to treat, regimens for complicated cystitis or pyelonephritis are reasonable

IV, Intravenous; *PO*, by mouth; *TMP/SMZ*, trimethoprim/sulfamethoxazole.

compelling reason to avoid antibiotics (allergy, recent *Clostridium difficile* infection, etc.). The patient described in the vignette could be treated with nitrofurantoin, trimethoprim–sulfamethoxazole, or fosfomycin, based on her preferences for multiday or single-dose therapy.

COMPLICATED CYSTITIS

A 55-year-old man presents to urgent care with a day of urinary frequency, dysuria, and voiding small amounts of urine. He was advised to take medication for an enlarged prostate, but has been reluctant to do so after researching side effects of the medication. He reports no fevers, flank pain, or other relevant symptoms. Examination is notable for an afebrile man with mild suprapubic tenderness and no costovertebral angle tenderness. Genital examination is normal; digital rectal examination shows a symmetrically enlarged prostate without nodules or tenderness. A postvoid bladder scan shows 300 mL of urine in the bladder.

Cystitis in a patient with one of the previously discussed complicating factors presents in a similar fashion as does cystitis in a patient without a complicating factor, often with the additional history of prior UTI episodes due to the underlying complicating condition(s). Just as in uncomplicated cystitis, symptoms are typically confined to those related to the bladder, without evidence of kidney involvement or systemic illness. A urinalysis and urine culture should be obtained from all patients based on the more varied microbiology of complicated cystitis. Treatment is also somewhat different for complicated versus uncomplicated cystitis. If prior urine cultures are available for review, selecting an agent active against the most recently isolated organism can increase the probability of selecting an appropriate agent for the current episode. Trimethoprim–sulfamethoxazole and nitrofurantoin are reasonable selections for empiric therapy; fosfomycin is less well studied, and most authorities would give more than the single dose recommended for uncomplicated cystitis. Therapy duration for the other agents is typically also extended relative to that used for uncomplicated cystitis (see Table 11.2). The more varied microbiology and the subsequent resistance profile lead to more fluoroquinolone therapy, although the risk of adverse events remains unchanged. In addition to treatment of the acute episode of cystitis, efforts should be made to address the underlying complicating factor. In this case, therapy for prostatic hypertrophy might relieve the bladder obstruction. Therapy for this episode could be initiated with nitrofurantoin or trimethoprim–sulfamethoxazole, with follow-up to ensure that the selected drug was active in 48 to 72 hours.

PYELONEPHRITIS

A 44-year-old woman is evaluated in the emergency department for 2 days of decreased appetite, malaise, chills, left flank pain, and subjective fevers. Her temperature is 102.3° F and blood pressure is 100/60, with a heart rate of 110. Examination is notable for flat neck veins and left costovertebral angle tenderness.

Pyelonephritis is infection and inflammation of the kidney, typically manifested by symptoms and examination findings, and sometimes confirmed with imaging studies. Localizing symptoms and signs of kidney involvement are flank pain and costovertebral angle tenderness. Systemic symptoms such as fevers, chills, and rigors are common, as are laboratory indications of systemic infection such as leukocytosis and an increase in the C-reactive protein. Nonurinary symptoms such as nausea and vomiting are common and play a role in the decision to treat in the ambulatory setting vs. admission to the hospital or an observation unit. Patients able to take oral medications and adequate fluid to maintain hydration can be treated as outpatients, provided that the patient has the ability or support system to reaccess care in a timely fashion in the event of clinical deterioration. Intravenous hydration and antiemetics can provide initial symptomatic relief and may facilitate successful outpatient management in patients who initially appear unsuitable for discharge. Diagnostic evaluation should include urine Gram stain, urinalysis, and blood and urine cultures. The urine Gram stain can help select empiric antimicrobial therapy, whereas the urinalysis can help increase the posttest probability of pyelonephritis. Urine cultures are almost uniformly positive unless antibiotics were administered before the sample was obtained, with blood cultures being positive in up to 30% of cases. Other tests such as a complete blood count and a basic metabolic panel are often obtained, which may help in stratifying disease severity and in determining whether renal dose adjustments are needed.

Empiric antimicrobial therapy for pyelonephritis should be based on local susceptibility patterns, with particular attention to *E. coli* and other enteric organisms (see Table 11.2). The urine Gram stain can help clinicians decide whether coverage for enterococci or other Gram-positive organisms is needed. Ideally empiric therapy should be active against >90% of likely pathogens, which in many areas of the United States means that there are no suitable oral agents, with 20% or more of *E. coli* isolates being resistant to fluoroquinolones or trimethoprim–sulfamethoxazole. Nitrofurantoin and fosfomycin may seem to be alternatives, because susceptibility to these agents often exceeds 90% to 95%, but it is important to note that these drugs are not appropriate for pyelonephritis. Both concentrate well in the bladder, but do not achieve sufficient renal or blood levels needed for an infection of the renal system with potential systemic involvement. Because there is often no oral option that has suitable pharmacokinetics and a favorable resistance profile, administration of a single dose of a parenteral agent with a course of oral therapy is one strategy to ensure active empiric therapy. Ceftriaxone and gentamicin can be dosed once daily, have good clinical efficacy in pyelonephritis, and most uropathogens have less than 10% resistance. Administering 1 g of ceftriaxone with a course of oral ciprofloxacin or trimethoprim–sulfamethoxazole is a reasonable option for ambulatory patients, with subsequent adjustment should urine or blood cultures reveal resistance.

Patients needing admission for pyelonephritis should have a similar diagnostic workup, but initial therapy should be parenteral until they are clinically stable and tolerating oral intake. An agent that has reliable activity against >90% of suspected uropathogens should be selected; for Gram-negatives, options include ceftriaxone, piperacillin–tazobactam, or aztreonam (typically used for those with β-lactam allergy), whereas for Gram-positive organisms vancomycin or ampicillin are suitable choices. For both ambulatory and hospitalized patients, positive blood cultures do not necessarily mean that parenteral therapy must be continued. Gram-negative bacteremia can be safely treated with oral therapy, as long as gastrointestinal function is normal and use of a highly bioavailable oral agent is possible (fluoroquinolones and trimethoprim–sulfamethoxazole are both highly bioavailable). Experts differ on whether Gram-positive bacteremia can be treated with oral therapy; oral linezolid may be an option for MRSA or VRE, but most clinicians would use intravenous therapy with vancomycin or daptomycin. Therapy duration can be as short as 5 to 7 days for women with pyelonephritis in the absence of complicating factors, whereas men are typically treated for 7 to 14 days.

Imaging is not typically needed for pyelonephritis, unless there is concern for urinary obstruction, signs of severe disease such as emphysematous pyelonephritis or urosepsis (discussed later), or continued fevers after 3 days of active antimicrobial therapy. The imaging modality of choice is computed tomography (CT) scanning with intravenous contrast, but ultrasonography can provide useful information if there are concerns with use of CT scanning (e.g., renal impairment making contrast administration undesirable, contrast allergy, or pregnancy). The patient described in the vignette should be treated empirically with ceftriaxone, with reevaluation of appropriateness for outpatient therapy with an oral antimicrobial after rehydration in the emergency department. If discharged on ciprofloxacin, she should be contacted in 24 hours to ensure she is improving, and antimicrobials should be adjusted as needed.

FEBRILE URINARY TRACT INFECTION

A 65-year-old man presents to his primary care clinic with complaints of dysuria, frequency, and subjective fevers. He reports no flank pain and is eating and drinking normally. Physical examination reveals a temperature of 101.8° F, blood pressure of 130/82 mmHg, and heart rate of 88 beats/min. He has no costovertebral angle tenderness, but does endorse mild suprapubic tenderness. A digital rectal examination is normal.

The patient described in this vignette falls into a category that does not neatly fit into prior classification systems of upper versus lower tract disease or pyelonephritis vs. cystitis. Unlike pyelonephritis, there is no localizing to the kidney with either symptoms or examination findings. And because of the fever, it does not fit the definition of cystitis, which typically is manifested by irritative symptoms that localize to the bladder, without evidence of systemic involvement. Whether there is renal infection present that is mild enough to not result in flank tenderness and costovertebral angle tenderness, or infection in other urinary structures, or simply a more robust inflammatory response to an infection that is contained to the bladder is unknown. Practically, management of febrile UTI parallels that used for pyelonephritis. This includes avoiding nitrofurantoin and fosfomycin, obtaining a urine culture to ensure active therapy, and considering a single dose of a long-acting parenteral agent such as ceftriaxone or gentamicin (in addition to an empiric course of oral therapy) when local resistance rates to fluoroquinolones and trimethoprim–sulfamethoxazole exceed 10%. Treatment duration is also similar—5 to 7 days for women, 7 to 14 for men. The patient described here could be treated with ciprofloxacin or levofloxacin for 7 days, with therapy adjusted based on urine culture results as needed.

UROSEPSIS

A 76-year-old woman is sent via ambulance to the emergency department when staff at her skilled nursing facility noticed that she was confused, febrile to 102.6° F, had a blood pressure of 88/60 mmHg, and had a heart rate of 115 beats/min. An indwelling catheter had been placed 2 weeks prior and had been draining clear urine, but no output was documented in the past 12 hours. Examination shows acute delirium, warm extremities, and distention in the suprapubic area that elicits pain. In the emergency department fluid resuscitation is initiated, blood cultures are drawn, and the indwelling catheter is replaced with return of over 1 L of cloudy urine.

The most serious manifestation of UTI is urosepsis, which is defined as sepsis physiology (hypotension, tachycardia, and organ system dysfunction) in response to a UTI. Many of the principles of treating urosepsis are similar to those that underlie the treatment of sepsis from any source: fluid resuscitation, circulatory support, identification of the site of infection, initiation of appropriate broad-spectrum antimicrobial agents, and obtaining source control. The details of fluid resuscitation and circulatory support are beyond the focus of this chapter, but source control and antimicrobial therapy will be covered.

Because the urinary tract is generally a self-draining system, source control is typically easier to obtain than, for instance, sepsis due to an obstructed biliary tree. In most instances insertion of an indwelling catheter (or removal of a previously obstructed catheter, as in the vignette) is sufficient to obtain source control. The evaluation of a patient with sepsis physiology in the presence of an indwelling catheter should include inspection of the drainage system to ensure no areas of tubing are kinked or externally compressed and flushing or replacement of the system if there is a suspicion of internal obstruction from clot, mineral encrustations, or other debris. Exceptions to these relatively simple methods for relieving obstruction include urosepsis in the presence of an obstructing stone and emphysematous pyelonephritis. Both of these necessitate emergent intervention, typically by urology for stone removal in the case of an obstructing stone, and either urology or interventional radiology for nephrectomy or percutaneous drainage in the case of emphysematous pyelonephritis.

In addition to source control, selection of active empiric therapy is crucial to the management of urosepsis. Because of high rates of antibacterial resistance among Gram-negative organisms plus a clinical scenario with little room for error, use of an agent(s) with low rates of resistance is imperative. In areas with minimal carbapenem resistance, carbapenem monotherapy is sufficient. But in a system with carbapenem resistance rates approaching 10% for any common Gram-negative organisms, use of a second agent such as an aminoglycoside or a fluoroquinolone is justified. This is not for theoretical synergy or enhanced bacterial killing with two agents, but rather to increase the odds that at least one of the drugs is active. Aminoglycosides are attractive options in this situation, because limited use over the past several years has resulted in little resistance, and they can hopefully be discontinued within the first 72 hours after the patient has improved and susceptibility testing has returned. If the patient has improved and can tolerate oral intake, is hemodynamically stable, and a highly bioavailable oral antimicrobial can be used, de-escalation to oral therapy is appropriate, similar to the strategy described for pyelonephritis. Blood and urine cultures should be obtained, in addition to routine laboratory investigations such as a complete blood count and a basic metabolic panel. The patient described in the vignette should receive meropenem or, alternatively, piperacillin/tazobactam plus gentamicin, along with fluid resuscitation and vasopressor support, if needed. Use of indwelling catheters should be avoided if at all possible.

ASYMPTOMATIC BACTERIURIA

A 90-year-old man is seen for his annual examination. He reports excellent health, walking several miles daily, and takes only atorvastatin and aspirin for medications. For unknown reasons, a urinalysis is ordered, which because of 11 leukocytes/high-powered field reflexes to a urine culture. Two days later >100,000 cfu/mL of Klebsiella oxytoca are isolated, with susceptibility to all tested antimicrobials. The patient is reached by phone and reports that he is feeling at baseline with no symptoms.

Asymptomatic bacteriuria (defined previously) is common, especially in nursing home residents, those with structurally abnormal urinary tracts, and those with indwelling catheters. Long-term indwelling catheters (those present for 2 weeks or longer) in particular should be recognized as nearly universally colonized, with positive results expected if a urine culture is obtained. Guidelines on ASB from the Infectious Disease Society of America have recently been updated, with various populations not previously addressed now having specific recommendations. These include patients undergoing nonurologic surgery, solid-organ transplant recipients, children, and patients with neutropenia. Fortunately, the take-home message from the updated guidelines is identical to prior guidelines: treatment for ASB supported by evidence in pregnant women and for patients about to undergo urologic surgery with anticipated urothelial bleeding. For all other patients, there is no evidence to support treating ASB. Because of the known harms or antimicrobial therapy (adverse drug events, *C. difficile* infection, resistance, and cost), evidence for benefit is needed before ASB should be treated (i.e., not merely the lack of data for a particular patient population). One point that bears emphasis is that ASB treatment decisions do not depend on the intrinsic virulence of the organism. A patient with a multidrug-resistant strain of *Pseudomonas aeruginosa* in the urine at >100,000 cfu/mL should be managed identically as if it were a pan-susceptible *E. coli* at 30,000 cfu/mL: if no symptoms, then no treatment is needed. The patient in the vignette should not receive antimicrobial therapy (and should not have had his urine tested).

BACTERIURIA AND PYURIA OF CLINICALLY UNDETERMINED SIGNIFICANCE

An 85-year-old man is brought to the clinic by a friend who checks in on him twice a week. The friend is concerned because he thinks the patient is eating less than usual and seems much less energetic than usual, falling asleep during their conversation and declining to go for their usual walk around the block. The patient endorses becoming fatigued after minimal exertion and feels "just all-around crummy." He denies urinary symptoms, and physical examination is unrevealing. Multiple laboratory studies are obtained in clinic. The patient is sent home with advice to get rest, try to increase oral intake, and that he will be called with the laboratory results. They are all within normal limits or at their prior baseline, except for a urinalysis with 45 leukocytes/high-powered field and a culture that grew *Enterobacter aerogenes* with resistance to ceftriaxone and ceftazidime. The patient is feeling better, remains without urinary symptoms, and thinks "I might have just been in a funk."

Management of UTI syndromes such as pyelonephritis and cystitis is made easier by clinical practice guidelines that give clear treatment recommendations; similarly, ASB guidelines provide recommendations for the two scenarios where ASB treatment is warranted, and otherwise recommend against antimicrobial therapy. Unfortunately, real-world patients do not always fit neatly into clinical syndromes. The patient described here does not report classic symptoms of any UTI syndrome and lacks any symptoms that seem plausibly linked to the urinary tract; however, the patient reports some symptoms (fatigue, malaise), and a caregiver corroborates that he is not at his baseline.

Nonspecific symptoms in a patient who is discovered to have pyuria or bacteriuria is exceedingly common but infrequently studied. One interpretation of this situation is that these nonspecific symptoms represent an atypical presentation of UTI—this can then result in a cycle where the patient presents with vague symptoms, the medical record and the patient report that these symptoms are typical for UTI, and the provider than accepts that this atypical presentation is the norm. This can result in frequent rounds of antimicrobial therapy, increasing bacterial resistance, and sometimes adverse events such as *C. difficile* infection. Another interpretation is that this represents a patient with nonspecific symptoms unrelated to the urinary tract, who also happens to have ASB. In this case, symptomatic therapy or watchful waiting may be just as effective as antimicrobials, without the associated adverse events. Because of increasing rates of resistance and the recognition regarding the harms of antimicrobial therapy, watchful waiting and supportive care may be a more appropriate course than empiric antimicrobials for clinically stable patients with bacteriuria and nonspecific symptoms. In this case, with the patient feeling better without antimicrobial therapy, watchful waiting is recommended. Were his nonspecific symptoms still present, a trial of antimicrobial therapy would be a reasonable next step, with the caveat that the diagnosis of UTI is not firmly established.

Common Conundrums

SAME STRAIN RECURRENCE

Same strain recurrence is when a patient experiences repeated episodes of UTI with the same causative organism and with full resolution between episodes. To truly determine whether the episodes are caused by the same organism, techniques such as sequence typing or pulse-field gel electrophoresis would be needed. Practically, isolation of the same organism with an identical pattern of antimicrobial susceptibility is reasonable evidence that the same strain is causing each episode—even more so if the susceptibility pattern is unique, such as a multidrug-resistant phenotype. Documenting same strain recurrence should prompt consideration of some nidus of infection where organisms are able to persist during what should be adequate courses of treatment. Commonly implicated culprits include renal or bladder calculi, bladder diverticula, indwelling ureteral stents, or prostatic involvement. Surgical correction of the diverticula, stone removal, and stent removal may resolve these foci of recurrence; prostate involvement can sometimes be addressed with a longer course of therapy (4 to 6 weeks), but may also require surgical source control.

RECURRENT URINARY TRACT INFECTION

Recurrent infections caused by different organisms typically occur in patients with one of the previously mentioned complicating factors, which increase the risk of UTI, make eradication of the infection more difficult, broaden the spectrum of causative organisms, or increase the risk of recurrence. When such factors can be alleviated, the risk of recurrence can be decreased. Examples include therapy to eliminate calculi, treatment of prostatic hypertrophy, and surgical correction of abnormal urinary tract anatomy, when feasible. Some factors cannot be alleviated, however, making management of recurrent UTI an ongoing challenge. Daily suppressive therapy is one option that has demonstrated efficacy in premenopausal women but has not been well studied in patients with complicating factors. There are good reasons to avoid this strategy, including that the variety of causative pathogens is too broad to cover with one agent, the increasing concerns regarding antimicrobial resistance, and the risk of adverse drug effects. Another option (which is not well studied) is to provide such a patient with a prescription or supply of an antimicrobial to take at the onset of symptoms, along with instructions and supplies to collect a urine sample for culture. The agent selected to have on hand should be based on the last available urine culture and be prescribed for a relatively short duration such as 7 days. Preventive strategies such as cranberry-containing products, probiotics, and hydration have mixed results, but ensuring intake of 1.5 L of water daily has minimal downsides for most patients and has some evidence of efficacy.

CONTINENCE AND RETENTION

Although slightly outside the scope of this chapter, urinary continence and retention are important (and challenging) aspects of UTI management. Incontinence can be socially distressing, and when poorly managed leads to skin maceration and breakdown. There are different varieties of incontinence, some of which respond more favorably to drug therapy than others. When pharmacologic therapy is insufficient, other options such as absorbent pads and garments, indwelling catheterization, and implantation of an artificial urethral sphincter may be considered. Similar comments apply to retention—pharmacologic therapy may relieve certain causes of retention such as prostatic hypertrophy, but catheterization (intermittent or indwelling) and surgery may be needed. Unfortunately, surgery to address obstruction may result in subsequent continence issues, and thus leave the patient with a new but related problem to manage.

CATHETERS

As discussed earlier, continence and retention problems may lead to the need for a urinary catheter. Catheterization for the management of incontinence is usually done with an indwelling catheter, either urethral or suprapubic. Both will be colonized with bacteria within a few weeks of insertion, and this colonized state typically is asymptomatic unless there is obstruction of the catheter or traumatic urethral injury. A suprapubic catheter may be easier for the patient to clean and maintain, and also can allow penile or vaginal intercourse. Rates of symptomatic infection between urethral and suprapubic catheters are similar, however. Intermittent catheterization may be more appealing for patients with urinary retention issues, allowing them to avoid the inconvenience of an indwelling catheter and the accompanying collection bag. Trauma from insertion may be more frequent with intermittent vs. indwelling catheters, and risk of UTI is still increased relative to patients without a urinary catheter. Both indwelling and intermittent catheters come with different antimicrobial coatings such as silver compounds or nitrofurazone, but the clinical efficacy of these coatings has not been defined. They decrease rates of bacteriuria short-term, but whether they prevent symptomatic UTI is unproven.

Conclusions

UTIs are a collection of different syndromes ranging in severity from bothersome to life-threatening. Asymptomatic bacteriuria, included here because it so often is treated as a UTI, is a major cause of unnecessary antimicrobial use and significantly inflates the number of reported UTIs in both ambulatory and hospital settings. Importantly, symptoms and examination findings are what differentiate ASB from cystitis, pyelonephritis, urosepsis, and other syndromes that fall under "UTI"—findings from urinalysis and urine culture cannot be used to differentiate different UTI syndromes (see Table 11.1). Biomarkers such as peripheral white cell count and C-reactive protein can be supportive of a more severe UTI syndrome, but they are ancillary to more crucial findings such as costovertebral angle tenderness, hypotension, and fever. Treatment for UTI has become more challenging, largely due to increasing antimicrobial resistance, and a working knowledge of local antimicrobial susceptibilities is needed to help choose optimal empiric therapy, particularly in more severely ill patients who require hospitalization.

Suggested Reading

Albert X, Huertas I, Pereiro II, Sanfelix J, Gosalbes V, Perrota C. Antibiotics for preventing recurrent urinary tract infection in non-pregnant women. *Cochrane Database Syst Rev*. 2004:CD001209.

Bleidorn J, Gagyor I, Kochen MM, Wegscheider K, Hummers-Pradier E. Symptomatic treatment (ibuprofen) or antibiotics (ciprofloxacin) for uncomplicated urinary tract infection?--results of a randomized controlled pilot trial. *BMC Med*. 2010;8:30.

Boucher HW, Talbot GH, Bradley JS, et al. Bad bugs, no drugs: No ESKAPE! an update from the infectious diseases society of america. *Clin Infect Dis*. 2009;48:1–12.

Cope M, Cevallos ME, Cadle RM, Darouiche RO, Musher DM, Trautner BW. Inappropriate treatment of catheter-associated asymptomatic bacteriuria in a tertiary care hospital. *Clin Infect Dis*. 2009;48: 1182–1188.

Drekonja DM, Kuskowski MA, Wilt TJ, Johnson JR. Antimicrobial urinary catheters: a systematic review. *Expert Rev Med Devices*. 2008;5:495–506.

Drekonja DM, Zarmbinski B, Johnson JR. Preoperative urine cultures at a veterans affairs medical center. *JAMA Intern Med*.173:71-72.

Filice GA, Drekonja DM, Thurn JR, Hamann GM, Masoud BT, Johnson JR. Diagnostic errors that lead to inappropriate antimicrobial use. *Infect Control Hosp Epidemiol*. 2015,36:949–956.

Foxman B. Epidemiology of urinary tract infections: incidence, morbidity, and economic costs. *Am J Med*. 2002;113(suppl 1A):5S–13S.

Gupta K, Grigoryan L, Trautner B. Urinary tract infection. *Ann Intern Med*. 2017;167:ITC49–ITC64.

Gupta K, Hooton TM, Naber KG, et al. International clinical practice guidelines for the treatment of acute uncomplicated cystitis and pyelonephritis in women: a 2010 update by the infectious diseases society of america and the european society for microbiology and infectious diseases. *Clin Infect Dis*. 2011;52: e103–e120.

Hooton TM, Vecchio M, Iroz A, et al. Effect of increased daily water intake in premenopausal women with recurrent urinary tract infections: a randomized clinical trial. *JAMA Intern Med*. 2018;178:1509–1515.

Johnson JR. Definition of complicated urinary tract infection. *Clin Infect Dis*. 2017;64:529.

Johnson JR, Drekonja DM. Bacteriuria/pyuria of clinically undetermined significance (BPCUS): common, but currently nameless. *Am J Med*. 2017;130:e201–e204.

Johnson JR, Porter S, Thuras P, Castanheira M. The pandemic H30 subclone of sequence type 131 (ST131) as the leading cause of multidrug-resistant escherichia coli infections in the United States (2011-2012). *Open Forum Infect Dis*. 2017;4:ofx089.

Johnson JR, Russo TA. Acute pyelonephritis in adults. *N Engl J Med*. 2018;378:1162.

Kunin CM, White LV, Hua TH. A reassessment of the importance of "low-count" bacteriuria in young women with acute urinary symptoms. *Ann Intern Med*. 1993;119:454–460.

Leuck AM, Wright D, Ellingson L, Kraemer L, Kuskowski MA, Johnson JR. Complications of Foley catheters--Is infection the greatest risk? *J Urol*. 2012;187:1662–1666.

McPhail MJ, Abu-Hilal M, Johnson CD. A meta-analysis comparing suprapubic and transurethral catheterization for bladder drainage after abdominal surgery. *Br J Surg*. 2006;93:1038–1044.

Nicolle LE, Gupta K, Bradley SF, et al. Clinical practice guideline for the management of asymptomatic bacteriuria: 2019 update by the infectious diseases society of america. *Clin Infect Dis*. 2019;268(10):e83–e110.

Ronald A. The etiology of urinary tract infection: traditional and emerging pathogens. *Am J Med*. 2002;113(suppl 1A):14S–19S.

Scholes D, Hooton TM, Roberts PL, Stapleton AE, Gupta K, Stamm WE. Risk factors for recurrent urinary tract infection in young women. *J Infect Dis*. 2000;182:1177–1182.

Schwenger EM, Tejani AM, Loewen PS. Probiotics for preventing urinary tract infections in adults and children. *Cochrane Database Syst Rev*. 2015:CD008772.

Talan DA, Stamm WE, Hooton TM, et al. Comparison of ciprofloxacin (7 days) and trimethoprim-sulfamethoxazole (14 days) for acute uncomplicated pyelonephritis in women: a randomized trial. *JAMA*. 2000;283:1583–1590.

Tambyah PA, Maki DG. Catheter-associated urinary tract infection is rarely symptomatic: a prospective study of 1,497 catheterized patients. *Arch Intern Med*. 2000;160:678–682.

Tamma PD, Conley AT, Cosgrove SE, et al. Association of 30-day mortality with oral step-down vs continued intravenous therapy in patients hospitalized with enterobacteriaceae bacteremia. *JAMA Intern Med*. 2019;179(3):316–323.

The prevention and management of urinary tract infections among people with spinal cord injuries. National institute on disability and rehabilitation research consensus statement. January 27–29, 1992. *J Am Paraplegia Soc*. 1992;15:194–204.

van Nieuwkoop C, van der Starre WE, Stalenhoef JE, et al. Treatment duration of febrile urinary tract infection: a pragmatic randomized, double-blind, placebo-controlled non-inferiority trial in men and women. *BMC Med*. 2017;15:70.

Wang CH, Fang CC, Chen NC, et al. Cranberry-containing products for prevention of urinary tract infections in susceptible populations: a systematic review and meta-analysis of randomized controlled trials. *Arch Intern Med*. 2012;172:988–996.

CHAPTER 12

Skin and Soft Tissue Infections

Silvano Esposito ■ Pasquale Pagliano ■ Anna Maria Spera

Introduction

Skin and soft tissue infections (SSTIs) are among the most commonly occurring bacterial infections, and their frequency approaches 10% of hospital admissions for infections in the United States. Many factors contribute to the increase in awareness of SSTIs: the aging of the general population, the growing number of critically ill or immunocompromised patients, and the emergence of multidrug-resistant (MDR) pathogens are commonly considered the main reasons for SSTI increase in frequency and severity.

SSTIs have variable presentation, as they can range from mild to severe, life-threatening infections. Healthy hosts or compromised hosts belonging to all age groups can be affected by SSTIs, and their severity and prognosis can be related to the host condition. Many differences can be observed with respect to etiology of SSTIs that can be influenced by a number of factors. Evidence deriving from common practice demonstrates that immunologic status, previous antimicrobial treatments, geographic localization, recent history of trauma or surgery, animal exposure, and bites have to be considered in the evaluation of diagnostic and therapeutic strategies for a patient reporting an SSTI. All these considerations warrant an accurate evaluation and clinical observation of each case either to avoid the severe, life-threatening complications of undertreatment or to avoid the severe complications with overdiagnosis of SSTIs, particularly in the setting of stasis dermatitis or after venom reactions, such as honeybee stings. On the basis of a large multicenter trial of patients presenting to an emergency department, a presumptive diagnosis of cellulitis—the most common skin infection, accounting for 650,000 hospitalizations in the United States annually—was not confirmed in 30% of the patients after dermatology consultation. In these cases, venous stasis dermatitis, erythema migrans, contact dermatitis, eczema, and erythema nodosum were the most common mimics of cellulitis.

Any study on the etiologic aspect of SSTIs is hampered by the low yields of blood and skin cultures that make the microbiologic findings available for less than 30% of the patients affected by cellulitis. As a general concept, *Staphylococcus aureus* and β-hemolytic streptococci (BHS) are considered the most frequent causative agents of SSTIs. The majority of SSTIs report a mono-microbial etiology, and a polymicrobial etiology can be demonstrated in about 20% of the cases.

Definitions and Classifications of SSTIs

Intact skin provides an effective protection from the external environment, acting as a physical barrier and maintaining a microbiologic environment that is not conducive to the growth of pathogenic organisms. SSTIs can occur after microorganisms invade otherwise healthy skin or when an underlying disease or trauma favors the infection of damaged skin. The damage is due to the destruction of affected tissues causing an inflammatory response clinically characterized by pain, local warmth, and erythema. In particular settings, such as in patients living with diabetes mellitus or neuropathies, the degree of skin damage can be high and the management can be more complicated. In these particular settings, recurrent episodes or the evidence of nonhealing lesions suggests the need for further investigations to assess vascular and lymphatic compromise.

SSTIs represent a heterogeneous array of disorders, and a number of classifications have been proposed. Every attempt at classification organizes SSTIs on the basis of a specific variable, such as anatomic localization, etiologic agent, skin extension, progression rate, clinical presentation, and severity. Each of them has its own usefulness, but in general what the clinician expects from classifications is to be driven toward the most appropriate management of the condition. On this basis, the Infectious Diseases Society of America (IDSA) classification has been the most useful and practical guidance to date by adopting three different distinctions: (1) skin extension: uncomplicated typically superficial infections (uSSTIs) and complicated infections (cSSTIs), usually with deep involvement; (2) rate of progression: acute and chronic wound infections; and (3) tissue necrosis: necrotizing and non-necrotizing infections. However, the need to standardize the definitions of SSTI to be adopted to patients involved in pivotal trials evaluating antibiotic treatments prompted the US Food and Drug Administration (FDA) to introduce the new definition of acute bacterial skin and skin-structure infection (ABSSSI) that includes cellulitis/erysipelas, wound infections, and major cutaneous abscesses. Thus an ABSSSI is defined as a bacterial infection of the skin with a lesion size area of ≥ 75 cm^2 (lesion size measured by the area of redness, edema, or induration). Table 12.1 provides a practical classification of SSTIs based on the anatomic structure involved, highlighting the different modality of transmission and clinical characteristics.

MICROBIOLOGY OF SSTI

The site of infection can influence microbiology. For example, facial infections are commonly caused by group A β-hemolytic streptococci (GABHS), and an increasing percentage of lower extremity infections is caused by non-GABHS such as *Streptococcus agalactiae*. *S. aureus* and BHS are the main etiologic agents of uncomplicated SSTIs; BHS is the primary cause of erysipelas.

Staphylococci sustain the majority of cases with skin abscesses, and the bacteria that constitute the normal skin flora boost their virulence. When we look at the patients affected by cellulitis, we find that GABHS or *S. aureus* is frequently involved. Patients with chronic venous stasis or with saphenous vein harvest for coronary artery bypass surgery experiencing recurrent cellulitis of the lower extremities report an infection caused by BHS. Similarly, recurrent episodes of cellulitis in patients with lymphedema are frequently sustained by BHS. Staphylococci and BHS are also the most common pathogens in bacterial infections among drug users. Gram-negative and anaerobic bacteria are more common in association with surgical site infections (SSIs) of the abdominal wall or infections of the soft tissue in the anal and perineal region due to the specific characteristic of the bacterial flora in these parts of the body.

TABLE 12.1 ■ Clinical Presentation of the Most Relevant SSTIs

SSTI	Conditioning Factors	Characteristics
Impetigo (Fig. 12.1)	**Subjects**: Children aged 2–5 yr (peak of incidence), newborns, adults in low-income areas. Atopic dermatitis is an important risk factor. **Transmission**: Person-to-person or via fomites. Clinically apparent 10 days after skin colonization. **Localization**: Exposed body areas, orifical areas, face, scalp, and the back of the hands (non-bullous impetigo); skin folds (bullous impetigo).	Nonbullous impetigo (contagious impetigo): Papules surrounded by erythema that become superficial vesicles and then pustules, which evolve to form characteristic thick, honey-colored crusts. Multiple spreading lesions (auto-inoculation). *S. aureus* is the most common pathogen; *Streptococcus pyogenes* is less common and can be either a single pathogen or in combination with *S. aureus*. Bullous impetigo: Caused by toxin-producing *S. aureus*, is a localized form of staphylococcal scalded skin syndrome. Vesicles that rapidly evolve into flaccid bullae filled with clear, yellow fluid that can become purulent.
Ecthyma	**Subjects**: Healthy people living in tropical areas or immunocompromised. **Pathogenesis**: Via small trauma, bacteria invade the skin barrier. **Localization**: Epidermal and dermal layers.	A vesicle or pustule overlying an inflamed area of skin that deepens into a dermal ulceration with overlying gray-yellow crust followed by a shallow, punched out ulceration that appears when crust is removed, evolving towards a hard brown-blackish crust. *Ecthyma gangrenosum*: Necrotic skin ulcer, which can be a primary or secondary infection; secondary infection set in course of sepsis caused by *P. aeruginosa*, among immunocompromised.
Erysipelas (Fig. 12.2)	**Subjects**: Peak of incidence in childhood and over 50 yr **Localization**: Lower extremities (adults); face (adults and children). **Course of infection**: Short.	Warm and aching erythema heralded by fever, heat, and shivering. The lesion extends to surrounding areas with a sharp border. Flaccid vesicles and bullae filled with purulent fluid may appear 2–3 days after infection with lymphangitis and regional lymph node inflammation.
Cellulitis (Fig. 12.3)	**Subjects**: No target population. **Localization**: Face and extremities. **Course of infection**: Long, with frequent recurrences and local complications; *S. aureus* and β-hemolytic streptococci commonly involved.	Erythema, edema, warmth, and tenderness of a poorly demarked area with lymphadenopathy and fever. *S. aureus* and *Bacteroides* spp.: Cellulitis in diabetic patients. *Pseudomonas* spp. and *Enterobacteriaceae*: In hospitalized patients. *Clostridium* spp.: In exposed fractures and penetrating trauma. *Streptococcus* spp. plus *Haemophilus influenzae*; Orbital cellulitis, in healthy children <5 yr.
Necrotizing fasciitis (NF) (Fig. 12.4)	**Population**: Those with an infected area after chickenpox, trauma, surgery, or illegal drug use. **Localization**: Extremities, abdomen, perineum. **Pathogenesis**: Streptococcal hemolytic toxins (streptolysin O and S). **Risk factors**: Immunosuppression, chickenpox.	NF type 1: Polymicrobial infection, destroys subcutaneous fat and muscular fascia. NF type 2: Caused by beta-haemolytic streptococci (BHS) of Lancefield groups A, C or G alone or associated with S. aureus.

Continued

TABLE 12.1 ■ Clinical Presentation of the Most Relevant SSTIs—cont'd

SSTI	Conditioning Factors	Characteristics
Myonecrosis (MN)	**Population**: Traumatologic or oncologic MN is an acute, life-threatening infection that can cause many complications, the most common being gangrene.	Gas gangrene: Slowly expanding ulceration confined to the superficial fascia; determines necrosis of muscle, gas in the tissues, and systemic toxicity; is caused by *Clostridium* spp. Traumatic gangrene: Presents with acute severe pain on the wound area, which becomes purple-reddish with bullae, edema, and crepitus within few days from trauma. It is associated with sepsis.

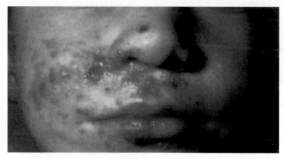

Fig. 12.1 Impetigo.

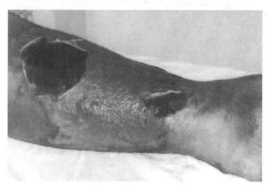

Fig. 12.2 Erysipelas.

Particular settings for SSIs and SSTIs can include those with cytotoxic therapy–induced granulocytopenia. In these cases, extended-spectrum β-lactamase (ESBL)–producing *Enterobacteriaceae* and carbapenem-resistant *Pseudomonas aeruginosa* constitute about 10% of the etiologic agents reported in those with SSI. Patients affected by hematologic malignancies or bone marrow transplant recipients can develop "ecthyma gangrenosum"—cellulitis caused by the hematogenous seeding of *P. aeruginosa*, *Stenotrophomonas maltophilia*, and other bacteria and fungi otherwise infrequently involved in SSTIs.

Immunocompromised patients after solid-organ transplantation represent another particular setting. They can develop cellulitis due to unusual organisms, including Gram-negative bacilli, anaerobes, and other opportunistic pathogens such as Mycobacteria and fungi. Cellulitis from uncommon bacterial species, including *Enterobacteriaceae*, *Enterococcus faecalis*, *Bacteroides* spp., and *Clostridium* spp., can be observed after subcutaneous injections of illegal drugs. Other uncommon causes of

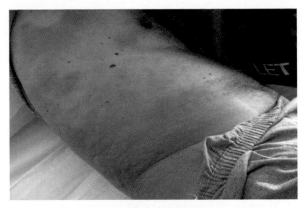

Fig. 12.3 Cellulitis.

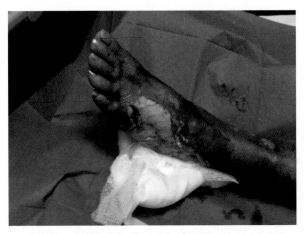

Fig. 12.4 Necrotizing fasciitis.

cellulitis include *Neisseria meningitidis*, *Mycobacterium avium*, *Pasteurella multocida* (which is associated with animal bites), *Aeromonas hydrophilia* (after contact with freshwater), *Chromobacterium violaceum*, *Vibrio vulnificus* (after contact with seawater), and several other pathogens.

When we look at hospital-acquired bacteria, focusing on patients requiring intensive care, we find that *Acinetobacter baumannii* is the main emerging MDR pathogen causing soft tissue infections, including cellulitis, after the use of invasive devices. Current data indicate that *A. baumannii* can be an important pathogen in patients with burn wounds, where a high percentage of resistant strains that significantly contribute to mortality has been observed.

Necrotizing fasciitis is frequently sustained by *S. aureus* and GABHS, alone or in combination. Most cases are polymicrobial, Gram-positive cocci, especially *S. aureus*, are the main pathogens causing diabetic foot infections, but Gram-negative pathogens can be reported in those with chronic infection receiving multiple antibiotic treatments. Infections in patients suffering foot ischemia or gangrene can be caused by obligate anaerobic pathogens.

Polymicrobial infections account for about 10% of cases of SSTI, and both Gram-positive and Gram-negative organisms can be the causative agent. According to general considerations, polymicrobial infections provide a complex environment in which a variety of interactions may occur between causal pathogens that may share virulence determinants and trigger the synergistic release of cytokines, adding to the severity of the infection. Most of the polymicrobial SSTIs can be included in the following: diabetes-related foot infections (DFIs), pressure ulcer infections, burn infections, and infected chronic ulcers. These distinct clinical entities have a common characteristic in that they can become chronic with a high degree of colonization from bacteria present in the surrounding environment that can interact to increase their pathologic effects and possibly lead to resistance.

MICROBIOLOGIC DIAGNOSIS

Even though microbiologic data do not play a role in the choice of initial empiric therapy, the need for etiologic tests depends on several factors, including the type of infection, severity of the clinical condition, and the underlying patient condition. As a general concept, uncomplicated SSTIs (cellulitis or small subcutaneous abscess) do not require microbiologic investigations; instead, when exudates and abscesses are evident in a patient with complicated SSTI, specimens have to be collected. Moreover, all immunosuppressed patients and injuries contaminated with soil or animal bites have to be investigated by cultures and microscopic examination of cutaneous aspirates or biopsies.

Diagnostic workup of SSTI differs with respect to patient condition and infection severity. Blood cultures have to be attempted for all cases with severe infection requiring hospitalization. Cultures and microscopic examination of cutaneous aspirates, pus, biopsies, or swabs should be considered in complex infection, septic and immunosuppressed patients, water- or soil-related injuries, and animal bites. It is important to emphasize that superficial swabs of open ulcers and drainage from fistulous material usually do not correctly identify the microbiologic etiology. In fact, in patients with deep tissue infections, the results of superficial techniques do not reflect the etiologic pathogen because of the presence of commensal microorganisms on the wound surface, which explains the low specificity of the diagnostic investigation. Quantitative cultures have been proposed to distinguish commensal microbiota from clinically significant bacterial growth, but the usefulness of this technique has been questioned by numerous prospective studies.

Blood cultures are positive in a percentage of cases, approaching 5%. Cultures attempted from materials derived from needle aspirations of the inflamed skin are positive in an extremely variable number of cases (<5% to 40%, on the basis of the different studies available by a literature analysis). Cultures of punch biopsy specimens yield an organism in 20% to 30% of cases. If an abscess is present, puncture and aspiration of fluid should be performed. SSTIs without any evidence of liquid collection have to be investigated by a small biopsy of skin or soft tissue after superficial disinfection and excision of necrotic tissue. Chronic wounds can be investigated by pus or fluid culture; alternative samples to biopsy include aspiration of saline that has just been infused into the wound depth.

Molecular technologies can be considered an effective, time-saving alternative to overcome the delay in the results associated with traditional bacterial culture. Polymerase chain reaction (PCR)–based techniques are equally sensitive as cultures, but can be useful for the diagnosis of SSTIs sustained by *S. aureus*, potentially providing crucial information as to the choice of appropriate antibiotic regimen, such as the rapid detection of Panton–Valentine leucocidin-encoding genes from pus samples or the identification of cryptic resistances.

IMAGING STUDIES

Imaging studies are sometimes required to establish an accurate diagnosis of SSTI. Plain radiography can help in detecting the presence of gas in the soft tissues, which is suggestive of a necrotizing infection, or in diagnosing an osteomyelitis. Computed tomography (CT) scans can give useful information and help to assess the extent of the infectious process, guiding fluid aspiration and revealing the presence of foreign objects or even small fluid–air collections in the soft tissues. Magnetic resonance imaging (MRI) has the advantage of a better definition of soft tissues and can be particularly helpful in differentiating cellulitis from pus and abscess formation. Moreover, MRI provides better accuracy than CT in detecting necrosis, inflammatory edema, and muscular fascia involvement, but its use is limited because of its cost. Ultrasonography can be a sensitive technique for SSTI diagnosis, reporting important advantages over other imaging studies, including MRI. In fact, ultrasonography provides useful information to differentiate cellulitis from abscess, therefore limiting more expensive imaging studies and unnecessary harmful procedures like incision and drainage. Moreover, ultrasonography is an easy and rapid technique without side effects and high costs that can be performed in many cases where MRI cannot be performed. Radionuclide scanning studies generally lack specificity in the acute situation, but the development of hybrid techniques (such as single-photon emission tomography [SPECT]/CT and positron emission tomography [PET]/MRI) can increase the specificity of nuclear medicine imaging techniques, eventually revealing the involvement of surrounding structures.

INDICATIONS FOR HOSPITAL ADMISSION

SSTIs are among the most common reasons for hospitalization of adults in the United States. Several authors have attempted to identify indications for hospital admission for patients with SSTI. Medical history, presence of fever or relevant comorbidities (e.g., vascular insufficiency, neuropathy, diabetes, and immunosuppression), the site of the lesion itself (the hand or head has the potential for more significant damage), particular aspects of laboratory investigations (e.g., elevated white blood cell count and lactate levels), and the degree of involvement of the body surface (>9%) have to be considered to establish the necessity for hospital admission. Overall, the large majority of patients with uncomplicated SSTIs can be managed as outpatients. However, complicated infections often require hospital admission, especially if muscle or fascial involvement is suspected, the process is rapidly progressing, signs of toxemia are developing, the diagnosis or prognosis is in doubt, exploratory surgery is contemplated, or the patient cannot adequately comply with outpatient treatment.

TREATMENT OF SSTI

Therapy for SSTIs should consider the following general aspects:
- Anatomic localization
- Etiologic agent
- Skin extension (localized or widespread infection)
- Rate of progression (acute or chronic disease)
- Clinical presentation (primary or secondary infection)
- Severity (presence of comorbidities)

In general, superficial infections are not complicated or severe, and they would need just oral antibiotic treatment or even topical treatment.

Deeper infections should be considered based on their severity, taking into consideration the skin extension, the rate of progression, and finally the necrotizing or non-necrotizing characteristics of the infection. This last consideration is extremely important for the choice of the antibiotic regimen, as the etiology of these infections is substantially different.

All these considerations are important not only for the choice of the most appropriate antibiotic regimen (oral versus parenteral treatment, broad- versus narrow-spectrum treatment) but also for the best site of care.

In general, SSTIs are a frequent reason for hospitalization of adults worldwide, and several authors have attempted to identify predictors for admission, as their correct evaluation would play a central role in choosing appropriately the best site of care. One of the best attempts comes from Eron et al. (2003), who took into consideration the general clinical conditions of the patient affected by an SSTI, considering four different classes, with each class corresponding to different needs regarding the site of care (Table 12.2). This kind of predictor allows also identify

TABLE 12.2 ■ SSTI Classification According to the Severity of Local and Systemic Signs

Class	Patient Criteria	Site of Care
1	Afebrile and healthy, other than cellulitis	Send home on oral antimicrobial therapy
2	Febrile and ill appearing, but no unstable comorbidities	OPAT with possibility to switch to oral therapy
3	Toxic appearance, or at least one unstable comorbidity, or a limb-threatening infection	OPAT with possibility of hospital admission
4	Sepsis syndrome or life-threatening infection (e.g., necrotizing fasciitis)	Hospital admission

OPAT, Outpatient parenteral antibiotic therapy; *SSTI,* skin and soft tissue infection.

the patients who need an outpatient parenteral antibiotic therapy (OPAT) approach instead of hospitalization.

OPAT is a treatment model widely utilized in the United States and several European countries and refers to antibiotic administration given in settings other than a traditional hospital stay, including the patient's home, the general practitioner's office, the hospital ambulatory unit, and public or private infusion centers.

SSTIs are a common indication for OPAT treatment. Several controlled trials comparing intravenous antibiotic treatment of cellulitis at home with hospital treatment not only showed no difference in outcome and greater patient satisfaction with home treatment but also a significant cost savings accrued from real or potential reductions in hospital stay. Antibiotics used for OPAT treatment of SSTI must be effective against common pathogens such as *S. aureus* and BHS and have a convenient once- or twice-daily dosing schedule. Ceftriaxone is most frequently used, with teicoplanin, vancomycin, and daptomycin reserved for SSTIs due to suspected or proven methicillin-resistant *S. aureus* (MRSA).

ACUTE NON-NECROTIZING INFECTIONS: THERAPY (TABLE 12.3)

Impetigo

Impetigo, which is most often due to *S. aureus*, can be usually treated topically with mupirocin or chlortetracycline twice daily for 5 days. Oral therapy can be a 7-day regimen with an anti-staphylococcal penicillin or cephalexin.

When MRSA is suspected or confirmed, doxycycline, minocycline, clindamycin, or sulfa-methoxazole–trimethoprim (SMX-TMP) can be used.

It remains unclear if oral antibiotics are superior to topical antibiotics, and the therapeutic choice remains an individual decision mostly based on the number of lesions and their location.

Furuncles and Carbuncles

Small furuncles can be treated with warm compresses to promote drainage, whereas larger furuncles and carbuncles and all abscesses require incision and drainage. If used, empiric antibiotic therapy with an anti-staphylococcal (and MRSA in areas of high prevalence) activity can be added.

Recurrence of furuncles can be prevented by using soap containing chlorhexidine gluconate with isopropyl alcohol and a 1- to 2-month course of low-dose oral clindamycin (1500 mg daily).

Animal and Human Bites

Antibiotic administration depends on the severity of lesion, its type, and location. Preemptive antibiotic therapy is generally recommended for those wounds at risk of infection. It must be done

TABLE 12.3 ■ Treatment of Non-necrotizing Infections

Diagnosis	Etiology	Antibiotic Choice	Note
Impetigo	Staphylococcus aureus, BHS	Local mupirocin or chlortetracycline Amoxicillin-clavulanate, Erythromycin	In case of suspected or proven MRSA: doxycycline, clindamycin, TMP-SMX
Furuncles and carbuncles	Staphylococcus aureus	As impetigo	As impetigo
Animal bytes	Gram-negative (Capnocytophaga canimorsus and Pasteurella multocida)	Oral amoxicillin ampicillin/sulbactam	In case of severe wounds: parenteral piperacillin/tazobactam or carbapenems
Cutaneous abscesses*	Staphylococcus aureus	Incision and drainage Amoxicillin/clavulanate	In case of suspected and proven MRSA: TMP-SMX, clindamycin, tetracyclines, linezolid, fusidic acid
Erysipelas*	Streptococcus pyogenes	Amoxicillin	As alternatives: first- and second-generation cephalosporins
Cellulitis*	Staphylococcus aureus, Streptococcus pyogenes Beta-haemolytic streptococci (BHS) of Lancefield groups A, C or G	Amoxicillin, clavulanate As alternatives: Fluoroquinolones, macrolides, and lincosamides	In case of Vibrio vulnificus: cefotaxime plus doxycycline. In case of Aeromonas hydrophila: ceftazidime plus gentamicin In case of MRSA: glycopeptides and newer antimicrobial options (linezolid, daptomycin, telavancin, and tigecycline)
Surgical site infections*	Staphylococcus aureus	Amoxicillin/clavulanate Ampicillin/sulbactam	In case of MRSA: glycopeptides and newer antimicrobial options, (linezolid, daptomycin, telavancin, and tigecycline)

*Whenever the lesion size is ≥75 cm² it is classified as ABSSSI. Dalbavancin and tedizolid have been approved for their empirical treatment.
BHS, β-Hemolytic streptococci; MRSA, methicillin-resistant S. aureus; TMP-SMX, trimethoprim-sulfamethoxazole.

with oral amoxicillin/clavulanate or ampicillin/sulbactam after accurate cleaning and copious irrigation. In the case of severe wounds, especially in patients with comorbidities (immunodepression, diabetes, end-stage liver disease) and/or patients with clinical signs of systemic infections (sepsis), parenteral therapy with piperacillin/tazobactam or carbapenem is recommended

Cutaneous Abscesses

Incision and drainage of pus and debris of cutaneous abscesses is strongly recommended as primary management; however, needle aspiration—even ultrasonographically guided—should not be performed due to its low rate of success.

Concomitant administration of antibiotics does not seem modify the patient's outcome for localized and small abscesses, but in case of major abscesses, the administration of antibiotics effective against S. aureus, which is the main pathogen responsible, such as amoxicillin/clavulanate, is recommended, especially in the presence of clinical symptoms such as temperature >38° C, tachypnea, tachycardia, or white blood cell count >12,000.

In cases of suspected or proven MRSA or in geographic areas with a high prevalence of community-associated MRSA (CA-MRSA), a variety of oral agents, such as TMP-SMX, clindamycin, tetracyclines, oxazolidinones, and fusidic acid, can be used in the outpatient setting.

Erysipelas

Erysipelas is almost always caused by *Streptococcus pyogenes*, which is the only pathogen responsible for this infection. Because *S. pyogenes* has remained sensitive to penicillin over time, this class of antibiotics remains the first choice in treatment. The route of administration—oral or intravenous—will be defined according to the severity of the infection. Amoxicillin is the best choice, but also first- and second-generation cephalosporins can be a good alternative.

Cellulitis

Cellulitis can be a serious infection requiring appropriate antibiotic treatment, such as amoxicillin/clavulanate (oral or intravenous, depending on the disease severity), and covering the most frequent responsible microorganisms (*S. aureus* and *S. pyogenes*). The therapy must be initiated promptly, monitoring the clinical evaluation and keeping in mind that other pathogens can be present. Fluoroquinolones and lincosamides can be an appropriate alternative even though the resistance to clindamycin is increasing. High rates of macrolide/azalide resistance among BHS already present in some areas of the world make use of these drugs a concern, unless susceptibility results are available in an individual case. If additional bacterial species are likely to be involved after unusual exposures, such as abrasion or laceration occurring after saltwater exposure, where *V. vulnificus* might be the pathogen, treatment with cefotaxime plus doxycycline is effective. Surgical intervention may also be required.

Similarly, in the setting of cellulitis after an abrasion or laceration occurring with freshwater exposure, where *A. hydrophila* might be involved, treatment with ciprofloxacin (along with an antimicrobial targeted to the common pathogens) is indicated or, as alternative, a combination of ceftazidime plus gentamicin.

If MRSA is suspected (both hospital-acquired [HA-MRSA] and CA-MRSA), glycopeptides, TMP-SMX, and newer antimicrobial options, including linezolid, daptomycin, telavancin (only available in the United States), and tigecycline, are suitable agents.

Surgical Site Infections

Similarly to cutaneous abscesses, for SSIs, incision and drainage remain the first and most important aspects of therapy.

Adjunctive systemic antimicrobial therapy can be beneficial, especially when a significant systemic response is present. Antibiotic treatment recommendations are based on the site of operation, but *S. aureus* remains the most frequent etiologic agent. Thus an anti-staphylococcal agent should be preferred, such as amoxicillin/clavulanate or ampicillin/sulbactam, with the route of administration depending on the general conditions of the patient. Whenever the prevalence of methicillin resistance is high, an anti-MRSA is mandatory, with glycopeptides being the gold standard of therapy.

ABSSSI

Recently, as noted earlier, the US FDA introduced the new definition of ABSSSI to more closely define cSSTI for the purpose of registration trials.

The new drugs for ABSSSI have important activity also against MRSA, especially dalbavancin and tedizolid. Consequently these new drugs can be used for prompt empirical treatment of ABSSSI. Tedizolid, thanks to its longer half-life, can be administered only once a day.

Dalbavancin was recently approved by the FDA and European Medicines Agency with a two-dose regimen of 1000 mg followed 1 week later by 500 mg administered intravenously over 30 minutes. One of the strengths of dalbavancin is the prolonged half-life which leads to the possibility of a single 1500-mg intravenous (IV) administration.

TABLE 12.4 ■ Empiric Antimicrobial Therapy for Chronic SSTIs

Infection	Route of Administration	Antibiotic/Dosage	Alternative/Dosage
Mild	Oral	Levofloxacin 500 mg od Amoxicillin/clavulanic acid 1000 mg BID/TID	TMP-SMX 800/160 mg BID/TID
Moderate	Intravenous (possible switch to oral)	Ampicillin/sulbactam 1000 mg QID	Piperacillin/tazobactam 4.5 g TID
		Ertapenem 1000 mg od	Linezolid 600 mg BID
		Tigecycline 50 mg BID (with loading dose)	Daptomycin 300/500 mg od
		Clindamycin 600 mg TID plus ciprofloxacin 500 mg BID	Clindamycin 600 mg TID plus Ceftazidime 2 g TID
Severe	Intravenous	Imipenem 500–1000 mg TID	Vancomycin 1 g BID
		Meropenem 1000 mg TID	Linezolid 600 mg BID
		Clindamycin 600 mg TID plus Amikacin 1g od plus Ampicillin mg^2 g TID	Linezolid 600 mg BID plus Aztreonam 2 g TID plus Metronidazole 500 mg TID

BID, Twice a day; *od,* once daily; *QID,* four times a day; *SSTI,* skin and soft tissue infection; *TID,* three times a day; *TMP-SMX,* trimethoprim-sulfamethoxazole.

CHRONIC NON-NECROTIZING INFECTIONS: THERAPY

DFIs, pressure ulcer infections, burn infections, and infected chronic ulcers are distinct clinical entities that have the common characteristic in that they can become chronic with a high degree of colonization from the bacteria present in the surrounding environment, which can multiply their pathologic effects and acquire resistance, which is often against multiple antibiotics and can limit the choices for both empiric and subsequent therapy.

Initial therapy has to be empirical and needs to be based on the severity of the clinical presentation and on the history of previous antibiotic treatment (Table 12.4). Because these infections are chronic, prior susceptibility data should be available in most patients to assist in the selection of initial empiric therapy. The spectrum of antibiotic therapy has to be broad, considering the possible polymicrobial etiology and should include coverage for *S. aureus,* considering an anti-MRSA in those areas with high prevalence of methicillin resistance. Moreover, coverage against Gram-negative bacilli has to be included in all cases with moderate to severe infection and in those failing narrower-spectrum treatment. After culture from tissue biopsy has been collected, the antibiotic spectrum can be narrowed on the basis of the results. The quality of the specimen has to be considered when deciding which isolates need to be covered.

In most cases, treatment of the most likely pathogens, such as *S. aureus,* streptococci, and any Enterobacteriaceae provides effective coverage. When cultures are obtained, therapy should be tailored with respect to microbiologic findings. When a fungal infection can be suspected on the basis of histopathology, cultures have to be attempted to identify those fungi whose coverage is not provided after amphotericin B administration.

Patients with a recent ineffective treatment are at highest risk of infection due to MDR microorganisms. In these cases alternative therapies should be considered: vancomycin, linezolid, or daptomycin for MRSA infections; colistin or tigecycline for MDR Gram-negative microorganisms. Antibiotic treatment can be administered in patients with pressure ulcers, but only on the basis of the presence of local or systemic clinical signs of sepsis; in addition, an indication for systemic antibiotic treatment has to be considered.

Treatment of burn injuries must consider early excision followed by grafting to reduce infection risk and length of hospital stay; these surgical procedures are an essential part of a burn patient's management. Topical antibiotics are currently employed; their utility can differ with respect to preparation, as demonstrated for silver–sulfadiazine. Antibiotic prophylaxis appears to have no significant value except in those with more severe injuries.

For chronic trophic ulcers, besides surgical treatment of vascular complications, control of underlying predisposing factors such as hyperglycemia ameliorates the outcome. Once infection is diagnosed, chronic ulcers must be treated aggressively. Treatment includes debridement, surgical drainage of abscesses, debridement of infected bone, and tissue culture–guided antimicrobial therapy. Although a lot of topical therapies/antimicrobials and dressings have been proposed for the treatment of chronic ulcers, very few have prospective data to support their effectiveness in promoting chronic ulcer repair.

NECROTIZING INFECTIONS: THERAPY

All necrotizing SSTIs (myositis, myonecrosis, necrotizing fasciitis, and Fournier gangrene) require immediate surgical debridement because prompt surgery ensures a higher likelihood of survival, and it must be continued until tissue necrosis ceases and the growth of fresh viable tissue is observed. In addition, early surgical treatment may minimize tissue loss, reducing the risk for amputation of the infected extremity. Surgical intervention may be required to ultimately confirm the diagnosis and the severity of illness, and its progression may require immediate surgery before a diagnosis is confirmed by other diagnostic interventions.

Empiric antibiotics should be started immediately as well (Table 12.5). Initial antimicrobial therapy should be broad-based to cover aerobic Gram-positive and Gram-negative organisms and anaerobes, with the highest possible doses of the antibiotics considering the patient's weight and liver and renal status (see Table 12.5).

Empiric antibiotic therapy can be employed until wound culture isolates are identified. Acceptable monotherapy regimens include a carbapenem, piperacillin/tazobactam, or tigecycline. However, an optimal choice in the management of necrotizing fasciitis can also be the association of ampicillin/sulbactam plus clindamycin and ciprofloxacin or gentamicin. In cases of suspected MRSA, TMP-SMX, vancomycin, or daptomycin can be used; alternatives include the newer compounds linezolid, tedizolid, dalbavancin, and ceftaroline. Clyndamycin

---

TABLE 12.5 ■ Empirical Antibiotic Treatment of Necrotizing Infection

Necrotizing Infection	Antibiotic Choice
Synergistic (aerobic and anaerobic pathogens)	Imipenem, meropenem, tigecycline, piperacillin/tazobactam,
Penicillin allergy (skin rash only)	Cefepime + metronidazole
Penicillin allergy (anaphylaxis)	Ciprofloxacin + metronidazole
If MRSA is suspected	Vancomycin or daptomycin
If CA-MRSA is suspected	Clindamycin, TPM-SMX
New anti-staphylococcal (including MRSA) alternatives	Linezolid, tedizolid, dalbavancin, ceftaroline
Difficult-to-treat Gram-negative bacteria	Ceftazidime/avibactam

CA-MRSA, community-acquired methicillin-resistant *S. aureus*; *TPM-SMX*, trimethoprim-sulfamethoxazole.

administration reports many advantages due to its action on suppression of bacterial toxins synthesis. Intravenous immunoglobulins can be considered in selected cases with septic shock.

The association of ceftazidime/avibactam with an antianaerobic agent (metronidazole or clindamycin) can be a useful option in the case of difficult-to-treat Gram-negative bacteria such as an ESBL-producing strain and/or MDR *Pseudomonas*.

Hyperbaric oxygen has been reported to reduce associated tissue loss and mortality, but well-controlled, randomized clinical trials demonstrating a statistically significant benefit of hyperbaric oxygen are lacking, and consequently, its use as an adjunctive therapy for necrotizing fasciitis remains controversial. Thus the mainstay of treatment remains surgical debridement, and this should never be delayed due to hyperbaric oxygen therapy–related activities.

Suggested Reading

Dryden MS. Complicated skin and soft tissue infection. *J Antimicrob Chemother*. 2010;65(suppl 3):35–44.

Eron LJ, Lipsky BA, Low DE, Nathwani D, Tice AD, Volturo GA. Expert panel on managing skin and soft tissue infections. Managing skin and soft tissue infections: expert panel recommendations on key decision points. *J Antimicrob Chemother*. 2003;52(suppl 1):i3–17.

Esposito S, Ascione T, Pagliano P. Management of bacterial skin and skin structure infections with polymicrobial etiology. *Expert Rev Anti Infect Ther*. 2019;17:17–25.

Esposito S, Bassetti M, Bonnet E, et al. Hot topics in the diagnosis and management of skin and soft-tissue infections. *Int J Antimicrob Chemother*. 2016;48:19–26.

Esposito S, Bassetti M, Concia E, et al. Diagnosis and management of skin and soft-tissue infections (SSTI). A literature review and consensus statement: an update. *J Chemother*. 2017;29:197–214.

Esposito S, De Simone G. Update on the main MDR pathogens: prevalence and treatment options. *Infez Med*. 2017;25:301–310.

Esposito S, Leone S, Noviello S, Ianniello F, Fiore M. Antibiotic resistance in long-term care facilities. *New Microbiol*. 2007;30(3):326–331.

Esposito S, Noviello S, Boccia G, De Simone G, Pagliano P, De Caro F. Changing modalities of outpatient parenteral antimicrobial therapy use over time in Italy: a comparison of two time periods. *Infez Med*. 2016;2:137–139.

Esposito S, Noviello S, De Caro F, Boccia G. New insights into classification, epidemiology and microbiology of SSTIs, including diabetic foot infections. *Infez Med*. 2018;26:3–14.

Esposito S, Noviello S, Leone S. Dalbavancin for the treatment of acute bacterial skin and skin structure infections. *Infez Med*. 2015;23:313–317.

Garau J, Ostermann H, Medina J, Avila M, Mc Bride K, Blasi F. Current management of patients hospitalized with complicated skin and soft tissue infections across Europe (2010-2011): assessment of clinical practice patterns and real-life effectiveness of antibiotics from the REACH study. *Clin Microbiol Infect*. 2013;19:E377–E385.

Jääskeläinen IH, Hagberg L, Forsblom E, et al. Microbiological etiology and treatment of complicated skin and skin structure infections in diabetic and nondiabetic patients in a population-based study. *Open Forum Infect Dis*. 2017;4:ofx044.

Lipsky BA, Berendt AR, Cornia PB, et al. 2012 Infectious diseases society of america clinical practice guideline for the diagnosis and treatment of diabetic foot infections. *Clin Infect Dis*. 2012;54:e132–e173.

Miller LG, Eisenberg DF, Liu H, et al. Incidence of skin and soft tissue infections in ambulatory and inpatient settings, 2005–2010. *BMC Infect Dis*. 2015;15:362.

Saeed K, Esposito S, Gould I, et al. Hot topics in necrotising skin and soft tissue infections. *Int J Antimicrob Agents*. 2018;52:1–10.

Saeed K, Gould I, Esposito S, et al. Panton-Valentine leukocidin-positive staphylococcus aureus: a position statement from the international society of chemotherapy. *Int J Antimicrob Agents*. 2018;51:16–25.

Stevens DL, Bisno AL, Chambers HF, et al. Practice guidelines for the diagnosis and management of skin and soft tissue infections: 2014 update by the Infectious Diseases Society of America. *Clin Infect Dis*. 2014;59:e10–e52.

US Food and Drug Administration. *Guidance for Industry. Acute Bacterial Skin and Skin Structure Infections: Developing Drugs for Treatment. Silver Spring, MD: US Department of Health and Human Services, Food and Drug Administration*. Center for Drug Evaluation and Research (CDER); 2013.

CHAPTER 13

Bone and Joint Infections

Talha Riaz ■ Aaron J. Tande

Infectious Arthritis

Infectious arthritis is defined as infection of one or more joints. It can be caused by bacteria, fungi, viruses, and parasites.

ACUTE BACTERIAL ARTHRITIS

Introduction

Native joint septic arthritis is an uncommon illness, with a reported incidence in the United States of 2 to 10 cases per 100,000 persons per year. However, the incidence appears to be rising, in part due to an increasing number of joint surgical procedures performed in the United States and because of a larger "at-risk population." The incidence of septic arthritis is higher in certain at-risk groups, including patients with rheumatoid arthritis and patients with a low socioeconomic status. Bacterial septic arthritis accounts for 8% to 27% of patients presenting with one or more acutely painful joints in the emergency room (ER). The knee joint is the most commonly affected joint. Septic arthritis is associated with significant morbidity; near half of the patients report decreased joint mobility after the infection. This, however, also depends on previous underlying joint disease and the type of microorganism involved. Bacterial arthritis is generally acquired hematogenously. Underlying joint architectural abnormality increases the risk of pyogenic arthritis. An important factor to consider is that the synovial membrane is a highly vascularized structure that lacks a basement membrane and is susceptible to hematogenous deposition of bacteria. Other routes of infection include trauma; animal bites; joint puncture from a nail, needle, or thorn; iatrogenic infection; and contiguous infection from adjacent soft tissue or bone. After knee arthroscopy, the infection risk is 0.04% to 0.4%, and after arthroscopic reconstruction, the risk is 0.14% to 1.7%. Rarely, septic arthritis has occurred in clusters after intraarticular injection of contaminated methylprednisolone.

Predisposing Factors

- Rheumatoid arthritis
- Old age
- Diabetes mellitus
- Renal insufficiency
- Penetrating joint trauma
- Intravenous (IV) drug use
- Endocarditis
- Immunocompromise
- Crystal-induced arthritis (gout and pseudogout), osteoarthritis, and Charcot arthropathy
- Chronic systemic diseases, including collagen vascular diseases, malignancy, chronic liver disease, sickle cell disease, and alcoholism
- Hypogammaglobulinemia
- Intraarticular injections
- Low socioeconomic status

Underlying joint disease especially due to rheumatoid arthritis is an important risk factor. Additionally, being treated with immunosuppressive medications such as penicillamine, sulfasalazine, anti–tumor necrosis factor alpha (anti-TNF) agents (doubles the risk according to one study), and corticosteroids further increase the risk. HIV infection, however, has not been associated with septic arthritis. In many cases, no predisposing risk factor is isolated.

Nongonococcal Arthritis

Pathogenesis. Adherence of bacteria to the synovial membrane followed by colonization and replication in synovial fluid is then followed by production of inflammatory cytokines and modulators. Bacteria such as *Staphylococcus aureus* have cell surface receptors that bind to joint extracellular matrix, promoting invasion. Joint damage results both directly from bacterial toxins and the host inflammatory response. Purulence is observed as a result of accumulation of acute and chronic inflammatory cells. This leads to destruction of joint cartilage. Joint effusion also leads to raised intraarticular pressure predisposing to decreased blood flow and tissue necrosis. Eventually, a joint space becomes narrow, and erosion of bone and cartilage occurs if arthritis is untreated.

Microbiology. In adults, Gram-positive cocci such as *S. aureus* or streptococci are responsible for the majority of native arthritis. *S. aureus* is responsible for 37% to 65% of the cases, with a higher incidence in patients with underlying rheumatoid arthritis.

Methicillin-resistant *S. aureus* (MRSA) is seen in elderly, those with recent orthopedic surgery, and those who are colonized with MRSA. Of the streptococci, *Streptococcus agalactiae* is a cause of bacterial arthritis in neonates, adults with malignancy, diabetes, and urogenital anatomic abnormalities and predisposes to polyarticular infection. *Streptococcus bovis* subgroup gallolyticus septic arthritis could be a manifestation of infective endocarditis; thus these patients should be evaluated for endocarditis and colonic malignancy.

Gram-negative rods account for 9% to 17% of all cases, and anaerobes are identified in 1% to 3%. Again, elderly and immunocompromised patients and IV drug users are at a higher risk. *Pseudomonas aeruginosa* is seen frequently in IV drug users and is also recognized as a cause of iatrogenic septic arthritis. In young infants, *Haemophilus influenzae* has now been replaced by *Kingella kingae*, a resident of oral flora.

Zoonotic pathogens such as *Pasteurella multocida* and *Capnocytophaga* spp. can occasionally cause contiguous septic arthritis after a dog or cat bite. *Streptobacillius moniliformis*, the cause of rat bite fever, can cause polyarticular arthritis after a rat bite. Cases of bacterial arthritis where a pathogen is not isolated from blood or joint fluid using conventional culture techniques are *Mycoplasma hominis, Ureaplasma urealyticum, Borrelia burgdorferi* and *Tropheryma whipplei.*

Clinical Presentation. The knee is the most common joint involved in nongonococcal septic arthritis followed by the hip, shoulder, wrist, and ankle. Arthritis of the small joints of the foot are seen generally in diabetics with adjacent skin and soft tissue ulceration. Polyarticular presentation may be seen in patients who are immunosuppressed (such as patients with rheumatoid arthritis [RA]) or patients with high-grade bacteremia (especially with *S. aureus*). In cases of *S. aureus* bacteremia, sacroiliitis can also be seen.

The typical presentation is one of progressive pain, loss of function, and loss of range of motion of the involved joint seen over a period of several days, up to 2 weeks, depending on the organism and patient. Other symptoms include joint swelling, redness, and warmth. Fever and malaise can also be seen, though high-grade fever with rigors is rare, unless accompanied by bloodstream infection. Physical examination typically demonstrates joint tenderness, effusion and limitation of active and passive range of motion, and painful weight bearing. However, in older and immunocompromised patients, these symptoms may be subtle, leading to a delay in diagnosis.

Laboratory Screening. There is no single laboratory finding that is sensitive or specific for native septic arthritis. Leukocytosis, elevated erythrocyte sedimentation rate (ESR), and C-reactive protein (CRP) are helpful when present.

Synovial Fluid Analysis/Microbiologic Diagnosis. Aspiration of the joint space will often yield synovial fluid that is low viscosity and purulent. Synovial fluid white blood cell (WBC) count is typically 50,000 cells/mm^3 with a neutrophilic predominance, although lower counts are regularly seen and should not be ignored. Gram staining lacks sensitivity for the diagnosis of septic arthritis and is only diagnostic in 50% of cases. On the other hand, among patients who have not received prior antibiotics, synovial fluid culture will yield bacterial growth more than 60% of the time in nongonococcal infection. Blood cultures should always be drawn, as they can be positive in 50% of the cases. The synovial fluid broad-range polymerase chain reaction (PCR) test holds promise but is not available in all clinical microbiology labs. It is particularly useful in cases of slow-growing microorganisms such as *K. kingae, Coxiella burnetii, Bartonella henselae,* and *Mycobacterium tuberculosis.* It can be helpful in situations where patients have already received systemic antibiotics.

Radiologic Evaluation. Early in the course of bacterial arthritis, plain radiography will show periarticular soft tissue swelling, but the bony structures are normal. Later, as the infection progresses, loss of joint space, periosteal reaction, periarticular osteoporosis, and subchondral bone destruction can be seen. Plain films help rule out the presence of any foreign body.

Ultrasound is another technique that can be used to assess for the presence of effusion and for assistance in joint aspiration. Computed tomography (CT) scan and magnetic resonance imaging (MRI) are additional and sensitive imaging modalities, especially in detecting early septic arthritis, as well as detecting periarticular fistulas, abscesses, and adjacent/periarticular cellulitis and tenosynovitis.

Gonococcal Arthritis

Native septic arthritis due to infection with *Neisseria gonorrhoeae* results from a complication of mucosal gonococcal infection. Risk factors associated with gonococcal arthritis are similar to those for genital gonococcal infection, including low socioeconomic status, men who have sex with men, illicit drug use, and having multiple sexual partners.

Pathogenesis. After mucosal inflammation and infection with *N. gonorrhoeae*, occult bacteremia results. Mucosal infection may be asymptomatic. Bacteremia can result in wide dissemination from the infected mucosa, resulting in several joints being involved (disseminated gonococcal infection). *N. gonorrhoeae* possesses several virulence factors that help in its attachment to the mucosal and synovial membranes, including a long pili. The pili also prevents it from undergoing host leukocyte phagocytosis.

Clinical Presentation. Generally, disseminated gonococcal infection is characterized by a triad of dermatitis, tenosynovitis, and a migratory polyarthralgia/polyarthritis. Patients present with fever, chills, and malaise, with painful tenosynovitis of fingers and hands and occasionally lower limb joints. Less than half of the patients will have true septic joint effusion. A rash involves the palms and soles and can range from macules to papules and a pustular rash as well. Isolated septic gonococcal arthritis without accompanying tendinopathy and skin manifestations is less common, with knees, wrists, and ankles being most commonly affected. This is characterized by an inflamed and swollen joint with an effusion.

Diagnostic Testing. ESR is raised in half of the patients, accompanied by mild leukocytosis. Joint aspiration reveals a pyogenic aspirate, with WBC count ranging from 50,000 to 100,000 WBCs/mm^3 (mainly neutrophils), but lower cell counts are seen in patients with disseminated gonococcal infection with less intense pyogenic process. Gram stain of the joint aspirate reveals intracellular and extracellular Gram-negative diplococci in 25% of the cases. PCR assay of the synovial fluid is another technique for detecting the presence of *N. gonorrhoeae*. It is also reasonable to perform mucosal swabs and send them for culture, as recovery of *N. gonorrhoeae* from the mucosal sites is higher than from synovial fluid or blood cultures. Nucleic acid amplification tests (NAATs) can also be performed on urine and swabs from cervical or urethral swabs.

Differential Diagnosis

It is important to differentiate bacterial arthritis from noninfectious causes. Situations such as an acute attack of gout, pseudogout, and other crystalline joint arthropathies can mimic acute bacterial arthritis, as symptoms and signs can overlap.

Presence of crystals in joint fluid does not rule out bacterial arthritis. Gram stain and culture along with cell count with differential should be performed on all joint aspirates. Recognition of bacterial arthritis in patients with underlying rheumatoid arthritis is important as well. Gonococcal arthritis (when it presents as part of disseminated gonococcal infection [DGI]) should be differentiated from reactive arthritis, which is typically seen after a recent gastrointestinal or genitourinary infection. The typical rash of DGI is not seen in reactive arthritis; these patients generally have concurrent sacroiliitis, conjunctivitis, and penile manifestations such as circinate balanitis and keratoderma blennorrhagica.

Treatment

Acute septic arthritis requires prompt joint drainage and is an infectious diseases emergency. Whether it requires arthroscopy or open arthrotomy depends on the clinical situation and on the surgeon. Another approach is to drain the joint through daily closed needle aspiration until clinical improvement is seen. For bacterial infections involving the knee, shoulder, and wrist,

TABLE 13.1 ■ Antibiotic Choices Based on Identified Pathogen

Microorganisms	Treatment of Choice (IV)	Alternatives (IV)
Gram-positive cocci	Vancomycin	Daptomycin[a]
Methicillin-susceptible S. aureus	Cefazolin, nafcillin, or oxacillin	Ceftriaxone or vancomycin[b]
Methicillin-resistant S. aureus	Vancomycin	Daptomycin or teicoplanin (where available)
Streptococcus spp.	Penicillin G	Ceftriaxone or vancomycin[b]
Gram-negative rods	Ceftriaxone or ceftazidime or cefepime[c]	Ciprofloxacin or levofloxacin or carbapenem
Anaerobes	Clindamycin	Metronidazole
Enterococci	Ampicillin, penicillin G	Vancomycin or daptomycin
Gonococcal arthritis	Ceftriaxone	
Gram-stain negative (but cell count consistent with septic arthritis)	Vancomycin[a] plus cefepime or ceftazidime	Daptomycin[a] plus piperacillin–tazobactam or fluoroquinolone or carbapenem

[a]For patients who are allergic or intolerant to vancomycin.
[b]For β-lactam hypersensitivity, vancomycin is the alternative.
[c]Cefepime, ceftazidime, ciprofloxacin, and levofloxacin have antipseudomonal activity.
[d]Vancomycin alone can be used if immunocompetent and in the absence of trauma.

arthroscopy is preferred; however, open arthrotomy is often required for the management of septic arthritis of the hip joint. In the published literature, there are no significant differences in the outcome between arthroscopy and arthrotomy for the initial drainage of the knee, hip, and other joints.

If infection has already destroyed the articular surface and underlying bone, then resection of the infected area is considered as well. In a case of severe hip septic arthritis, this would mean resection of the femoral head (Girdlestone procedure). Alternatively, arthrodesis may be performed, in which surgical fusion of the bones across former synovial space occurs, typically performed after septic arthritis of the knee or ankle. Amputation is indicated only in overwhelming and life-threatening infections or persistent local infection with significant bone loss, where the functional benefit after amputation is superior to limb salvage.

Along with joint drainage, concomitant antimicrobial therapy is must (Table 13.1). In general, parenteral therapy or use of highly bioavailable therapy is preferred over the use of other oral agents. Whether or not Gram stain reveals Gram-positive cocci, given increasing prevalence of health care–associated MRSA and community acquired (CA)–MRSA, vancomycin should be included in the initial empirical therapy. If the Gram stain is noted for Gram-negative rods (or if Gram-negative organisms are suspected), then patients should also be started on an antipseudomonal cephalosporin. If specific epidemiologic or clinical factors raise concern for β-lactamase–producing pathogens, then a carbapenem antibiotic is indicated. If methicillin-susceptible S. aureus is identified, vancomycin can be de-escalated to an antistaphylococcal penicillin such as nafcillin or a first-generation cephalosporin such as cefazolin. Alternatives to vancomycin for MRSA septic arthritis include daptomycin, ceftaroline, and linezolid. These alternatives are used when a patient has an allergy or is intolerant to vancomycin. If vancomycin-resistant Enterococcus is recovered in cultures, then daptomycin or linezolid may be used. Adverse effects of daptomycin include muscular toxicity, evident by elevated creatine kinase or, rarely, eosinophilic pneumonia. Linezolid inhibits ribosomal proteins and can be given intravenously or orally at equivalent doses. Adverse effects of linezolid include peripheral or optic neuropathy, anemia, thrombocytopenia, and lactic acidosis. Other drugs with Gram-positive activity include tigecycline, ceftaroline, trimethoprim/sulfamethoxazole, and doxycycline or minocycline. In cases of septic arthritis due to human or animal bites, ampicillin–sulbactam or amoxicillin–clavulanate are preferred due to their activity against oral anaerobes. In cases of gonococcal arthritis, ceftriaxone 1 g IV daily is preferred. Fluoroquinolones are also used due to their Gram-negative spectrum. In all situations, definitive therapy should be chosen based on the antimicrobial susceptibility testing, with input based on cost and adverse effects, individualized to the patient.

There is a lack of consensus with regard to the optimal duration of therapy for septic arthritis. Generally, 2 weeks IV therapy for streptococci, 3 to 4 weeks IV therapy for staphylococci and Gram-negative bacteria, and greater than 4 weeks may be needed for immunocompromised patients and other host comorbidities such as extent of joint damage. For gonococcal arthritis, 7 to 14 days of therapy with ceftriaxone is the standard.

FUNGAL ARTHRITIS

Generally, fungal arthritis affects immunocompromised patients, such as patients with RA or inflammatory bowel disease who are on high-dose corticosteroids or TNF-alpha inhibitor therapy. Common pathogens include *Candida* spp., *Cryptococcus* spp., *Aspergillus* spp., and other molds. Except for *Candida* species, most of these fungal pathogens have primary pulmonary infection with secondary hematogenous seeding of a joint in the setting of augmentation of immunosuppression. Occasionally, healthy hosts can develop fungal arthritis; this is typically seen in endemic mycoses and include *Blastomyces dermatitidis*, *Histoplasma capsulatum*, *Coccidioides* spp., and *Sporothrix* spp.

Candidal Arthritis

Risk factors for candidal arthritis include diabetes, malignancy, hemodialysis, IV drug abuse, and immunosuppressive medications, as well as prolonged use of broad-spectrum antibiotics. Infection is mostly acquired hematogenously. *Candida albicans* is the most common species, and the knee joint is most commonly affected. Synovial fluid analysis reveals low glucose and polymorphonuclear leukocytes, typically in excess of 50,000 cells/mm^3.

Cryptococcal Arthritis

The causative organism is *Cryptococcus neoformans*, with arthritis typically seen concomitantly with cryptococcal osteomyelitis. The knee joint is commonly affected, and immunosuppression is the main risk factor. In addition to synovial fluid fungal cultures needed for diagnosis, serum cryptococcal antigen must be sent.

Coccidioidal Arthritis

This is typically seen in the southwestern regions of the United States. Causative fungi are *Coccidioides immitis* and *Coccidioides posadasii*. Infection generally is introduced via inhalation, followed by pneumonitis and polyarticular arthritis seen in one-third of the patients. Disseminated coccidioidomycosis is seen in ≈1%. Patients typically present with chronic granulomatous infection of bones and joints. The knee joint is the most commonly affected, and many times, infection is indolent in its course. Synovial fluid has a lymphocytic predominance, and spherules can be seen as well. Serologic testing includes serum coccidioides antibody testing and is confirmed on fungal culture of synovial fluid.

Blastomycosis

This primary infection due to *B. dermatitidis* usually involves the pulmonary tract and can disseminate, with joint involvement seen in patients with subjacent osteomyelitis. Occasionally, draining sinus tracts are seen as well. Diagnosis is made by cytologic examination of synovial fluid and confirmed upon performing synovial fluid fungal cultures.

Other Fungi

Fungal arthritis due to *Histoplasma capsulatum* is rare, but should be considered in patients from endemic areas with chronic joint infection. Arthritis due to *Sporothrix* is generally seen in the setting of traumatic injury with a foreign body contaminated with soil. Diabetes and immunosuppression are risk factors, and diagnosis is often challenging due to synovial fluid cultures being frequently negative. Other fungal species that cause arthritis include *Aspergillus*, *Fusarium* spp., and *Scedosporium* spp., organisms that are typically seen in immunocompromised hosts.

Treatment of Fungal Arthritis

The surgical approach varies from case to case. Patients may need open versus arthroscopic debridement. Treatment of *Candida* arthritis should be based upon antifungal susceptibility testing. An echinocandin is appropriate treatment, pending susceptibility testing, but oral triazole therapy is appropriate once susceptibilities return. For the endemic mycoses (*Coccidioides, Histoplasma, Sporothrix, Blastomyces* spp.), treatment is with itraconazole 200 mg twice daily for up to a year. Finally, for *Aspergillus* species, voriconazole is generally preferred.

VIRAL ARTHRITIS

Viral arthritis tends to be acute in presentation and accompanied by a systemic febrile illness.

Parvovirus

This is the most common form of viral arthritis. It presents with a classic facial rash in children, whereas in adults, it presents with a febrile illness accompanied by polyarthralgia. It is more common in females; patients can have involvement of knees, wrists, ankles, and metacarpophalangeal and interphalangeal joints. In addition to clinical examination, diagnosis is made by positive serology and peripheral blood PCR. Treatment is with nonsteroidal antiinflammatory drugs (NSAIDs), and rarely, IV immunoglobulin is used.

Rubella

Arthritis due to rubella virus can result after natural infection or after immunization with live-attenuated vaccine. It affects small joints of the hands, followed by knees, wrists, and ankles. Treatment is generally supportive and NSAIDs.

Hepatitis B and C

Both infections have been associated with an inflammatory arthritis syndrome, better described with hepatitis B. This tends to mimic RA, with a predilection for the small joints of the hand and feet. Management requires treating underlying hepatitis B and C infections along with providing supportive care.

MYCOBACTERIAL ARTHRITIS

Tuberculous Arthritis. *M. tuberculosis* spreads to the bones and joints hematogenously, typically from a pulmonary focus. It presents as an oligoarticular arthritis, typically affecting weight-bearing joints such as the hip, knee, and ankle but can involve any joint. Joints are generally involved from adjacent tuberculous osteomyelitis. Pathogenesis involves local inflammation that evolves into formation of granulation tissue followed by destruction of cartilage, demineralization, and bone necrosis.

In advanced stages, periarticular cold abscesses and fistulas may be seen. Although *M. tuberculosis* is endemic throughout countries in the developing world, in nonendemic areas, the high-risk population includes homeless people from inner cities, immigrants, persons with a substance abuse disorder, and malnourished individuals. Diagnosis of tuberculous arthritis involves, first of all, a high index of suspicion. Radiologic findings typically reveal "Phemister triad," characterized by juxtaarticular osteoporosis, gradual narrowing of joint space, and peripherally located osseous erosions.

Synovial tissue biopsy has a yield of 90% via arthroscopic biopsy, whereas culture has a yield of 80%. *M. tuberculosis* grows slowly, so newer techniques involving PCR-based tests that use amplification of parts of the bacterial genome have shown promise. Treatment of tuberculous arthritis is similar to treatment of pulmonary tuberculosis and includes combination antituberculous therapy and, depending on the clinical situation, surgical debridement. Antituberculous therapy involves two phases, with an intensive bactericidal phase in which four medications are typically used, followed by 4 to 8 months of a continuation phase, typically with two medications. The first-line medications include isoniazid, streptomycin, rifampin, pyrazinamide, and ethambutol.

Nontuberculous Mycobacterial Arthritis. These infections are uncommon. Most patients have preexisting joint disease and predisposing factors, with HIV infection/AIDS historically being the most common. Infection with many of the more than 120 species of Mycobacteria has been reported. As with tuberculous septic arthritis, management includes combination antimycobacterial therapy, often in conjunction with surgical debridement.

Osteomyelitis

Osteomyelitis, infection of bone, can develop hematogenously or as a result of contiguous spread from adjacent soft tissues in the setting of vascular insufficiency or neuropathy. It can also result after trauma or surgery.

CLASSIFICATION

The Lew and Waldvogel classification system takes into account duration of infection, route of infection (hematogenous vs. contiguous), and presence of vascular insufficiency. Acute osteomyelitis develops over days to weeks. Subacute osteomyelitis can be caused by *Brucella* species or *M. tuberculosis* or low-virulence organisms such as *Cutibacterium acnes* in the presence of an implant. Chronic osteomyelitis is a smoldering form of osteomyelitis characterized by dead bone and can persist for years.

Finally, as further outlined in this chapter, osteomyelitis can also be classified by location. It can involve the vertebral column (axial skeleton) or the appendicular skeleton (including long bones). In adults, the vertebral column is the most common site for hematogenous osteomyelitis, whereas the appendicular skeleton is the most common site for contiguous osteomyelitis.

VERTEBRAL OSTEOMYELITIS

Infection of the vertebral endplate and the adjacent vertebral body is often referred to as *spondylodiscitis*. An associated disk space infection is often also present, and an epidural or psoas abscess may or may not be present as well. The intervertebral disk is cartilaginous in origin and lacks blood supply of its own. Microorganisms arrive via arterial blood supply, invade the adjacent endplates, and then may go on to infect the disk cartilage. Hematogenous seeding can result from primary infection of skin and soft tissues, urogenital infections, infective endocarditis in IV drug users, and in patients with respiratory tract infections. Infection can also result iatrogenically, after spine surgery, via epidural injections, or spinal trauma.

Microbiology

Acute vertebral osteomyelitis is typically caused by *S. aureus* and coagulase-negative staphylococci, *Streptococcus* spp., and aerobic Gram-negative rods such as *Escherichia coli* and *P. aeruginosa*.

Candida species can also cause osteomyelitis, which is often diagnosed late; typically patients are IV drug users or immunosuppressed patients. Subacute and chronic vertebral osteomyelitis are caused by *M. tuberculosis* and *Brucella* species and are seen in regions endemic for those organisms or among patients with suggestive exposure history. Osteomyelitis due to viridans group streptococci has a subacute presentation as well and occurs in the setting of endocarditis. Spinal hardware–associated osteomyelitis can be caused by *S. aureus* (which typically occurs within 30 days of surgery) or can also be caused by coagulase-negative staphylococci or *C. acnes*.

Clinical Presentation

Patients present with localized back pain and tenderness. Fever is seen in only half of the patients. The lumbar spine is the most frequently affected anatomic region, followed by the thoracic spine and then cervical spine. Typically, two contiguous vertebrae and the interposed disk are affected. In a minority of patients, motor and sensory deficits can be seen as well. These deficits may be a result of abscess formation leading to cord compression, cauda equina syndrome, or nerve root compression or compression of the femoral nerve due to psoas abscess. Of note, psoas abscesses are common in patients with tuberculous vertebral osteomyelitis.

Blood Chemistry

WBC counts are elevated in less than 50% of the patients. Normochromic anemia has been reported in three-quarters of the patients. ESR elevation is seen in more than 90% of the cases. CRP can be elevated as well. The levels of CRP may be higher in patients with pyogenic infection, rather than those with *Brucella* or tuberculous spinal. CRP is useful to monitor the response to therapy, as it is more closely related. CRP appears to decrease more rapidly after initiation of ultimately successful treatment for acute vertebral osteomyelitis compared with the rate of decline for ESR.

Microbiologic Diagnosis

When a diagnosis of acute vertebral osteomyelitis is entertained, blood cultures should be obtained before antibiotics are initiated. At least two sets of blood cultures should be done. If blood cultures are negative and radiographic appearance is consistent with osteomyelitis, then CT-guided biopsy and aspiration, which has a sensitivity of 38% to 60%, is the next diagnostic step. Bone and disk space contents should be sent for Gram stain, aerobic and anaerobic bacterial cultures, fungal cultures, and histopathology. A second image-guided biopsy increases the diagnostic yield and can be performed if the first biopsy is negative. Alternatively, depending on the clinical scenario, empiric antibiotic therapy may be initiated in the case of a negative biopsy. Among patients with negative CT-guided biopsy or in those not responding to empiric antibiotics, an open surgical biopsy may be pursued in coordination with a spine surgeon.

Broad-range PCR of the aspirated contents is considered in scenarios when the blood cultures and disk biopsy cultures are negative.

Radiology

Imaging is important not only in localizing the site of infection but also to identify other alternative diagnoses such as metastasis to the bone and osteoporotic fractures. Pyogenic complications such as epidural and psoas abscess can be visualized as well. It is reasonable to start with a plain film; however, MRI is the test of choice. It holds greater than 90% accuracy in diagnosing vertebral osteomyelitis. Normally, on the T2-weighted imaging sequences, high signal intensity is seen. When MRI cannot be done or is inconclusive, CT scan or Ga-67 citrate scanning are the alternative modalities. Positron emission tomography (PET) is a highly accurate modality that can be used in cases of patients with multifocal infection and those with spinal implants, but is limited by cost and availability.

TABLE 13.2 ■ Antibiotic Therapy for Chronic Osteomyelitis, Including Vertebral Osteomyelitis

Microorganism	Antibiotic – First Choice	Antibiotic – Alternative Choice
Staphylococcus species		
Oxacillin susceptible	Nafcillin or oxacillin or cefazolin for 6 wk	Vancomycin for 6 wk; some add rifampin PO
Oxacillin-resistant (MRSA)	Vancomycin or daptomycin for 6 wk	Linezolid PO, or levofloxacin PO/ IV daily, plus rifampin PO for 6 wk if susceptible to both
Penicillin-sensitive streptococci	Penicillin G or ceftriaxone for 6 wk	Vancomycin for 6 wk
Enterococci or streptococci with penicillin MIC ≥0.5 ug/mL or *Abiotrophia* or *Granulicatella* spp.	Aqueous crystalline penicillin G or ampicillin sodium IV for 6 wk; the addition of gentamicin sulfate for 1–2 wk is optional	Vancomycin for 6 wk; the addition of gentamicin sulfate for 1–2 wk is optional
Enterobacteriaceae	Ceftriaxone or ertapenem for 6 wk	Ciprofloxacin or levofloxacin PO for 6 wk
Pseudomonas aeruginosa	Cefepime or meropenem or imipenem for 6 wk	Ciprofloxacin or ceftazidime for 6 wk

IV, Intravenous; *MIC,* minimum inhibitory concentration; *MRSA,* methicillin-resistant *S. aureus*; *PO,* oral.

Treatment

The goals of treatment include infection eradication, to provide relief from back pain, and to prevent complications. In general, an initial 6-week course of parenteral or highly bioavailable antibiotic therapy is the standard of care. In a recently published randomized controlled trial, a 6-week course of therapy was not inferior to a 12-week course, with a cure rate above 90% in both groups. IV therapy is generally extended if there are undrained paravertebral abscesses or in patients with spinal hardware. Surgery is generally not needed, except in patients with large abscesses, patients with spinal implants, and those with spinal instability and/or progressive neurologic deficits.

Response to antimicrobial therapy should be monitored with periodic CRP values. Among patients with improvement in pain and inflammatory markers, a follow-up MRI is not recommended, as it may lead to a false impression of disease progression. However, among patients who have worsening pain, new neurologic deficits, and/or persistently elevated inflammatory markers, MRI is the appropriate radiographic study. Given the delay in response to therapy of the bony changes on MRI, focus should be on the soft tissue component of the infection.

In cases of hardware associated vertebral osteomyelitis, surgical debridement is almost always required. Infections occurring within a month of surgery are treated with debridement, retention, and a 6-week course of parenteral antibiotic therapy followed by oral suppressive therapy until the spine fuses. This may take up to 2 years. For late postsurgical hardware–associated vertebral osteomyelitis, explantation of hardware and a 6-week course of antibiotics are recommended (Table 13.2).

OSTEOMYELITIS OF THE APPENDICULAR SKELETON

Osteomyelitis of the appendicular skeleton (which includes the long bones of the limbs) can develop secondary to contiguous infection of the adjacent tissues, hematogenous seeding, or as a consequence of fracture of the long bone with subsequent contamination. Long bones can also be infected perioperatively during orthopedic repair surgeries.

After an open, contaminated fracture, the risk of developing osteomyelitis is 3% to 25%, depending on the extent of musculoskeletal damage and contamination. These are generally young men, and lower extremity bones are typically involved such as the tibia and fibula. Complications, if left untreated, include persistent nonunion of the fracture site and chronic osteomyelitis with dead bone that could potentially require amputation.

Microbiology

S. aureus is the most commonly implicated pathogen. Aerobic Gram-negative bacteria such as *P. aeruginosa* are also commonly encountered. Depending on the geographics and endemicity, fungi such as *B. dermatitidis*, *Cryptococcus* species, *Coccidioides* species, or *Sporothrix schenckii* can also be involved (after exposure to soil in contaminated fractures or hematogenous seeding). Nontuberculous Mycobacteria can also be implicated. Among patients with implant-associated osteomyelitis, coagulase-negative staphylococcal species are frequently encountered.

Clinical Presentation

Similar to vertebral osteomyelitis, patients may present with pain and low-grade fever. Local swelling and erythema overlying the involved bone can be seen as well. A draining sinus tract over the infected bone is highly suggestive of chronic osteomyelitis. Patients who have underlying implants can have secondary seeding of the hardware at any time after device placement, manifesting as new-onset pain. Typically, late-onset infection in the presence of orthopedic hardware is caused by low-virulence pathogens such as *C. acnes* and coagulase-negative staphylococcal species.

Diagnosis

Blood chemistry typically reveals elevated CRP and sedimentation rate. WBC count can be elevated or normal. Just as in vertebral osteomyelitis, a plain film can first be obtained. MRI and CT scan are highly sensitive tests to help delineate the extent of infection and underlying necrotic bone (sequestrum). Three-phase bone scans which include technetium-99m methylene diphosphonate, gallium scan, and indium-labeled white cell scan can be used for the diagnosis, but they lack specificity and can give false-positive results in cases of bone tumors and recent surgery. They are, however, useful in cases of late recurrence of osteomyelitis.

Microbiologic diagnosis is critically important to help guide antimicrobial therapy. Image-guided bone biopsy or an open biopsy may be pursued and sent for cultures and histopathology. In patients with draining sinus tracts, a swab obtained from the sinus tract is neither sensitive nor specific for identifying the causative pathogen. However, the identification of *S. aureus* correlates with deep cultures and may provide useful information.

Treatment

A combination of medical and surgical intervention is needed to address osteomyelitis of the appendicular skeleton. In cases that are acquired hematogenously, antimicrobial treatment is similar to that of vertebral osteomyelitis, as outlined in Table 13.1. After surgical debridement and collection of cultures, antibiotics should be started, except if a patient is suffering from sepsis, in whom treatment of sepsis should be done immediately and before diagnostic and surgical procedures are performed. Duration of therapy is typically 4 to 6 weeks.

In a patient who suffers an open contaminated fracture, management requires early wound irrigation and debridement, stabilization of the fracture and soft tissue coverage of the exposed bone, and prompt initiation of empiric antimicrobial prophylaxis to prevent development of osteomyelitis. Osteomyelitis typically presents late (months) after open fracture with signs of poor wound healing and pain at the site of fracture, with radiographic evidence of nonunion. Management includes irrigation and debridement and deliberate management of the implant. Depending on the stability of the implant, it may be kept or removed. If retained, patients require antibiotic suppression orally until the fracture heals. In staphylococcal implant-associated infection, a combination of fluoroquinolone and rifampin has been shown to cure infection in a 3- to 6-month course, such that the device can be retained. If infection recurs after discontinuation of suppressive antibiotic therapy, then hardware should be removed and another course of antimicrobial therapy is warranted.

OSTEOMYELITIS IN DIABETICS AND PATIENTS WITH VASCULAR DISEASE

Of all patients who suffer from diabetes mellitus, it is projected that 15% to 25% develop foot ulcers during their lifetime. Poor glycemic control, peripheral neuropathy, and vascular insufficiency all contribute to the formation of a diabetic foot ulcer, which may lead to the development of contiguous osteomyelitis. Emphasis should be placed on prevention of formation of these ulcers. Patients with diabetes must have a regular complete foot examination, including assessment of pedal pulses. An additional noninvasive vascular modality being utilized at our institution is the measurement of transcutaneous oxygen pressures that may provide further information about the microvascular status of the foot, in addition to the information provided by duplex ultrasound. Efforts should be made to help patients quit smoking.

With regard to diagnosis of osteomyelitis, a chronic ulcer measuring more than 2 cm^2 or a positive probe-to-bone test has a high positive predictive value. The probe-to-bone test, in which a sterile metal probe is used to attempt to contact underlying exposed bone, is also highly specific for diagnosing contiguous osteomyelitis. MRI of the foot is the standard of care to confirm the diagnosis. Microbiology of diabetic wounds reveals that they are generally polymicrobial. However, there is a poor correlation between cultures obtained from superficial wound swabs and bone biopsy cultures, except when S. aureus is isolated. Thus deep surgical cultures should ideally be obtained via techniques such as transcutaneous bone biopsy or open debridement. Common pathogens include S. aureus, Gram-negative rods, and anaerobes.

Ideally, antimicrobial therapy should be based on deep tissue cultures and should be withheld until cultures are obtained. If bone biopsy cannot be performed, then the antimicrobial regimen should be constructed based on the likely organisms that could be present. Patients who have poor blood flow to the feet should undergo revascularization, if appropriate. Orthopedic surgeons or podiatrists are consulted to help with debridement of the wound.

Antimicrobial therapy is generally broad-spectrum, as these wounds are typically infected with several organisms. However, underlying risk factors for specific organisms should also be given consideration. Vancomycin should be chosen when patients are considered at risk for MRSA. For patients with risk factors for P. aeruginosa, such as in warm climates or moist environments, cefepime or piperacillin–tazobactam is used. Empiric therapy with a β-lactam antibiotic combined with metronidazole is an appropriate choice. Combination of metronidazole or clindamycin with a fluoroquinolone may also be considered in select cases, as these are highly bioavailable. After surgical debridement, treatment duration depends on whether there is residual osteomyelitis or not. If debridement was not definitive and infected bone remains, patients should be treated with a 4 to 6 weeks of antimicrobial therapy. In cases where surgical debridement is not done, a prolonged course of antimicrobials of 3 months or longer can be curative. If the infected bone is removed in its entirety through amputation, antibiotics can be discontinued, provided soft tissue infection, if present, has been sufficiently treated.

Periprosthetic Joint Infections

Joint arthroplasties or prosthetic joints are used to replace joints that have been damaged due to underlying inflammatory arthritis, degenerative arthritis, or as a result of trauma. As the population continues to age, the number of patients with joint arthroplasties continues to increase. Periprosthetic joint infection (PJI) is one of the most devastating complications after joint arthroplasty, with the rate of PJI between 0.5% and 2.0%, depending on location of the joint.

DEFINITION

A clinical suspicion of PJI is essential to diagnosis. The presence of a sinus tract or persistent wound drainage over a joint prosthesis, acute onset of painful prosthesis, or chronically painful prosthesis any time after joint implantation should prompt consideration of a PJI. Acute inflammation consistent with infection on histopathologic examination of periprosthetic tissue supports the diagnosis of PJI. Other criteria include elevated leukocyte count and/or predominance of neutrophils in the synovial fluid. The growth of an identical microorganism in at least two intraoperative cultures or a combination of preoperative aspiration and intraoperative cultures in case of a low-virulence pathogen (*C. acnes* and coagulase-negative *Staphylococcus* species) supports a diagnosis of PJI. A single culture with a pathogen unlikely to be a contaminant, such as *S. aureus*, is highly suggestive of PJI. ESR and CRP levels individually lack sensitivity and specificity, so these should be used in combination with other diagnostic criteria.

CLASSIFICATION

Generally, based on the route of acquisition, PJIs can be hematogenously or exogenously acquired. They are also classified as being early (<3 months after surgery), delayed (3 to 12 months), and late infections (>1 year after surgery).

Hematogenously acquired infection is typically caused by virulent bacteria, most often *S. aureus*, and may occur during any period. Exogenously acquired infections in the setting of poor wound healing may be caused by any organism. Symptoms of exogenous infection typically first become apparent during the early or delayed time period. The route of acquisition and the temporal classification have implications for medical/surgical management.

PATHOGENESIS

Formation of biofilm is key to the process of pathogenesis. Bacteria and fungi within biofilms are difficult to treat with antibiotics and the innate immune system. Bacteria in biofilms are 1000-fold resistant to antibiotics and become protected from phagocytosis. Additionally, granulocyte function has been reported to get impaired at the surface of implants (nonphagocytable surface). In experimental mice models, it has also been noted that this leads to granulocyte degranulation and release of collagenase, which would then lead to joint loosening.

RISK FACTORS

These can be classified into three categories: host-specific factors, intraoperative factors, and postoperative risk factors.

Host-Related Factors

Patient-related comorbid conditions include poorly controlled diabetes mellitus, obesity with body mass index (BMI) >30 kg/m^2, underlying immunosuppressive diseases such as RA, and the use of disease-modifying antirheumatic drugs. Preoperative anemia, hypoalbuminemia, peripheral vascular disease, smoking, and congestive heart failure are additional comorbid conditions. History of previous joint infection or previous PJI at the involved site is considered a risk factor too.

Operating Room–Related Factors

Length of an operation and duration of tourniquet time are important associated risk factors. American Society of Anesthesiologists (ASA) score greater than 2, reflecting a cumulative level of systemic disease, is also considered a risk for PJI. Need for blood transfusions and intraoperative blood loss and suboptimal administration of perioperative antimicrobial prophylaxis is an additional risk factor. Traffic in the operating room is associated with increased bacterial air counts and may lead to increased risk of surgical site infection.

Postoperative Factors

These include formation of hematoma, wound dehiscence, poor wound healing and drainage, and stitch abscess formation. Postoperative bacteremia and subsequent hematogenous seeding of the prosthesis arising from an oral, urologic, skin, or gastrointestinal focus is an additional risk factor. Thus identification of a distant infection and prompt treatment are necessary. Of note, the rate of PJI after *S. aureus* bacteremia is approximately 35%. Prolonged hospital stay is recognized as another associated risk factor (Fig. 13.1).

MICROBIOLOGY

Of all the microorganisms, *S. aureus* is the most frequently isolated. The common microorganisms in order of frequency of occurrence (in the context of total hip arthroplasty [THA] and total knee arthroplasty PJIs) are as follows:

- *S. aureus*
- Coagulase-negative staphylococci
- *Streptococcus* species
- *Enterococcus* species
- *C. acnes*
- Aerobic Gram-negative rods
- Miscellaneous (including *Candida* spp.)
- Polymicrobial
- Culture-negative

CLINICAL PRESENTATION

Pain is the most common symptom. Presentation generally differs if infection is acquired exogenously versus hematogenously. Exogenously acquired infections are seen early in the postsurgical period and generally present with signs of local wound breakdown, redness, and drainage. If infection is caused by a low-virulence pathogen, patients generally have a more smoldering presentation with joint effusions and occasional formation of sinus tract and joint loosening. Pain that is acute in onset often occurs in the context of hematogenously acquired infection. In the majority of cases, patients will be systemically ill if they develop a bloodstream infection.

DIAGNOSTIC INVESTIGATIONS

CRP and sedimentation rates are sensitive tests, but lack specificity. Occasionally, in the context of infection due to a low-virulence pathogen, CRP and ESR levels may be normal. Peripheral WBC count does not have a correlation with PJI. Procalcitonin also has a low sensitivity in localized PJI (with absence of sepsis syndrome).

Microbiology, Histology, and Molecular Techniques for Diagnosis

As a rule, the cutoff number for leukocyte counts is much lower for the diagnosis of PJI than for native septic arthritis. For hip PJIs, the thresholds are 4200 WBCs per microliter or greater

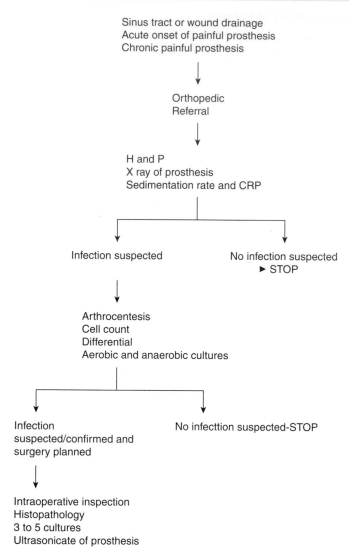

Fig. 13.1 Algorithm for the diagnosis of prosthetic joint infection (PJI). (Adapted from Infectious Diseases Society of America. IDSA Guidelines 2012.)

than 80% polymorphonuclear cells, or both. For knee PJIs, a lower cutoff of 1700 WBCs/uL or greater than 65% neutrophils, or both seems to be ideal. Culture of synovial fluid is more than 85% sensitive and specific for PJI. Synovial fluid specimens can be obtained via aspiration before surgery or intraoperatively as well. Superficial sinus tract cultures may be performed, but can often be misleading, except in cases of *S. aureus.* Intraoperatively, synovial membrane should be sent for histopathology. Acute inflammation, defined as a high-power field with at least five neutrophils, strongly suggests infection. Frozen intraoperative specimens correlate well with infection and allow for rapid diagnosis of infection. Biopsy is also useful in scenarios where cultures are negative, and histologic results are then used to help guide therapy. Synovial fluid PCR is a novel technique that is currently being studied and may provide more rapid diagnostic information. This test may have a role in culture-negative PJIs or aid in the diagnosis of low-virulent pathogens such as *C. acnes*.

Ultrasonication of explanted prosthetic joints allows for detection of microorganism trapped in biofilms by dislodging them from the joint surface. This increases sensitivity, especially when patients have been treated with antibiotics in the preceding 2 weeks. Other tests that are being studied and hold promise are synovial fluid alpha-defensin level and synovial fluid CRP levels. False-positive results, however, may be seen in the presence of metallosis.

Radiography

Different radiologic modalities are used to aid in the diagnosis of PJI. Joint loosening and radiolucency can be detected on a plain film, but may also be seen in cases of aseptic loosening. Ultrasound is utilized to help guide aspiration of the joint space. CT scan and MRI help in the detection of the extent of hardware-associated osteomyelitis and for the detection of abscesses and sinus tracts. Radionuclide imaging techniques such as three-phase bone scans using technetium-99m–labeled methylene diphosphonate (^{99m}Tc-MDP), detect infection even before anatomic changes develop. However, false-positive results may be seen in cases of heterotopic (abnormal) ossification and aseptic loosening. ^{18}F-fluorodeoxyglucose (FDG) PET is yet another technique that has the potential of being utilized in diagnostically challenging cases.

TREATMENT

Treatment of PJI entails a multidisciplinary approach, including collaboration with orthopedic surgeons, infectious diseases specialists, and occasionally, plastic surgeons, among others. Surgical management is generally recommended in all situations. Nonsurgical management should only be considered in patients who are unable or unwilling to undergo even a single surgical procedure. Goals of treatment should include control or cure of the infection, preservation or restoration of joint function, and minimization of adverse effects related to treatment.

Central to successful treatment is having a high index of suspicion in diagnosing PJI. Antibiotics should be withheld until microbiologic specimens have been obtained, except in scenarios when patients are septic or hemodynamically unstable.

SURGICAL MODALITIES

Following are the common surgical approaches:
1. Debridement and implant retention (DAIR): This is for patients who have an acute infection, with symptom duration <3 weeks or infection within 4 weeks after implantation, provided that the implant is stable, there is no sinus tract, and the pathogen is susceptible to available oral antimicrobial therapy. Typically, the polyethylene liner is exchanged.
   After DAIR, patients receive a prolonged course of pathogen-directed IV therapy for up to 6 weeks. It is important to note that for PJI due to *S. aureus*, rifampin is used in addition to parenteral therapy (during the initial 6 weeks), followed by transition to an oral antistaphylococcal agent along with rifampin to complete a total of 3 to 6 months of therapy. The antistaphylococcal oral agents routinely used in combination with rifampin include levofloxacin, trimethoprim–sulfamethoxazole, doxycycline, and minocycline as well as first-generation cephalosporins. In circumstances where patients are not able to tolerate rifampin or have issues with drug–drug interactions, they may require indefinite long-term oral suppression with an antistaphylococcal agent. A lack of a rifampin-based regimen has been reported to be a risk factor associated with treatment failure. For all other nonstaphylococcal pathogens, duration of therapy with parenteral antibiotics or highly bioavailable oral therapy after DAIR is generally 4 to 6 weeks, followed by suppressive oral antimicrobial therapy.

Patients who do not meet the criteria for debridement and retention would then be considered for resection arthroplasty with one- or two-stage exchange.

2. One-stage exchange (OSE): OSE involves removal of all the hardware, including any wires or cement; thorough irrigation; and debridement followed by implantation of a new artificial joint, all in the same operation. This technique is not commonly performed in the United States, and typically THA infections are treated via this approach. After OSE, patients are typically treated for a duration of 4 to 6 weeks of IV antibiotics, followed by 3 to 12 months of oral antimicrobial therapy. For staphylococcal infection, rifampin-based therapy is utilized similar to DAIR (as described earlier).

3. Two-stage exchange (TSE): This is the more commonly employed approach in the United States and has been reported to have a success rate of close to 85%. The first stage involves removal of the infected prosthesis along with thorough debridement of soft tissues as well as bony debridement. Microbiologic specimens are collected, and the joint space is maintained with an antibiotic-impregnated cement spacer. The spacer can be static or articulating. This is then followed by 4 to 6 weeks of IV antimicrobial therapy based on the culture data. Antibiotic-laden cement releases antibiotics locally via diffusion. Spacers are typically impregnated with vancomycin and an aminoglycoside. After completion of parenteral antibiotics, patients are then clinically observed off of antibiotics for at least 2 weeks. Inflammatory markers such as CRP and ESR are also used to help in decision-making. Persistently elevated inflammatory markers may suggest ongoing infection, and synovial fluid cell count and cultures may be obtained to help guide decision-making. These patients may need further debridement and exchange of the spacer. For those patients for whom infection is thought to have been eradicated, the second stage involves intraoperative inspection of the joint space, collection of frozen sections, and culture collection, and if there are no intraoperative signs of infection, patients then have implantation of a new joint prosthesis. Patients who have positive cultures at the time of reimplantation will need another course of antimicrobial therapy followed potentially by long-term oral suppressive therapy.

4. Resection arthroplasty with no implantation: This treatment approach may be chosen in cases of PJIs where a TSE is not possible due to poor bone stock, patients have a baseline and anticipated functional status that would not be improved by a new prosthesis, or with infections with multidrug-resistant organisms. These patients undergo complete resection of the joint prosthesis without placement of a spacer. In cases of hip resection arthroplasty (also called the *Girdlestone procedure*), a vastus lateralis muscle transfer may be used to fill this dead space. Patients are typically treated for 4 to 6 weeks of parenteral antimicrobials after resection arthroplasty. Definitive resection of a knee arthroplasty may be followed by an arthrodesis or fusion procedure, either utilizing an external fixator or intramedullary rod.

5. Amputation: Amputation is the last resort after patients have failed past attempts at controlling infection, including prior TSE procedures and/or failed attempt at resection arthroplasty. After amputation, if there is residual osteomyelitis depending on the level of lower limb amputation, patients may need an additional 4 to 6 weeks of pathogen-directed antibiotic therapy.

PROPHYLACTIC ANTIBIOTICS BEFORE DENTAL PROCEDURES AND RISK OF PJI

Typically, oral antibiotics are not indicated before dental procedures in patients with prosthetic joints, and there is lack of evidence to support it. The decision to administer oral antibiotics before a dental procedure in such patients should be made on a case-by-case basis. Patient undergoing extensive oral surgery and reconstruction and those with several comorbidities would be considered high risk. The decision to give antibiotics to high-risk patients should be made after a discussion with the oral and orthopedic surgeon.

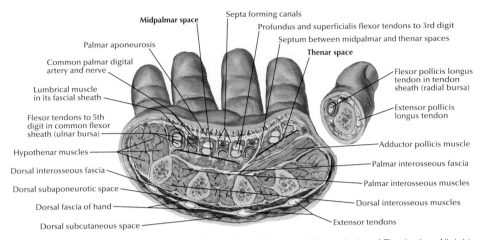

Septa forming canals
Midpalmar space
Profundus and superficialis flexor tendons to 3rd digit
Septum between midpalmar and thenar spaces
Palmar aponeurosis
Thenar space
Common palmar digital artery and nerve
Lumbrical muscle in its fascial sheath
Flexor pollicis longus tendon in tendon sheath (radial bursa)
Extensor pollicis longus tendon
Flexor tendons to 5th digit in common flexor sheath (ulnar bursa)
Hypothenar muscles
Adductor pollicis muscle
Dorsal interosseous fascia
Palmar interosseous fascia
Dorsal subaponeurotic space
Palmar interosseous muscles
Dorsal fascia of hand
Dorsal interosseous muscles
Dorsal subcutaneous space
Extensor tendons

Fig. 13.2   Regional hand and wrist anatomy. (Netter illustration used with permission of Elsevier, Inc. All rights reserved. www.netterimages.com.)

Infectious (Suppurative) Tenosynovitis

INTRODUCTION

Tenosynovitis is inflammation of the tendon and the associated synovial sheath. Infection of the tendons and synovial sheaths commonly involves the hand and/or the wrist. It is therefore important to have an understanding of the regional hand and wrist anatomy (Fig. 13.2). Both the extensor and flexor tendon sheaths are lined with an inner visceral and outer parietal layer with a potential space between the two layers. During infectious tenosynovitis, this space fills with purulent fluid. The hand has many small anatomic compartments, and infectious tenosynovitis can spread via adjacent anatomic spaces. Occasionally, infection can spread to adjacent soft tissues that can be complicated by compartment syndrome.

MICROBIOLOGY AND MECHANISM

Direct Inoculation due to Trauma

The most common route of acquisition of infection occurs via direct inoculation after trauma. Typical pathogens are Gram-positive cocci, including *S. aureus* and streptococci. Polymicrobial infection may also occur, especially in cases of lacerated wounds or after animal bites. In diabetics, tenosynovitis tends to be polymicrobial, including Gram-negative rods. A similar microbiologic spectrum can also be implicated in immunocompromised patients.

Aquatic exposure, including fish tanks, is the leading cause of *Mycobacterium marinum* tenosynovitis. According to one study, it was found to be the causative agent in 82% of the 241 cases of nontuberculous mycobacterial hand infections worldwide (Table 13.3).

Hematogenous Spread

N. gonorrhoeae can spread to tendons hematogenously; tenosynovitis due to this organism is typically seen in young, sexually active patients as part of the classic triad of tenosynovitis, pustular dermatitis, and polyarthralgia. It can also be seen in DGI. Tuberculous tenosynovitis also occurs via hematogenous spread, although this is uncommon, and has been reported in areas where *M. tuberculosis* is endemic. However, cases of *M. tuberculosis* tenosynovitis have also been reported in nonendemic areas, including the United States. Finally, *H. capsulatum*, *C. posadasii/immitis*, and *C. neoformans* can all cause subacute tenosynovitis. Infection may be a result of either local inoculation or as part of a disseminated infection.

TABLE 13.3 ■ Type of Trauma and Associated Pathogens

Cat and dog bites	• Polymicrobial • *Pasteurella multocida*
Puncture wounds	• After injury due to thorns or plants resulting in fungal tenosynovitis and due to *Sporothrix schenckii*
Intravenous drug use (IVDU)	• β-Hemolytic streptococci, *Staphylococcus aureus, Eikenella corrodens,* and *Anaerobes* spp.
Water-related injuries	• *Mycobacterium marinum* and other nontuberculous *Mycobacteria* • *Aeromonas* spp. via traumatic (especially immunocompromised) and *Vibrio vulnificans* and *parahaemolyticus* species • *Erysipelothrix rhusiopathiae*

CLINICAL PRESENTATION

In cases of flexor tenosynovitis, patients typically present with signs including tenderness along the flexor sheath, fusiform swelling of the involved digit, and pain with passive extension of the finger. Patients may also have fever. For slow-growing organisms such as the nontuberculous *Mycobacteria*, the presentation can be subacute. Extensor tenosynovitis commonly involves the ankle (around the extensor retinaculum) and the wrist. Patients often lack typical findings such as those seen in flexor tenosynovitis and sometimes lead to delay in diagnosis. Of note, extensor tendons lack a retinacular system, and therefore infection tends to be less loculated.

DIAGNOSIS

Diagnosis is based on clinical presentation in an appropriate clinical context. Obtaining a thorough history, including patient hobbies, geography, sexual history, pet/animal exposure, and comorbid conditions (including immune compromise) is of paramount importance.

Physical examination findings are an important component of diagnosis. Patients who have flexor tenosynovitis typically have tenderness along the course of the tendon sheath, spindle-shaped swelling of the digit, and pain along the tendon with passive flexion. On the contrary, extensor tenosynovitis should be kept in the differential diagnosis when patients present with soft tissue swelling/infection involving extensor surfaces of the wrist and ankles that does not improve with antibiotics.

After a thorough clinical examination, further investigational studies include tendon sheath aspiration and biopsy. Specimens should be sent for histopathology as well as microbiology, including bacteria, mycobacterial, and fungal cultures. In patients who have systemic signs of infection such as fever, blood cultures should also be obtained. Radiographic modalities include x-rays (to rule out foreign body), as well as more sophisticated modalities such as CT scan and/or MRI to delineate the extent of infection and whether osteomyelitis is present. Ultrasound may play an important role if the diagnosis is in doubt and may guide aspiration. Osteomyelitis can be seen, typically in chronic cases of tenosynovitis.

TREATMENT

Optimal therapy consists of appropriate antimicrobials with surgical debridement. Generally, surgical debridement in cases of suppurative tenosynovitis is needed to prevent tendon necrosis and rupture. Extensive tenosynovectomy may be required in immunocompromised patients, which can be performed at the time of initial tendon biopsy.

Understanding the circumstances in which trauma took place helps guide antimicrobial therapy against a likely pathogen. Empiric antibiotic therapy should be based on antecedent exposure history. An initial empiric regimen of vancomycin along with a third-generation cephalosporin is recommended in the context of trauma or if the mechanism of injury is not known. In cases of bite wounds (humans or animals), a β-lactam/β-lactamase inhibitor such as ampicillin–sulbactam is often the first choice because of its broader Gram-positive, Gram-negative, and anaerobic coverage. In cases of water-borne injury, an initial regimen comprising vancomycin along with an antipseudomonal agent such as cefepime or ceftazidime is reasonable. Once microbiologic data are available, the antimicrobial spectrum should be adjusted accordingly. The optimal duration of therapy for bacterial tenosynovitis, however, ranges from 2 to 3 weeks. Initial parenteral therapy can be switched at an appropriate time to oral antibiotics, depending on the patient's situation. For gonococcal tenosynovitis (which can typically present in combination with arthralgia and dermatitis, a 7-day course of ceftriaxone (dosing dependent on patient's weight) is generally recommended as per the Centers for Disease Control and Prevention (CDC).

Treatment of mycobacterial tenosynovitis requires a prolonged course of antimicrobial therapy, and surgical debridement may be needed as well. Of note, mycobacterial cultures can take weeks to finalize due to slow-growing *Mycobacteria*. Therefore clinical suspicion with supportive histopathologic examination of resected tissue that shows granulomatous inflammation and/or acid-fast bacilli (seen on mycobacterial stains) should be used to guide therapy. Treatment of mycobacterial tenosynovitis is based on combination antimycobacterial therapy (monotherapy is not advised), and the duration of therapy ranges from 3 months to more than a year, depending on the causative mycobacteria. For *M. marinum*, antibiotics of choice include two among a selection of azithromycin–clarithromycin, ethambutol, and rifampin for 3 to 4 months.

Duration of therapy for fungal tenosynovitis depends on whether it is a manifestation of a disseminated infection or a result of local inoculation. Disseminated infection may need more than a year of antifungal treatment, whereas localized infection may be treated in 3 to 6 months.

Suggested Reading

Berbari EF, Kanj SS, Kowalski TJ. 2015 Infectious Diseases Society of America (IDSA) clinical practice guidelines for the diagnosis and treatment of native vertebral osteomyelitis in adults. *Clin Infect Dis*. 2015;61(6):e26–e46.

Hyatt BT, Bagg MR. Flexor tenosynovitis. *Orthop Clin N Am*. 2017;48:217–227.

Osmon DR, Berbari EF, Berendt AR, et al. Diagnosis and management of prosthetic joint infection: clinical practice guidelines by the infectious diseases society of america. *Clin Infect Dis*. 2013;56:e1–e25.

Ross JJ. Septic arthritis of native joints. *Infect Dis Clin North Am*. 2017;31(2):203–218.

Tande AJ, Gomez-Urena EO, Berbari EF, Osmon DR. Management of prosthetic joint infection. *Infect Dis Clin North Am*. 2017;31(2):237–252.

CHAPTER 14

Diagnostic Approach to a Patient with Suspected Central Nervous System Infection

Adarsh Bhimraj

A diagnostic hypothesis for a suspected central nervous system (CNS) infection has two components: an anatomic and a microbiologic or etiologic diagnosis. The anatomic diagnosis localizes the inflammation to a specific part of the CNS. The microbiologic or etiologic diagnosis identifies the pathogen or etiology that is causing the CNS inflammation. An accurate anatomic and microbiologic hypothesis requires a detailed history (including symptoms, duration, exposure, and epidemiologic risk factors); a complete physical examination, including a thorough neurologic examination; and an appropriate diagnostic workup, including imaging and cerebrospinal fluid (CSF) laboratory tests. Prognosis and management depend on an accurate diagnosis. For instance, if the diagnosis is pneumococcal meningitis, the anatomic site of inflammation is the pia–arachnoid layer of the meninges, and the etiology is *Streptococcus pneumoniae*. The antimicrobial treatment is ceftriaxone, which penetrates the anatomic site (subarachnoid space) and has activity against *S. pneumoniae*.

A practical approach to the patient with suspected CNS infection would be to answer the following questions to make a diagnosis and asses the prognosis:

1. Where is the "-itis" or inflammation (anatomic site)?
2. How long has it been going on (duration of illness)?
3. Is it community acquired or health care acquired?
4. What is the exposure or epidemiologic history?
5. Is the patient a "normal host" or an " immunocompromised host"?
6. Is it an acute severe infection or a chronic stable infection?
7. What is the type of CSF inflammatory response on routine analysis?

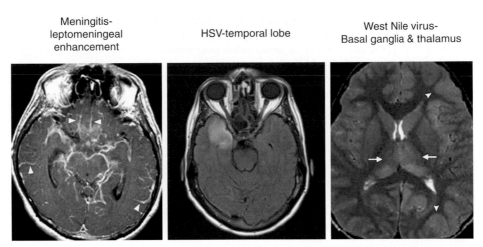

Fig. 14.1 Where is the inflammation (anatomic location in the CNS)? MRI brain imaging.

Question 1: Where Is the Inflammation?

Microorganisms have a tropism to certain anatomic sites both in the CNS and outside. So anatomic localization helps identify the etiology or organism. *S. pneumoniae* and *Neisseria meningitidis* have tropism to the leptomeninges or pia-arachnoid layer. Herpes simplex virus-1 (HSV-1) has tropism to the medial temporal lobe, and West Nile virus has tropism to the basal ganglia. At a cellular level, poliovirus infects the anterior horn cells, and JC virus infects the oligodendrocytes, which produce myelin in the CNS. Anatomic localization can be done based on history, neurologic examination, imaging—especially with magnetic resonance imaging (MRI) of the CNS, and CSF analysis. A patient with meningitis can have headache, meningeal signs, leptomeningeal enhancement on a T1 post-contrast MRI of the brain, and increased white blood cells, with a low glucose on routine CSF analysis. The patient with HSV-1 encephalitis can present with amnesia and temporal lobe changes on brain MRI. Often clues to the diagnosis can be present at anatomic sites outside the CNS. *Nocardia* causes brain abscesses and lung nodules. Sarcoidosis causes basilar leptomeningeal meningitis, but a clue to the diagnosis could be bilateral hilar lymphadenopathy. Classifying the patient into the following anatomic syndromes is diagnostically useful, as that gives clues about the etiology or organism:

- *Meningitis:* Leptomeningeal meningitis is inflammation of the pia–arachnoid layer, and pachymeningitis is inflammation of the dura.
- *Encephalitis or meningo-encephalitis:* This is inflammation within the brain parenchyma with or without meningeal involvement.
- *Myelitis or myelo-radiculitis:* This is inflammation of the spinal cord with or without involvement of the spinal nerve roots.
- *Space-occupying, ring-enhancing lesions* in the brain on post-contrast CNS imaging.
- *Stroke or strokelike syndromes* involving vascular territories of the brain (Fig. 14.1).

Question 2: How Long Has It Been Going On?

Some microorganisms cause acute infections that progress over days, and some cause chronic infections that progress over weeks to months. Subacute infections, which are generally around 2 to 3 weeks in duration, could be either an acute infection that has lingered longer or a chronic infection that was diagnosed earlier. Virulent fast-growing bacteria like *S. pneumoniae* or *N.*

meningitidis cause severe acute meningitis, but indolent slow-growing organisms like fungi and *Mycobacterium tuberculosis* cause chronic meningitis. A patient can also have recurrent acute CNS infections. This could be because of an immunodeficiency making one prone to a CNS infection multiple times. An example would be recurrent meningococcal infection with terminal complement deficiencies. Recurrent acute meningitis could also be from recurrent reactivation of a latent virus like HSV-2, which causes Molleret meningitis or benign recurrent lymphocytic meningitis.

Question 3: Is It Community Acquired or Health Care Acquired?

In the CNS, unlike other anatomic sites, hospital- or health care–acquired infections usually occur in the context of either neurotrauma or neurosurgery. The skull and the meninges are an effective barrier and defense against nosocomial pathogens entering the CNS. Only when the skull and dura are breached by trauma or surgery do hospital-acquired pathogens like *Escherichia coli* and *Staphylococcus aureus* find a portal of entry into the CNS. These organisms, unlike organisms that cause community-acquired bacterial meningitis like *S. pneumoniae* or *N. meningitidis,* lack the capacity to directly invade the CNS. It would be unusual to have a nosocomial pathogen causing CNS infection in a patient on the non-neurosurgical or non–critical care wards.

Question 4: What Is the Exposure or Epidemiologic History?

The following three factors are essential for the pathogenesis of a CNS infection:
1. The organism should be capable of not only infecting a human host but also have tropism to the CNS.
2. The host should be susceptible to an infection by a particular organism. *S. pneumoniae* is a highly virulent organism capable of causing an infection even in a normal host and is also neurotropic. On the contrary, *Listeria monocytogenes* usually causes meningitis in the elderly and hosts with deficient T-cell immunity.
3. A conducive environment and host behavior for transmission (exposure or epidemiology) is necessary in addition to the host and pathogen factors. For instance, a patient should have traveled to a tropical country and been bitten by a female *Anopheles* mosquito to get cerebral malaria. On the contrary, anyone can sporadically get HSV encephalitis.

Obtaining a tailored exposure history is important in establishing the etiology and ordering appropriate diagnostic tests. A few examples are provided here:
- **Travel:** Travel to Arizona puts the patient at risk for chronic meningitis from coccidioidomycosis.
- **Insect bites:** Tick bites are a risk factor for neuroborreliosis and mosquito bites for West Nile virus.
- **Animal bites:** Raccoon bites or bat contact puts one at risk for rabies.
- **"Sick contacts":** Close contact with someone with meningococcal meningitis (in a college dorm or military barrack) increases risk for acquiring it. Health care workers and prison inmates are at a higher risk for chronic meningitis from tuberculosis.
- **Sexual history:** An acute lymphocytic meningitis in a patient with recent unprotected sexual intercourse could be acute retroviral syndrome from HIV or neurosyphilis.

Question 5: Is the Patient Immunocompetent or an Immunocompromised Host?

The susceptibility of a patient to different infections depends on which arm of the immune system is compromised and the net state of immunosuppression. Opportunistic pathogens are organisms that are usually nonpathogenic in a normal host but are pathogenic in an immunocompromised host. Hematopoietic stem cell transplant patients are at a higher risk for opportunistic infections pre-engraftment and subsequently if they need to be treated with immunosuppressive medications for graft-versus-host disease. Solid-organ transplant patients are at highest risk immediately after transplantation and subsequently if they need to be treated for transplanted organ rejection. Patients with HIV and patients with hematologic and rheumatologic conditions requiring treatment with biologics and other immunosuppressive medications are also more prone to opportunistic infections. Treatment with eculizumab, a terminal complement inhibitor, is associated with an increased risk of meningococcal meningitis.

The differential diagnosis for the same anatomic syndrome changes significantly based on the host. For example, ring-enhancing lesions or abscesses on brain imaging (post-contrast MRI or computed tomography [CT]) in an immunocompetent host are usually bacterial abscesses. However, in an HIV patient with a CD4 count of less than 100/μL, cerebral toxoplasmosis should be considered. In a solid-organ transplant recipient, invasive molds are higher on the differential.

Question 6: Is It an Acute Severe Infection or a Chronic Stable Infection?

Differentiating a life-threatening CNS infection from a chronic stable infection is vital. Clinicians should act fast if a patient has acute worsening of mental status or rapidly progressive neurologic deficits within hours. A 3-hour delay in treatment of critically ill patients with pneumococcal meningitis can increase mortality by about 14 times.[1] A patient with a spinal epidural abscess who develops sudden lower extremity weakness and incontinence needs emergent surgery. On the contrary, there is no rush to treat a patient who presents with headaches for weeks and no focal neurologic features from chronic stable lymphocytic meningitis.

Question 7: What Is the Type of CSF Inflammatory Response?

Routine cell counts and chemistry analysis of the CSF can be done quickly and can provide valuable diagnostic information. CSF can be obtained either by lumbar puncture from the subarachnoid space or from the cerebral ventricles via an external ventricular drain or ventricular shunt.

- **CSF total nucleated white blood cell (WBC) count and differential:** If the CSF WBC count/μL is in the thousands and is predominantly neutrophilic, it is suggestive of a bacterial meningitis from a virulent organism like *S. pneumoniae*. If the CSF WBC count/μL is close to 100,000 and is neutrophilic, it is suggestive of intraventricular rupture of a brain abscess. The differential diagnosis for a mild to moderate lymphocytic CSF pleocytosis is very broad, including viral, fungal, mycobacterial, neoplastic, and immune-mediated meningitis or encephalitis. The differential diagnosis for a predominantly eosinophilic CSF pleocytosis (greater than 10%) is very narrow and includes parasitic worm infections, coccidioidomycosis, or an adverse reaction to intrathecally administered drugs. Certain CNS infections like Creutzfeldt–Jakob disease (CJD) and progressive multifocal leukoencephalopathy (PML) do not usually cause CSF pleocytosis.
- **CSF:blood glucose ratio** is another discriminatory test. A very low ratio (0.4 or less) is suggestive of a bacterial, fungal, mycobacterial, or neoplastic meningitis. It is important not to rely just on the CSF glucose level and to obtain a blood glucose level at 30 to 45 minutes around the time of CSF sampling. CSF glucose levels usually equilibrate with blood levels in less than an hour. CSF glucose of 60 mg/dL is "normal," but the CSF:blood glucose ratio would be very low if the patient's blood sugar were 600 mg/dL.

DIAGNOSTIC TESTING IN A PATIENT WITH A CNS INFLAMMATORY OR INFECTIOUS SYNDROME

It is beyond the scope of this chapter to go into the details of diagnostic testing, but we will briefly discuss general principles of testing. Diagnostic imaging, especially MRI brain with and without contrast, is not just useful for anatomic localization—the radiographic pattern on different sequences can give clues about etiology. For example, a ring-enhancing lesion on T-1 post-contrast MRI with restricted diffusion in the center on diffusion-weighted images is more suggestive of an abscess than a tumor.

Tests for organism detection can be performed in the blood, serum, CSF, or tissue from a biopsy of the brain or meninges. Traditional stains and cultures for bacteria, fungi, and *Mycobacteria* still play an important role, though the yield might be low, especially when the CSF or tissue sample is of an inadequate volume. There are newer CSF molecular diagnostic tests like multiplex polymerase chain reactions (PCRs), universal 16S or 18S ribosomal RNA PCRs, and unbiased metagenomic sequencing available for organism detection. The same principles of diagnostic testing that apply to traditional stains and cultures are also relevant when interpreting molecular diagnostic tests. There could be false-positive tests from contamination during specimen collection, both with traditional and molecular tests. An example would be of a single colony of *Staphylococcus epidermidis* that grows from the CSF bacterial culture or is detected by a molecular test. Both these "positive CSF tests" are suggestive of a contamination. Latent viruses like Epstein–Barr virus (EBV), cytomegalovirus (CMV), and human herpesvirus 6 (HHV-6) can reactivate in the context of another CNS inflammatory disease, and a positive test from the CSF does not necessarily mean they are the cause of the disease.

Serum and CSF antibodies, both for infectious and immune-mediated etiologies, are also problematic to interpret. Antibodies to infectious organisms often remain positive for months and years after the resolution of the infection, and a positive test does not always mean that the patient has an active infection. Borderline positive antibody tests are often false positive. The clinician should be extremely cautious in interpreting these "positive" tests, especially in the workup of chronic meningitis and chronic encephalitis, as the false-positive rate increases with the number of tests ordered.

A CLINICAL SYNDROME-BASED APPROACH TO CNS INFECTIONS

- **Acute meningitis:** This is inflammation of the meningitis, which occurs rapidly within hours to days. Acute neutrophilic meningitis in adults is usually from community-acquired bacterial pathogens like *S. pneumoniae, N. meningitidis,* and *Listeria.* Acute lymphocytic meningitis is usually from enteroviruses or arboviruses like West Nile virus. In the postcraniotomy patient, virulent pathogens like *E. coli* and *Staphylococcus aureus* can cause an acute meningitis or cerebral ventriculitis. It is also important to note that postcraniotomy meningitis from indolent pathogens like *Staphylococcus epidermidis* can present as chronic meningitis.
- **Recurrent acute meningitis:** The differential diagnosis depends on the type of CSF pleocytosis. The causes of recurrent lymphocytic meningitis are:
  - Mollaret meningitis from recurrent HSV-2 reactivation in the pia–arachnoid layer.
  - Intermittent leaking into the subarachnoid space from epidermoid cysts or craniopharyngiomas.
  - Recurrent episodes of autoimmune disease (Bechet, sarcoid, or granulomatous polyangiitis).
  - Drug-induced meningitis from recurrent use of the same medication (nonsteroidal anti-inflammatory drugs [NSAIDs], trimethoprim, or intravenous immunoglobulin [IVIG]).

The causes of recurrent neutrophilic meningitis are:

- Recurrent bacterial meningitis secondary to anatomic communication of the subarachnoid space with a nonsterile surface (mucosa or skin). This could be secondary to congenital defects or from trauma to the face, head, or spine. If the patient has clear rhinorrhea or otorrhea, test the fluid for beta-2 transferrin. Its presence in the fluid is highly suggestive that it is CSF.
- IG deficiency or asplenia can lead to recurrent infections from encapsulated organisms like *S. pneumoniae, N. meningitidis,* and *Haemophilus influenza.* These organisms are neurotropic and cause meningitis.
- **Chronic meningitis:** This is meningitis that has an indolent presentation and lasts weeks to months. Often an etiologic diagnosis is difficult, requiring multiple lumbar punctures and extensive testing. A few of the causes to consider in the differential diagnosis are:
  - *Cryptococcus*
  - Coccidioidomycosis, histoplasmosis, blastomycosis
  - Spirochetes (syphilis, Lyme, leptospirosis)
  - *Mycobacterium tuberculosis*
  - Leptomeningeal carcinomatosis (adenocarcinomas of the lung, breast, and melanoma)
  - Lymphomatous leptomeningitis (non-Hodgkin lymphoma [NHL], acute lymphoblastic leukemia [ALL])
  - Leptomeningeal gliomatosis

The differential diagnosis for chronic meningitis that predominantly involves the basilar leptomeninges includes fungal meningitis, tuberculous meningitis, neoplastic meningitis, and neurosarcoidosis. If there is concomitant uveitis (inflammation of the iris, ciliary body, or choroid of the eye), consider the following etiologies:

- Sarcoidosis
- Bechet syndrome, which can also involve the brainstem
- Vogt–Koyanagi–Harada syndrome, which presents with meningitis; deafness; granulomatous uveitis; alopecia; vitiligo; and poliosis of eyelashes, eyebrows, and hair
- Wegner granulomatosis
- Sjogren syndrome
- *Tropheryma whippeli*

- **Encephalitis:** This is inflammation of the brain parenchyma. Like chronic meningitis, making an etiologic diagnosis for chronic encephalitis is often difficult. It can linger like smoldering embers, evading a diagnosis and testing a clinician's acumen and perseverance. Most commonly known etiologies are either infections (usually viral) or immune-mediated encephalitis. The most common infectious etiology for acute sporadic encephalitis is herpes simplex, which has a predilection to involve the medial temporal lobes. Episodes of encephalitis involving deep gray matter (basal ganglia) during the summer and fall in the United States is suggestive of West Nile viral infection. Japanese B encephalitis, which is more common in Asia, can have a presentation similar to West Nile encephalitis.

Autoimmune encephalitis can often mimic infectious encephalitis, so it is important for infectious disease clinicians to be aware of them. It was initially described as a paraneoplastic syndrome, but is now reported without any association with tumors as well. It is either associated with antibodies against neuronal cell-surface synaptic proteins or with antibodies against intracellular proteins. Please see Table 14.1 for details about autoantibodies associated with autoimmune encephalitis. Even today, a significant number of encephalitis cases remain undiagnosed. In most published series around 40% or more of cases do not have an etiologic diagnosis[2-4] (see Table 14.1).

TABLE 14.1 ■ Antibodies Associated with Autoimmune Encephalitis

	Association with Malignancies	Clinical Findings	Imaging Findings
Anti-Hu (ANNA-1)	Small cell lung cancer	Encephalomyelitis, subacute sensory neuropathy, cerebellar degeneration	T2-FLAIR hyperintensity in limbic system, cerebellum, brainstem
Anti-Ma (Ma1/Ma2/Ma3)	Testicular cancer, small cell lung cancer, breast cancer	Brainstem dysfunction, ophthalmoplegia, limbic encephalitis uncommon	Variable T2 hyperintense signal in thalamus and brainstem
Anti-GAD (glutamic acid decarboxylase)	Type I diabetes	Stiff-person syndrome, limbic encephalitis	T2 hyperintensity in the limbic system
Anti-Yo (PCA-1)	Breast cancer, ovarian cancer	Cerebellitis (ataxia), vertigo, nystagmus	Cerebellar degeneration
Anti-CV2	Small cell lung cancer, thymoma	Choreiform movements	T2-FLAIR hyperintensity in the striatum; relative sparing of the medial temporal lobes
Anti-NMDAr		Viral prodrome, psychiatric symptoms; amnesia, seizures, and encephalopathy	Often normal; variable transient cortical T2 hyperintensity and enhancement
Anti-VGKC (voltage-gated potassium channel)		Epilepsy (early and intractable), limbic encephalitis	T2-FLAIR hyperintensity in medial temporal lobes progressing to mesial temporal sclerosis
Anti-GABA (two subtypes:anti–GABA-A, anti–GABA-B)	Anti–GABA-B associated with small cell lung cancer	Similar to anti-VGKC but with better prognosis	Anti–GABA-A often shows extralimbic abnormalities
Anti-GluR3 (glutamate receptor 3)		Rasmussen encephalitis, intractable epilepsy	Holohemispheric diffuse tissue loss and T2-FLAIR hyperintensity
Anti-GluR1 (glutamate receptor 1)	Lymphoma	Cerebellar ataxia	Cerebellar degeneration
Anti-AMPAr (alpha-amino-3-hydroxy-5-methyl-4-isoxazolepropionic acid receptor)	Breast, lung, and thymic tumors	Subacute psychiatric symptoms	T2-FLAIR signal abnormality isolated to the hippocampi
Anti-LGI1 (leucine-rich, glioma-inactivated 1)		Epilepsy (early and intractable), limbic encephalitis	T2-FLAIR hyperintensity in medial temporal lobes progressing to mesial temporal sclerosis

FLAIR, Fluid-attenuated inversion recovery.
Adapted from Yu FF, Small JE. Autoimmune encephalitis. In JE Small, DL Noujaim, DT Ginat, HR Kelly, PW Schaefer, eds. *Neuroradiology.* Elsevier: 2019:96-103. https://doi.org/10.1016/B978-0-323-44549-8.00011-0.

- **Myelitis or myelo-radiculitis:** Myelitis is inflammation of the spinal cord, and myelo-radiculitis is inflammation of both the spinal cord and spinal nerve roots. The causes are infectious, postinfectious or postvaccination, and noninfectious immune mediated. Depending on the part of the spinal cord and level of the spinal cord involved, the symptoms could be weakness; sensory disturbances; and bowel, bladder, or sexual dysfunction. Infectious organisms that usually cause extensive transverse and vertical myelitis are herpes simplex and varicella zoster virus (VZV). CMV usually causes myeloradiculitis in immunocompromised patients, especially in HIV patients with CD4 counts of 100/μL or less. Certain viruses have a predilection to infect anterior horn cells and cause acute flaccid paralysis. These viruses are West Nile virus, nonpolio enterovirus like enterovirus D68, and Japanese B encephalitis virus. Among the noninfectious etiologies of extensive myelitis, the most important is neuromyelitis optica, which can cause significant CSF pleocytosis and can mimic an infectious myelitis.
- **Space-occupying, rim-enhancing lesions in the brain** on post-contrast T-1 MRI can be caused by brain abscesses, demyelinating lesions, tumors, or hematomas. Multiple brain abscesses in different vascular territories of the brain are usually from hematogenous spread and are caused by a single organism like *S. aureus* or *Streptococcus* species. Solitary brain abscesses are usually infections that spread from a contiguous focus like mastoiditis or paranasal sinusitis and are polymicrobial with Gram-positive cocci, anaerobes, and sometimes Gram-negative rods. "Complete" ring enhancement of the lesions is usually seen in brain abscesses and tumors, whereas "incomplete" ring enhancement or the C-shaped enhancement is usually seen in demyelinating lesions like acute demyelinating encephalomyelitis (ADEM) or in tumefactive demyelinating lesions.
- **Stroke or strokelike syndromes from infectious and inflammatory etiologies:** Infections of the CNS can cause ischemic strokes either by direct invasion of the vessel wall to cause vasculitis or when meningeal inflammation in meningitis spreads to the Virchow–Robin spaces surrounding the blood vessels and eventually to the cerebrovascular arterial wall to cause strokes. Infectious and inflammatory causes of stroke are:
  - Varicella zoster vasculitis
  - Meningovascular syphilis
  - Basilar meningitis from yeasts like *Cryptococcus, Candida* and dimorphic fungi, or *Mycobacterium tuberculosis*
  - Secondary to systemic vasculitis like granulomatous polyangiitis, giant cell arteritis, or Takayasu arteritis
  - Primary CNS angiitis, which is a diagnosis of exclusion of other secondary causes
  - Intravascular lymphoma

Suggested Readings

Auburtin M, Wolff M, Charpentier J, et al. Detrimental role of delayed antibiotic administration and penicillin-nonsusceptible strains in adult intensive care unit patients with pneumococcal meningitis: the PNEUMOREA prospective multicenter study. *Crit Care Med.* 2006;34:2758–2765.

Bloch KC, Glaser CA. Encephalitis surveillance through the emerging infections program, 1997–2010. *Emerg Infect Dis.* 2015;21:1562–1567.

Mailles A, Stahl JP. Steering Committee and Investigators Group. Infectious encephalitis in France in 2007: a national prospective study. *Clin Infect Dis.* 2009;49:1838–1847.

Granerod J, Ambrose HE, Davies NW, et al. Causes of encephalitis and differences in their clinical presentations in England: a multicentre, population-based prospective study. *Lancet Infect Dis.* 2010;10:835–844.

Vector-Borne Infections

Raj Palraj

Introduction

Vector-borne infections include diseases caused by diverse pathogens (bacteria, viruses, parasites) that are transmitted to humans by a variety of vectors such as ticks, mosquitoes, lice, tsetse flies, sandflies, triatome bugs, blackflies, mites, and snails. Vectors are typically blood-sucking insects that ingest the pathogen from an infected host reservoir (human, animal, bird) and then transmit them to a susceptible human during their next bloody meal. Globally, infections caused by mosquitoes contribute to a significant burden of diseases, especially in tropical and subtropical regions. In the United States, tick-borne infections constitute the majority of the diseases transmitted by vectors. However, the unprecedented increase in global travel and trade over the past decades has resulted in a higher number of Americans at risk of travel-related mosquito-borne infections.

It is important that primary care physicians are able to provide appropriate pretravel counseling and other preventive measures to their patients to reduce their risk of acquiring vector-borne infections during their travel outside the United States.

Tick-Borne Infections in the United States: Lyme Disease

EPIDEMIOLOGY

Lyme disease is the most common vector-borne infection reported in the United States, contributing to more than 60% of reported cases.[1] The common vector-borne infections in the United States are listed in Table 15.1. Lyme disease is caused by the spirochete *Borrelia burgdorferi* and transmitted by the *Ixodes* tick. In 1977, an investigation of a cluster of juvenile rheumatoid arthritis among children in Connecticut led to the recognition of Lyme disease.[2] The Centers for Disease Control and Prevention (CDC) estimates that approximately 300,000 people in the United States acquire Lyme disease annually.[3,4] Almost all Lyme disease cases are reported from a dozen states in certain geographic regions of the United States, emphasizing the importance of environmental and ecologic factors in the transmission of vector-borne infections. The proportion of ticks infected with *B. burgdorferi* and other pathogens varies across different regions of the country.[5] Climate

TABLE 15.1 ■ **Common Vector-Borne Infections in the United States**

Vector-Borne Disease	Pathogen	Vector	Endemic Regions in United States
Lyme disease	*Borrelia burgdorferi*	Blacklegged deer tick *(Ixodes scapularis, Ixodes pacificus)*	Northeast, upper Midwest, northern California
Human granulocytic anaplasmosis	*Anaplasma phagocytophilum*	Blacklegged deer tick *(Ixodes scapularis, Ixodes pacificus)*	Northeast, upper Midwest
Babesiosis	*Babesia microti*	Blacklegged deer tick *(Ixodes scapularis, Ixodes pacificus)*	Northeast, upper Midwest
Human monocytic ehrlichiosis	*Ehrlichia chaffeensis*	Lone Star tick *(Amblyomma americanum)*, black-legged deer tick *(Ixodes scapularis)*	Southeast and southcentral United States
Rocky Mountain spotted fever	*Rickettsia rickettsii*	American dog tick *(Dermacentor variabilis)*, Rocky Mountain wood tick *(Dermacentor andersoni)*	Southcentral United States
West Nile virus infection	West Nile virus	*Culex* mosquito	All states in continental United States
Tularemia	*Fransicella tularensis*	American dog tick *(Dermacentor variabilis)*, Lone Star tick *(Amblyomma americanum)*, deer flies *(Chrysops* spp.)	Southcentral United States
Powassan virus infection	Powassan virus (Flavivirus)	Black-legged deer tick *(Ixodes scapularis)*, *Ixodes cookie*, *Ixodes marxi*	Northeast, upper Midwest
Plague	*Yersinia pestis*	Rodent fleas	Rural Western United States

change that enables ticks to expand their geographic home, an increase in deer population, and a rise in the number of homes near forested areas have all contributed to the rise in the number of Lyme disease cases in the United States. The causative pathogen—*B. burgdorferi*—is transmitted primarily by black-legged ticks, *Ixodes scapularis*, in the northeastern and upper Midwest regions, whereas *Ixodes pacificus* ticks are the predominant vectors for Lyme disease in northern California and Oregon.[6] During its life cycle, *I. scapularis* goes through larval, nymph, and adult stages over a period of 2 years.[7] The primary reservoir of *B. burgdorferi* is the white-legged mouse, from which the larval stage of *I. scapularis* ticks get infected after taking a bloody meal. Ticks do not fly, but quest on tall grass and get attached to the exposed skin of humans as they pass by. Once attached, the nymphs may go unnoticed by the human host, as they are very small and their bite is painless. If the tick is removed early, Lyme disease can be prevented, as it takes approximately 48 hours for transmission of the spirochete to occur. The nymphal stage of black-legged ticks is the most efficient in transmitting *B. burgdorferi*.[8] The incidence of Lyme disease peaks in the summer months, corelating with the time period of peak activity of *Ixodes* nymphs. Adult female *I. scapularis* ticks feed on deer, and hence they are also called *deer ticks*. Even though deer is not a reservoir for *B. burgdorferi*, the deer population is important for survival of adult female *I. scapularis* ticks and hence for the transmission of Lyme disease.

Clinical Manifestations of Lyme Disease

Lyme disease can present with a variety of clinical symptoms and often involve multiple systems. The clinical presentations can be divided into three states: (1) early localized, (2) early disseminated, and (3) late Lyme disease. It should be noted that the clinical features may overlap between the three stages, and patients may also present with a late disease manifestation without previous history of early Lyme disease.

Early Localized Lyme Disease

Patients with early localized Lyme disease usually present with a characteristic erythema migrans skin rash and may have accompanying constitutional symptoms, including fatigue, arthralgias, myalgias, headache, fever, and anorexia.[9] Classic erythema migrans has a target-like or bull's-eye appearance. The rash starts at the site of the tick bite, usually after 7 to 14 days, and then slowly expands over days with a zone of central clearing. Although the classic erythema migrans is considered diagnostic of early Lyme disease, it is seldom seen among patients when they present to their primary physicians. During the first few days of the rash, it is usually homogenously red or has central erythema. The rash is warm to the touch and may itch or burn rarely, but is not painful. Thorough body skin examination is important, as the rash is commonly found in "hidden" parts such as axilla, popliteal fossa, inguinal region, or belt line. Biopsy of the skin lesion is not needed, and it may show signs of vascular endothelial injury.

DIAGNOSIS

Erythema migrans is present in approximately 80% of patients with early Lyme disease, despite only a small minority (around 25%) remembering a history of tick bite.[10,11] In the appropriate epidemiologic setting, early localized Lyme disease is diagnosed clinically based on erythema migrans skin rash.[12] Patients may have mild, nonspecific abnormalities in total white blood cell count, erythrocyte sedimentation rate, red blood cell count, platelet and count, so these are not useful in making the clinical diagnosis. Abnormalities in hepatic transaminase levels, thrombocytopenia, and anemia may suggest the presence of coinfections transmitted by the same *Ixodes* tick bite, such as anaplasmosis or babesiosis. Serology is not a useful diagnostic tool in early Lyme disease and may be misleading, as false-negative results are quite common.[13] Newer molecular methods may be helpful in identifying the coinfections.

TREATMENT

The important goals of antimicrobial therapy for early localized Lyme disease are to reduce the duration of clinical disease and lower the risk of subsequent occurrence of late Lyme disease manifestations. The first-line antibiotics include oral doxycycline, amoxicillin, and cefuroxime–axetil. Small randomized clinical trials conducted in the United States have shown that three first-line antibiotic regimens have equivalent efficacy in the treatment of early localized Lyme disease.[14–16] Oral doxycycline, however, is the preferred antibiotic, given its activity against possible coinfecting pathogens such as *Anaplasma phagocytophilum*, *Ehrlichia* spp., and *Borrelia miyamotoi*. Because of its effectiveness, oral doxycycline may also be used in children less than 8 years of age, as endorsed by the CDC and American Academy of Pediatrics.[17] The preferred antibiotic regimens for different clinical presentations of Lyme disease are listed in Table 15.2. Although most clinical trials used 21 days of antibiotic treatment, a shorter duration of treatment (10 to 14 days) appears to be equally effective. Many experts prefer shorter regimens (10 days of oral doxycycline or 14 days of oral amoxicillin) for the treatment of early localized Lyme disease. For pregnant women, doxycycline should be avoided due to potential adverse effects, and either a course of oral amoxicillin or cefuroxime–axetil is the preferred regimen.[18] Macrolides such as azithromycin were noted to be not as effective as amoxicillin and are reserved only for patients who cannot tolerate any of the first-line antibiotic agents.[19] Among patients treated with oral macrolides, chances of treatment failure, relapse, or progression to the late stage is significant, and close clinical monitoring is essential. Of note for primary care physicians is that first-generation oral cephalosporins such as cephalexin have no activity against *B. burgdorferi* and are not recommended for the treatment

TABLE 15.2 ■ **Antibiotic Regimens for Lyme Disease**

Clinical Syndrome	Antibiotic Regimen for Adults
Early Lyme Disease	
Localized Erythema Migrans	• Oral doxycycline 100 mg twice daily for 10–21 days • Oral amoxicillin 500 mg three times daily for 14–21 days • Oral cefuroxime–axetil 500 mg twice daily for 10–21 days
Early Disseminated Disease	
Multiple Erythema Migrans	• Oral doxycycline 100 mg twice daily for 10–21 days • Oral amoxicillin 500 mg thrice daily for 14–21 days • Oral cefuroxime–axetil 500 mg twice daily for 10–21 days
Early Lyme Carditis	• IV ceftriaxone 2 g every 24 hours for symptomatic patients, PR interval >300 ms, second- and third-degree atrioventricular block • Once improved, transition to oral regimens to complete 21- to 28-day course
Early Lyme Facial Nerve Palsy	• Oral doxycycline 100 mg twice daily for 10–21 days
Early Lyme Meningitis	• IV ceftriaxone 2 g every 24 hours for 21–28 days
Late Lyme Disease	
Late Lyme Arthritis	• Oral doxycycline 100 mg twice daily for 28 days • Oral amoxicillin 500 mg thrice daily for 28 days • Oral cefuroxime–axetil 500 mg twice daily for 28 days
Late Lyme Central Nervous System Manifestations	• IV ceftriaxone 2 g every 24 hours for 21–28 days

of Lyme disease.[20] This is clinically relevant, as a common diagnostic dilemma faced by primary physicians in endemic regions is to differentiate between atypical homogenously erythematous early Lyme skin lesion and cellulitis. If it is difficult to separate the two entities, a reasonable approach might involve using oral cefuroxime–axetil that has activity against both *B. burgdorferi* and common pathogens involved in cellulitis.

Most patients with early localized Lyme disease have complete resolution of symptoms with appropriate antibiotic therapy. However, a small percentage of patients may have persistent subjective symptoms like fatigue, headache, arthralgias, myalgias, and fatigue for several weeks to months after treatment. These patients require reassurance that these symptoms usually resolve spontaneously and do not need further antibiotics, as they do not have active infection. If symptoms persist beyond 6 months, patients are categorized as post–Lyme disease syndrome.

Early Disseminated Lyme Disease

Early disseminated Lyme disease is characterized by hematogenous spread of the spirochete to distant sites such as the skin, heart, and nervous system that present within a few weeks to months after the initial tick bite.

Multiple Erythema Migrans Lesions

The presence of multiple erythema migrans skin lesions is usually a sign of hematogenous dissemination rather than multiple concurrent tick bites (Figs. 15.1 to 15.3). In one study, patients with spirochetemia were more likely to have multiple skin lesions and be symptomatic.[21] In these patients, careful clinical evaluation is indicated to detect involvement of other systems such as the heart and nervous system. Oral doxycycline 100 mg twice daily for 21 days is the recommended

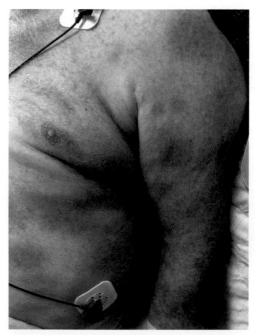

Fig. 15.1   Disseminated erythema migrans involving the trunk.

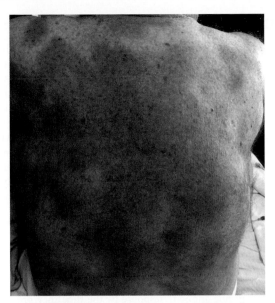

Fig. 15.2   Large area of erythema due to the confluence of multiple erythema migrans lesions.

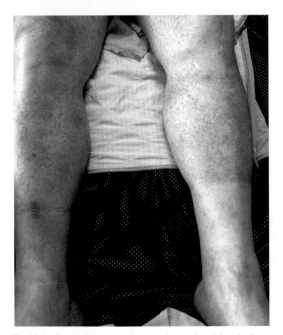

Fig. 15.3   Disseminated erythema migrans involving the legs.

antibiotic regimen for patients with multiple erythema migrans and without any evidence of Lyme meningitis or severe Lyme carditis requiring hospitalization.[22] A significant proportion of patients with multiple erythema migrans lesions develop worsening of symptoms in the first 24 hours of antibiotic therapy due to an immune response to antigens released by dying spirochetes, called *Jarisch–Herxheimer reaction.*[15]

Early Lyme Carditis

Lyme carditis occurs in approximately 1% to 10% of patients diagnosed with Lyme disease in the United States.[23] Early Lyme carditis usually occurs within the first 2 months and may present alone or overlap with erythema migrans and/or early neurologic symptoms. The most common cardiac manifestation is the varying degrees of atrioventricular (AV) block due to dysfunction of the conduction system. Depending on the severity of cardiac involvement, patients may be asymptomatic or have symptoms such as palpitations, lightheadedness, or syncope. A report of three sudden cardiac deaths among otherwise healthy young adults and postmortem evidence of Lyme carditis raised the alarm of this potentially lethal presentation.[24] Rarely patients may also develop mild forms of myopericarditis with nonspecific ST-T changes in the electrocardiogram (ECG) and usually without significant clinical symptoms. Lyme disease does not cause valvular endocarditis or aortitis.

DIAGNOSIS

The CDC recommends two-tier serology testing: initial screening with enzyme-linked immunosorbent assay (ELISA) and confirmatory Western blot analysis for the diagnosis of Lyme carditis. Although serology may be negative during the early few weeks of infection, most patients would have developed a Lyme-specific antibody response by the time they present with symptoms of Lyme carditis.[25] Positive two-tier serology testing in the appropriate epidemiologic risk factors and ECG findings is helpful in the diagnosis of Lyme carditis. Patients with negative Lyme serology are unlikely to have cardiac Lyme disease, and alternative diagnostic evaluation for cardiac conduction abnormalities should be pursued.

TREATMENT

Symptomatic patients and those with a high degree AV block require close monitoring with cardiac telemetry, as the degree of AV conduction block can fluctuate rapidly. Intravenous (IV) ceftriaxone 2 g daily in adults is the preferred initial regimen for symptomatic patients and those with first-degree AV block with a PR interval more than 300 milliseconds or second- or third-degree AV block.[26] A third-generation cephalosporin (IV cefotaxime) or IV penicillin G are acceptable alternative regimens, and desensitization should be considered for patients with a history of severe immunoglobulin E (IgE)–mediated anaphylaxis to penicillin. Consultation with a cardiac electrophysiologist is helpful, as patients may require implantation of a temporary pacemaker. It is reasonable to continue an IV antibiotic until the high-degree AV block has resolved and then transition to one of the oral antibiotics (oral doxycycline, amoxicillin, cefuroxime axetil) to complete a total of a 21- to 28-day course. With appropriate antibiotic therapy, complete AV block usually improves within a week, and hence, patients do not need permanent pacemaker placement.[27] Minor conduction abnormalities may last up to 6 weeks before resolution.

Early Lyme Neurologic Manifestations

Patients with early disseminated Lyme disease involving the nervous system may present with lymphocytic meningitis, facial nerve palsy, or motor or sensory radiculoneuropathy.[28] Early neurologic symptoms typically occur weeks to several months after the tick bite. A high degree of clinical suspicion is important for diagnosis, as these may be the only and first symptoms of Lyme disease. Abrupt onset of facial nerve palsy is the most common neurologic manifestation of early disseminated Lyme disease. Lyme disease is one of the very few causes of bilateral facial nerve palsies. In endemic regions, Lyme neuritis may constitute up to a quarter of all facial nerve palsies during the summer season.[29] Other cranial nerves may rarely be involved. Severe radicular pain involving one or more dermatomes may be a presentation of Lyme radiculoneuritis involving peripheral nerves. Patients may also rarely present with acute brachial and/or lumbosacral plexopathies.

Early dissemination of spirochetes to the meninges can result in lymphocytic meningitis that may mimic viral meningitis with symptoms of headache, fever, neck stiffness, and photosensitivity. Signs of meningeal irritation may also accompany other clinical manifestations of early Lyme disease, such as erythema migrans, Lyme carditis, facial nerve palsy, or peripheral neuropathy.

DIAGNOSIS

Two-tier serology testing with initial ELISA followed by confirmatory Western blot is the recommended initial test. A positive or equivocal ELISA result should be followed by confirmatory Western blot. If serology is negative, the likelihood of early disseminated Lyme disease affecting the nervous system is very low. Cerebrospinal fluid (CSF) analysis in patients with Lyme meningitis shows lymphocytic pleocytosis (a few hundred lymphocytes per microliter), moderate protein elevation, and relatively normal glucose level.[30] The sensitivity of CSF Lyme antibodies is unclear, and negative CSF antibodies do not eliminate central nervous system (CNS) Lyme disease.[31] Similarly, CSF polymerase chain reaction (PCR) for *B. burgdorferi* has variable sensitivity and specificity, limiting its utility in clinical diagnosis.[32] Magnetic resonance imaging (MRI) of the brain is usually normal, as brain parenchymal infection is uncommon. In patients with suspected peripheral neuropathy, electromyography and nerve conduction studies are indicated to evaluate the type and distribution of peripheral nerve damage.

TREATMENT

Patients with isolated facial nerve palsy or peripheral neuropathy may be treated with oral doxycycline 100 mg twice daily for 14 to 28 days.[26] Oral amoxicillin and cefuroxime–axetil have not been tested for this clinical entity. Antimicrobial therapy does not usually accelerate clinical resolution of facial nerve palsy, but helps prevent other complications from disseminated Lyme disease. If there is concurrent meningitis with CSF abnormalities, IV ceftriaxone is recommended. Glucocorticoids have not been shown to be a beneficial adjunctive therapy in patients with Lyme facial nerve palsy. For patients with Lyme lymphocytic meningitis or encephalomyelitis, IV ceftriaxone 2 g daily for 21 to 28 days is the preferred regimen.[26] Some patients may have persistent nonspecific neurologic symptoms such as fatigue and cognitive or memory difficulties for several weeks to months, despite appropriate antimicrobial therapy and microbiologic cure.

Late Lyme Disease

During the early stage of Lyme infection, spirochetes may disseminate hematogenously to different distant sites such as the joints, nervous system, and heart. Appropriate antibiotic therapy given during the early stage of Lyme disease is curative and prevents progression to late Lyme disease. Late Lyme disease develops in a significant proportion of patients who did not receive first-line antibiotic therapy for their early Lyme disease. However, in some patients, late Lyme disease may present even without any clinically significant manifestation of early Lyme disease. Late symptoms usually develop several months to a few years after the tick bite and predominantly involve the joints and/or the nervous system.

Late Lyme Arthritis

Most patients with late Lyme disease present with arthritis involving the knee, usually several months to years after the initial tick bite.[33] Patients usually do not recall a tick bite and may not have experienced clinically apparent early Lyme disease. Among patients with potential exposure to ticks, clinical evaluation of arthritis should include the possibility of late Lyme arthritis. Monoarthritis involving the knee joint is the most common clinical syndrome, but other large joints such as the shoulder, ankle, and wrist may be infected. Patients usually have a large swollen joint that is warm to the touch and minimal pain. Systemic symptoms such as fever, chills, and night sweats are usually absent, and Lyme arthritis may mimic mechanical injury/arthritis. In children, asymmetric oligoarticular Lyme arthritis may resemble juvenile rheumatoid arthritis. [2]

DIAGNOSIS

Synovial fluid analysis usually has an elevated white blood count in the range of 10,000 to 25,000 cells per microliter, consistent with inflammatory arthritis.[34] Two-tier Lyme serology using CDC criteria is the established initial test for the evaluation of patients with suspected Lyme arthritis. Because Lyme arthritis is a late clinical manifestation, the sensitivity of two-tier serology testing is high and has a high negative predictive value. Another fact to remember is that Lyme serology may remain positive for years, even after successful antibiotic treatment for Lyme arthritis. A persistently positive Lyme serology does not mean active/chronic infection and does not necessitate a longer course of antibiotic therapy. Synovial fluid PCR for *B. burgdorferi* can be tested to help in the diagnosis of Lyme arthritis, but has not been validated for widespread clinical use.[35]

TREATMENT

Infectious Diseases Society of America (IDSA) guidelines recommend 28 days of oral doxycycline 100 mg twice daily or amoxicillin 500 mg three times daily or cefuroxime–axetil 500 mg twice daily for treatment of Lyme arthritis without concomitant neurologic manifestations.[26] In some patients, clinical resolution may be slow or incomplete with the first course of antibiotics and may require another 28 days of oral antibiotic therapy. For patients who had very minimal or no improvement with the oral regimen, IV ceftriaxone 2 g daily for 14 to 28 days is recommended.[26] Intraarticular steroid injections should be avoided, as they may adversely affect the resolution of Lyme arthritis. If active synovitis persists despite 2 to 3 months of antibiotics, patients might benefit from disease-modifying antirheumatic drugs (DMARDs) used in the treatment of chronic inflammatory arthritis, as the ongoing inflammation is thought to be due to retained spirochetal antigens or autoimmunity triggered by initial infection.[36] In antibiotic-refractory Lyme arthritis, further prolonged antibiotic therapy is of little use, as there is no evidence of active spirochetal infection.

Late Lyme Neurologic Disease

The most common late neurologic syndrome is Lyme encephalopathy that can present with nonspecific symptoms such as fatigue, cognitive slowing, or memory difficulties. Because the symptoms are nonspecific, it is important to identify patients with true Lyme encephalopathy due to active infection. CSF analysis and brain MRI are indicated, and IV ceftriaxone 2 g daily for 21 to 28 days is recommended for those with objective findings.[26] In the absence of objective evidence of active brain infection, presence of nonspecific symptoms alone does not suggest late Lyme disease, and prolonged IV antibiotics have not been helpful. Other uncommon neurologic symptoms associated with late Lyme disease include mononeuritis multiplex, sensory axonal peripheral neuropathy, and encephalomyelitis.

Post–Lyme Disease Syndrome

Although the majority of patients with early Lyme disease have resolution of clinical symptoms with appropriate antibiotic therapy, approximately 5% to 15% of patients have persistent symptoms such as fatigue, musculoskeletal pain, and cognitive and/or memory difficulties.[37] If symptoms persist for more than 6 months, patients may have post–Lyme disease syndrome. The risk factors, pathogenesis, and biologic mechanisms that contribute to persistent symptoms are still unclear, and scientific research to answer these important questions is sorely needed. Microbiologic treatment failure with current first-line antibiotic regimens is very rare, and no resistant strains of *B. burgdorferi* have been described so far.[38] An alternative term—*chronic Lyme disease*—which may inaccurately imply chronic persistent infection, has been used by some physicians and patient advocacy groups who have supported longer courses of antibiotics for these patients. However, available current scientific evidence does not support the hypothesis of persistent bacterial infection, and current guidelines from IDSA and American Association of Neurology (AAN) do not recommend additional longer courses of antibiotics for persistent subjective symptoms.[26,39] Randomized controlled trials have shown that longer courses of antibiotics did not improve the subjective symptoms.[40–42] Alternatively, prolonged antibiotics have been reported to have caused serious adverse reactions, including anaphylaxis, catheter-related bloodstream infections, and severe *Clostridium difficile* infections.[43] Patients with persistent symptoms should be thoroughly evaluated for other alternative medical conditions such as fibromyalgia, underlying malignancy, and depression.

LYME DISEASE ACQUIRED IN EUROPE

Lyme disease in Europe can be caused by *B. afzelli* and *B. garinii* in addition to *B. burgdorferi*, the predominant strain in the United States. Certain skin presentations such as borrelial lymphocytoma, acrodermatitis, chronic atrophicans, and morphea-like lesions are seen only among patients who acquired the infection in Europe during their travel.[44] Infections due to *B. garinii* in Europe have also been associated with rare late neurologic manifestations, including chronic encephalomyelitis, cranial neuropathy, and cognitive impairment.[45]

Coinfections Associated with Lyme Disease

The *I. scapularis* ticks prevalent in the Northeastern and Midwestern parts of United States may also carry other pathogens such as *Anaplasma phagocytophilum* and *Babesia microti*. Approximately up to a third of patients with Lyme disease in these regions have coinfections.[46,47]

HUMAN GRANULOCYTIC ANAPLASMOSIS

Anaplasmosis is an infection of human granulocytes with obligate intracellular bacteria, namely *Anaplasma phagocytophilum*. Around 3% to 15% of patients infected with *B. burgdorferi* can also have *A. phagocytophilum* infection transmitted by the same tick bite.[48] White-footed mice are the primary reservoir in the endemic regions. In patients diagnosed with Lyme disease, the presence of leukopenia, thrombocytopenia, and mild-to-moderate elevation in hepatic transaminases suggests coinfection with anaplasmosis. Leukopenia is a common feature and may be either due to lymphopenia or neutropenia, depending on the stage of infection. If untreated, patients may progress to severe disease with multiorgan dysfunction and septic shock physiology. Fortunately,

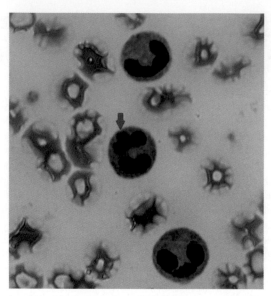

Fig. 15.4   Anaplasmosis: Peripheral smear showing intracellular inclusion (arrow).

oral doxycycline commonly used for the treatment of Lyme disease is effective against *A. phagocytophilum*. The other first-line Lyme antibiotics (amoxicillin and cefuroxime) are not effective, and persistent fever beyond 48 hours should prompt evaluation for coinfections. In endemic regions, febrile illness associated with leukopenia and thrombocytopenia with mild elevation of hepatic transaminases during summer or spring are highly suggestive of human granulocytic anaplasmosis (HGA), and prompt antibiotic treatment should be initiated without waiting for confirmatory diagnostic evaluation. Peripheral blood smear may show intracellular inclusions in the granulocyte but lack sensitivity (Fig. 15.4). It takes 2 to 3 weeks for the development of specific antibodies against the infecting organism. Initial ELISA or indirect fluorescent antibody (IFA) test may be negative. A fourfold rise in titer between acute and convalescent IFA is diagnostic of infection. Some laboratories may also offer PCR-based molecular tests for the detection of coinfections. Oral doxycycline 100 mg twice daily for 10 days is the recommended regimen for adults[26] (Table 15.3). Potential benefits of doxycycline exceed the risk of dental staining, and the American Academy of Pediatrics (AAP) recommends its use for patients less than 8 years of age.[49] The use of tetracycline in pregnant women has been associated with maternal hepatotoxicity and adverse effects on fetal bone and teeth development. However, the benefits of doxycycline use outweigh risks for the treatment of HGA in pregnant women.

BABESIOSIS

Babesiosis is another common coinfection of Lyme disease, especially in the northeastern part of the United States. The causative pathogen is an intraerythrocytic parasite, *B. microti*. Patients usually present with febrile illness and anemia. Additional testing may show evidence of intravascular hemolysis such as anemia, increased red blood cell distribution width, increased reticulocyte count, high level of serum indirect bilirubin, elevated lactose dehydrogenase, and low serum haptoglobin. Peripheral blood smear may show intraerythrocytic parasite forms (Fig. 15.5). In patients with asplenia and/or immunosuppressive conditions, severe disease with high-grade parasitemia, severe intravascular hemolysis, dark-colored urine, and multiorgan dysfunction may

TABLE 15.3 ■ **Antibiotic Regimens for Other Common Vector-Borne Infections in the United States**

Disease	Common Clinical Presentations	Treatment
Anaplasmosis	Febrile illness, leukopenia, thrombocytopenia, mild elevation in hepatic transaminases	Oral doxycycline 100 mg twice daily for 10–14 days
Babesiosis	Febrile illness, intravascular hemolytic anemia, jaundice, dark-colored urine, severe life-threatening illness in asplenic patients	• Oral atovaquone 750 mg twice daily plus azithromycin (initial 500 mg followed by 250 mg daily) for 7–10 days • Oral clindamycin 600 mg three times daily plus quinine 650 mg three times daily for 7–10 days
Ehrlichiosis	Febrile illness, leukopenia, thrombocytopenia, mild elevation in hepatic transaminases	Oral doxycycline 100 mg twice daily for 5–7 days
Rocky Mountain Spotted Fever	Febrile illness, rash that spreads from periphery (wrists, ankles including palms, soles) to trunk, fatal illness if not treated promptly	Oral doxycycline 100 mg twice daily for 5–7 days
Tularemia	Febrile illness, skin ulcer at the site of bite with regional lymphadenopathy	IV streptomycin for 10 days (alternatives include IV gentamycin, oral tetracyclines)
West Nile Virus Infection	Majority are asymptomatic, febrile illness in approximately 20%, meningitis in less than 1%	Supportive care

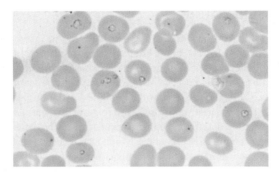

Fig. 15.5 Babesiosis: Peripheral smear showing intraerythrocytic parasitic form.

be present.[50] None of the first-line antibiotic regimens used for Lyme disease are effective for babesiosis. A combination of oral azithromycin and atovaquone for 7 to 10 days is the preferred antimicrobial regimen.[26] Patients with a high degree of parasitemia may benefit from exchange transfusion aimed at removing infected red blood cells. Parasitemia may be prolonged for several weeks in asplenic patients and require a longer course of antimicrobial therapy.

Other Uncommon Tick-Borne Infections in the United States

HUMAN MONOCYTIC EHRLICHIOSIS

The clinical presentation of human monocytic ehrlichiosis (HME) is similar to that of anaplasmosis (HGA).[51] *Ehrlichia chaffeensis* is an obligate intracellular bacterium that primarily infects the monocytes. It is transmitted by the Lone Star tick, *Amblyomma americanum*, and the white-tail deer is the principal animal reservoir. In the United States, it is endemic in the southeastern, southcentral, and Mid-Atlantic regions. The treatment regimen is the same as that of anaplasmosis, and doxycycline is the preferred agent.[26]

ROCKY MOUNTAIN SPOTTED FEVER

Rocky Mountain spotted fever (RMSF) is a tick-borne infection caused by an intracellular bacterium, *Rickettsia rickettssi*.[52] It is transmitted mainly by American dog ticks *(Dermacentor variabilis)* and Rocky Mountain wood ticks *(Dermacentor andersoni)*. The majority of cases occur in the summer months in the southwestern region of the United States. The clinical presentation may be indistinguishable from ehrlichiosis in the first few days followed by appearance of a skin rash. The classic rash is erythematous macules that start in the wrist and ankles, spread inward to the truck, and involve the palms and soles. If doxycycline is not initiated promptly, the clinical picture deteriorates rapidly to multiorgan failure, pulmonary edema, acute respiratory distress syndrome, limb necrosis, and cerebral edema with a high fatality rate. Antibiotic therapy should begin with initial clinical suspicion, as delay increases the mortality rate.[52] A fourfold rise in convalescent antibody titer is diagnostic, but does not help timely diagnosis. Doxycycline is the drug of choice in adults, pregnant women, and children, as the use of alternative antibiotics has been associated with high mortality rates.

Mosquito-Borne Infections in the United States

WEST NILE VIRUS INFECTION

In the continental United States, the most common mosquito-borne infection is due to West Nile virus (WNV). The initial case of WNV in the United States was discovered in 1999, and the virus has spread to all 48 contiguous states. WNV also infects a variety of birds, and sightings of dead birds may be the initial sign of the onset of WNV season. Most patients with WNV infection are asymptomatic, and only about 20% develop febrile illness with nonspecific symptoms such as headache, arthralgias, body ache, gastrointestinal symptoms, and/or maculopapular rash.[53] Severe manifestations such as viral meningitis, encephalitis, and acute flaccid paralysis occur in less than 1% of infected patients. CSF analysis may show lymphocytic pleocytosis in patients with meningitis. MRI brain may show abnormalities in patients with encephalitis, but findings are nonspecific. Detection of WNV-specific immunoglobulin M (IgM) antibodies in serum and/or CSF supports the diagnosis. Plaque-reduction neutralization tests are more specific and are available in reference laboratories. No specific drug has shown to be beneficial, and treatment is generally supportive care. Even though patients with WNV febrile illness improve spontaneously, recovery from severe infection involving the nervous system may take months with residual deficits.[54] No vaccine is available, and the main preventive measures include mosquito control and avoidance.

Travel-Related Vector-Borne Infections

Global travel has become much easier in the past decades, and more Americans travel to regions of the world where they may be exposed to vector-borne infections that are rarely seen in the United States (Table 15.4). Primary care physicians will play an increasing role in providing pretravel counseling, vaccinations, and prophylactic medications to ensure the safety and health of their patients during their travel. Mosquitoes are the most common vectors that transmit the majority of travel-related infections such as malaria, yellow fever, Japanese encephalitis, dengue, chikungunya, and Zika virus infections.

TABLE 15.4 ■ Vector-Borne Infections Related to Global Travel

Disease	Pathogen	Vector	Risk Areas	Common Clinical Presentations	Preventive Measures
Malaria	Plasmodium falciparum, P. ovale, P. vivax, P. malariae, P. knowlessi	Female Anopheles mosquito	West Africa, Asia, South America	Febrile illness, severe cerebral malaria with P. falciparum, Relapse in P. ovale and P. vivax	• Nighttime mosquito bite prevention • No vaccine available • Chemoprophylaxis depending on itinerary
Yellow Fever	Yellow fever virus (flavivirus)	Aedes aegypti	South America, sub-Saharan Africa	Febrile illness, jaundice, severe liver disease, bleeding	• Daytime mosquito bite prevention • Live-attenuated vaccine that provides lifelong immunity
Dengue	Dengue virus (flavivirus)	Aedes aegypti	Urban parts of Asia, South America, sub-Saharan Africa	Febrile illness, possible severe illness with thrombocytopenia and bleeding	• Daytime mosquito bite prevention • No vaccine or chemoprophylaxis available
Chikungunya	Chikungunya virus (alphavirus)	Aedes aegypti	Urban parts of Asia, sub-Saharan Africa	Febrile illness, severe arthralgia ("that which bends up")	• Mosquito bite prevention • No vaccine or chemoprophylaxis available
Zika	Zika virus (flavivirus)	Aedes aegypti	South America, Central America	Febrile illness, infection during pregnancy may cause microcephaly	• Daytime mosquito bite prevention • No vaccine or chemoprophylaxis available
Chagas Disease	Trypanosoma cruzi	Kissing bug (triatomine)	Rural parts of South America, Central America, Mexico	Acute febrile illness, chronic dilated cardiomyopathy, chronic dilated esophagus	• Insect bite prevention • No vaccine or chemoprophylaxis available
African Sleeping Sickness	Trypanosoma brucei	Tsetse flies	Sub-Saharan Africa	Acute febrile illness, subacute or chronic central nervous system manifestations	• Insect bite prevention • No vaccine or chemoprophylaxis available
African Tick Bite Fever	Rickettsia africae	African Tick	Sub-Saharan Africa	Second most common cause of febrile illness among travelers to sub-Saharan Africa	• Insect bite prevention • No vaccine or chemoprophylaxis available
Japanese Encephalitis	Japanese Encephalitis virus (flavivirus)	Culex species mosquito	Rural parts of Asia	Febrile illness, encephalitis	• Mosquito bite prevention • Live-attenuated vaccine for travelers spending more than one month in at-risk rural areas

MALARIA

Malaria is a parasitic infection caused by *Plasmodium* species, transmitted by female *Anopheles* mosquitoes. Female *Anopheles* mosquitoes bite only from dusk to dawn, and the risk of malaria transmission is mainly during the nighttime. Five species *(P. falciparum, P. vivax, P. ovale, P. malariae, P. knowlessi)* are known to cause infection in humans. The risk of malaria infection is highest among travelers to West Africa, followed by those to the Indian subcontinent and South America.[55] *P. falciparum* is most common in West Africa and can cause severe illness, including cerebral malaria, that may be life-threatening if not appropriately treated.[56] *P. vivax* and *P. ovale* have a clinically silent hypnozoite phase in the liver and can cause a relapsing illness several months to years after the initial infection.[57] Avoidance of mosquitoes is the most important preventive measure that travelers can take to protect themselves. Wearing protective permethrin-treated clothing with minimal skin exposure, mosquito repellants such as DEET (*N,N*-diethyl-3-meta-toluamide), and sleeping in air-conditioned rooms or permethrin-treated bed nets are recommended to prevent mosquito bites. No effective malaria vaccine is available for travelers. Chemoprophylaxis for malaria prevention is recommended to travelers based on their travel itinerary and the risk of malaria acquisition. The CDC Traveler's Health website is a good resource that provides country-specific malaria distribution maps and can help clinicians determine if chemoprophylaxis is warranted. For most travelers spending less than 3 weeks in a malaria-endemic region, a daily oral atovaquone–proguanil regimen, initiated 2 days before travel and continued for 7 days after leaving the endemic region, is the most preferred regimen with a low risk of adverse effects.[58] Alternative regimens include daily oral doxycycline or weekly mefloquine, but they are limited by their adverse effect profile. It should be noted that the chemoprophylaxis regimens do not kill the dormant forms of *P. vivax* and *P. ovale*. Relapse may occur several months later despite chemoprophylaxis, and malaria should be considered for any febrile illness after travel to endemic regions.[59]

YELLOW FEVER

Yellow fever is a virus infection transmitted by *Aedes* mosquitoes with the highest risk of transmission in tropical/subtropical parts of South America and sub-Saharan Africa. It usually presents as fever, myalgia, and body ache but can cause jaundice, severe liver disease, and bleeding. There is no curative medical treatment, and thus prevention is important. In addition to mosquito-bite prevention measures, an effective and safe vaccine is available. Yellow fever vaccine is a live-attenuated virus vaccine that is available in travel medicine clinics and CDC-designated vaccination clinics. Yellow fever vaccine is safe but can cause rare, severe reactions such as anaphylaxis, encephalitis, meningitis, organomegaly, and Guillain–Barré syndrome. The risk is estimated to be around 1 per 250,000 vaccinations and is highest among those who are above 60 years of age. Careful analysis of the risk–benefit ratio based on travel itinerary and host factors is important.[60] Booster doses of yellow fever vaccine is no longer recommended, as a single dose appears to produce long-lasting immunity with more than 80% of vaccine recipients having virus-neutralizing antibodies at 20 years.[61] Certain countries may require mandatory yellow fever vaccination for travelers.

JAPANESE ENCEPHALITIS

Japanese encephalitis (JE) is a serious infection involving the CNS caused by JE virus, transmitted by *Aedes* mosquitoes. It is endemic in rice-producing rural parts of Southeast Asia. The risk of acquisition of JE for tourists during their travel to urban areas or short travel to rural parts of Asia is low.[62] An inactivated Vero-cell culture JE vaccine is available and is recommended only for those who plan to stay longer than 1 month in rural areas during the transmission season.

OTHER MOSQUITO-BORNE INFECTIONS

Dengue is a systemic viral febrile infection transmitted by *Aedes* mosquitoes that is endemic in tropical and subtropical regions. Transmission occurs in crowded urban centers during the daytime, as *Aedes* mosquitoes bite during the day. No dengue vaccine is commercially available for US travelers, and avoidance of mosquito bites is the key preventive measure.[63] Other mosquito-borne viral infections with similar clinical presentations include chikungunya and Zika virus infection. Zika virus infection is an emerging infectious disease that has been associated with an epidemic of newborns with microcephaly in Brazil.[64] Pregnant women and those of reproductive age traveling to areas with active Zika virus transmission should be counseled about the risks of Zika virus infection and its associated complication to the newborn. Guillain–Barré syndrome and other neurologic manifestations have been associated with Zika virus infections in adults. Chikungunya virus infection has been characterized by rare but debilitating arthralgias, and its name is derived from an African word translated as "that which bends up."[65]

OTHER ARTHROPOD VECTOR-BORNE INFECTIONS

Ticks, mites, and fleas can transmit many infections, and insect bite prevention measures are the main available strategy available for travelers. *Rickettsia africae*, transmitted by tick bites, is a common cause of febrile illness among travelers to sub-Saharan Africa.[66] African trypanosomiasis, or African sleeping sickness, is a parasitic infection of the CNS caused by the parasite *Trypanosoma brucei*. It is transmitted by tsetse flies found in rural parts of sub-Saharan Africa.[67] American trypanosomiasis, or Chagas disease, is prevalent in rural parts of Mexico and Central and South America. The causative parasite, *Trypanosoma cruzi*, is transmitted through the feces of an infected kissing bug (triatomine bug). Acute infection may cause nonspecific febrile illness, and about a third of patients may progress to chronic Chagas disease with dilated cardiomegaly and/or dilated esophagus.[68]

Summary

- Vector-borne infections are caused by diverse pathogens transmitted to humans by arthropod vectors during their bloody meal.
- Ticks are the most important vectors in transmitting diseases to humans in the United States, whereas mosquitoes are responsible for the majority of vector-borne infectious diseases worldwide, especially in the tropical and subtropical regions
- In the United States, Lyme disease is the most common tick-borne infection, affecting more than 300,000 people annually.
- Lyme disease is caused by the spirochete, *B. burgdorferi*, transmitted by black-legged deer ticks primarily in the Northeastern and upper Midwestern United States.
- Clinical presentations of Lyme disease often involve multiple organ systems and can be categorized as early localized, early disseminated, and late Lyme disease.
- Appropriate diagnosis and antibiotic treatment during the early stage of Lyme disease are effective and prevent progression of disease to the late stage.
- Early localized Lyme disease is diagnosed clinically based on the appearance of a characteristic erythema migrans rash.
- Two-tier serology testing based on CDC criteria is the recommended initial diagnostic test for patients suspected to have early disseminated Lyme carditis, Lyme meningitis, or late Lyme disease.
- A small but significant proportion of patients may have persistent nonspecific symptoms such as fatigue and memory and cognitive difficulties lasting several months despite appropriate

antibiotic therapy. Multiple studies have shown that prolonged antibiotic therapy has not been beneficial and is instead potentially harmful for these patients with post–Lyme disease syndrome

- In the upper Midwest and Northeast United States, up to a third of patients diagnosed with Lyme disease may have coinfections such as anaplasmosis and/or babesiosis transmitted by the same deer tick bite.
- Depending on the region of endemicity, febrile illness with leukopenia, thrombocytopenia, and mild elevation of hepatic transaminases are suggestive of either anaplasmosis or ehrlichiosis.
- A clinical syndrome of fever, anemia, jaundice, and dark-colored urine and laboratory abnormalities such as increased reticulocyte count, low serum haptoglobin level, and elevated indirect bilirubin that are suggestive of intravascular hemolysis point toward babesiosis, a parasitic infection of red blood cells. Severe life-threatening infection and prolonged parasitemia have been seen in asplenic and other immunosuppressed individuals.
- RMSF is characterized by a petechial rash that spreads from the periphery to the trunk. It is one of the few infections with rash involving the palms and soles. It is a life-threatening illness, and prompt initiation of appropriate antibiotic therapy upon clinical suspicion is necessary, as delay is associated with a high fatality rate.
- WNV is the most common mosquito-borne infection in the United States. It is now prevalent in all 48 contiguous states in the continental United States. Most patients with infection are asymptomatic, and less than 1% develop viral meningitis.
- Unprecedented global travel in recent decades has led to an increasing number of travelers at risk of mosquito-borne infections such as malaria, dengue, Zika, chikungunya, yellow fever, and JE.
- Insect bite avoidance and protective measures are essential for travelers to protect themselves against vector-borne infections, especially for those infections where no effective vaccine or chemoprophylaxis is available.
- Vaccines are available as preventive tool only for yellow fever and JE. Careful risk–benefit analysis based on individual travel itinerary and host factors is essential.
- For malaria prevention, chemoprophylaxis is recommended based on risk of transmission during travel.

Suggested Reading

American Academy of Pediatrics. Lyme disease. In: Kimberlin DW, Brady MT, Jackson MA, Long SS, eds. *Red Book*. 31st ed. Atlanta, GA: Coordinating Center for Health Information and Service, Centers for Disease Control and Prevention; 2018:515.

American Academy of Pediatrics. Tetracyclines. In: Kimberlin DW, Brady MT, Jackson MA, Long SS. SS, eds. *Red Book: 2018 Report of the Committee on Infectious Diseases*. 31st ed. Itasca, IL: American Academy of Pediatrics; 2018:905.

Bakken JS, Krueth J, Wilson-Nordskog C, Tilden RL, Asanovich K, Dumler JS. Clinical and laboratory characteristics of human granulocytic ehrlichiosis. *JAMA*. 1996;275(3):199.

Belongia EA. Epidemiology and impact of coinfections acquired from Ixodes ticks. *Vector Borne Zoonotic Dis*. 2002;2(4):265.

Berende A, ter Hofstede HJ, Vos FJ. Randomized trial of longer-term therapy for symptoms attributed to Lyme disease. *N Engl J Med*. 2016;374(13):1209–1220.

Bern C. Chagas' disease. *N Engl J Med*. 2015;373(5):456.

Boggild AK, Parise ME, Lewis LS, Kain KC. Atovaquone-proguanil: report from the CDC expert meeting on malaria chemoprophylaxis (II). *Am J Trop Med Hyg*. 2007;76(2):208.

Centers for Disease Control and Prevention (CDC). Three sudden cardiac deaths associated with Lyme carditis - United States, November 2012-July 2013. *MMWR Morb Mortal Wkly Rep*. 2013;62(49): 993–996.

Chapman AS, Bakken JS, Folk SM. Diagnosis and management of tickborne rickettsial diseases: Rocky Mountain spotted fever, ehrlichioses, and anaplasmosis--United States: a practical guide for physicians and other health-care and public health professionals. *MMWR Recomm Rep.* 2006;55(RR-4):1.

Chen LH, Wilson ME, Schlagenhauf P. Controversies and misconceptions in malaria chemoprophylaxis for travelers. *JAMA.* 2007;297(20):2251.

Dantas-Torres F. Rocky Mountain spotted fever. *Lancet Infect Dis.* 2007;7(11):724.

Dattwyler RJ, Luft BJ, Kunkel MJ. Ceftriaxone compared with doxycycline for the treatment of acute disseminated Lyme disease. *N Engl J Med.* 1997;337(5):289.

Dattwyler RJ, Volkman DJ, Conaty SM, Platkin SP, Luft BJ. Amoxicillin plus probenecid versus doxycycline for treatment of erythema migrans borreliosis. *Lancet.* 1990;336(8728):1404.

Davis LE, DeBiasi R, Goade DE. West Nile virus neuroinvasive disease. *Ann Neurol.* 2006;60(3):286.

Eisen L, Lane RS. Vectors of Borrelia burgdorferi sensu lato. In: Gray JS, Kahl O, Lane RS, et al., eds. *Lyme Borreliosis Biology, Epidemiology and Control.* Wallingford, Oxfordshire, UK: CABI Publishing; 2002:91.

Feder Jr HM, Johnson BJ, O'Connell S, Shapiro ED, Steere AC, Wormser GP. A critical appraisal of "chronic Lyme disease". *N Engl J Med.* 2007;357(14):1422.

Gotuzzo E, Yactayo S, Córdova E. Efficacy and duration of immunity after yellow fever vaccination: systematic review on the need for a booster every 10 years. *Am J Trop Med Hyg.* 2013;89(3):434.

Guzman MG, Harris E. Dengue. *Lancet.* 2015;385(9966):453–465.

Halperin JJ, Golightly M. Lyme borreliosis in Bell's palsy. Long Island Neuroborreliosis Collaborative Study Group. *Neurology.* 1992;42(7):1268.

Halperin JJ, Shapiro ED, Logigian E. Practice parameter: treatment of nervous system Lyme disease (an evidence-based review): report of the Quality Standards Subcommittee of the American Academy of Neurology. *Neurology.* 2007;69(1):91.

Halperin JJ. Nervous system Lyme disease. *Infect Dis Clin North Am.* 2008;22(2):261.

Hills SL, Griggs AC, Fischer M. Japanese encephalitis in travelers from non-endemic countries, 1973-2008. *Am J Trop Med Hyg.* 2010;82(5):930.

Hinckley AF, Connally NP, Meek JI. Lyme disease testing by large commercial laboratories in the United States. *Clin Infect Dis.* 2014;59(5):676–681.

Hojgaard A, Eisen RJ, Piesman J. Transmission dynamics of Borrelia burgdorferi s.s. during the key third day of feeding by nymphal Ixodes scapularis. *J Med Entomol.* 2008;45(4):732.

Hu LT. In the clinic. Lyme disease. *Ann Intern Med.* 2012;157(3):ITC2-2–ITC2-16.

Hunfeld KP, Ruzic-Sabljic E, Norris DE, Kraiczy P, Strle F. In vitro susceptibility testing of Borrelia burgdorferi sensu lato isolates cultured from patients with erythema migrans before and after antimicrobial chemotherapy. *Antimicrob Agents Chemother.* 2005;49(4):1294.

Klempner MS, Hu LT, Evans J. Two controlled trials of antibiotic treatment in patients with persistent symptoms and a history of Lyme disease. *N Engl J Med.* 2001;345(2):85.

Kostić T, Momčilović S, Perišić ZD. Manifestations of Lyme carditis. *Int J Cardiol.* 2017;232:24–32.

Krupp LB, Hyman LG, Grimson R. Study and treatment of post Lyme disease (STOP-LD): a randomized double masked clinical trial. *Neurology.* 2003;60(12):1923.

Lakos A. CSF findings in Lyme meningitis. *J Infect.* 1992;25(2):155.

Ljøstad U, Skarpaas T, Mygland A. Clinical usefulness of intrathecal antibody testing in acute Lyme neuroborreliosis. *Eur J Neurol.* 2007;14(8):873.

Luft BJ, Dattwyler RJ, Johnson RC. Azithromycin compared with amoxicillin in the treatment of erythema migrans. A double-blind, randomized, controlled trial. *Ann Intern Med.* 1996;124(9):785.

Luger SW, Paparone P, Wormser GP. Comparison of cefuroxime axetil and doxycycline in treatment of patients with early Lyme disease associated with erythema migrans. *Antimicrob Agents Chemother.* 1995;39(3):661.

Mareedu N, Schotthoefer AM, Tompkins J, Hall MC, Fritsche TR, Frost HM. Risk factors for severe infection, hospitalization, and prolonged antimicrobial therapy in patients with babesiosis. *Am J Trop Med Hyg.* 2017;97(4):1218.

Marzec NS, Nelson C, Waldron PR. Serious bacterial infections acquired during treatment of patients given a diagnosis of chronic Lyme disease—United States. *MMWR Morb Mortal Wkly Rep.* 2017;66(23):607.

McAlister HF, Klementowicz PT, Andrews C, Fisher JD, Feld M, Furman S. Lyme carditis: an important cause of reversible heart block. *Ann Intern Med.* 1989;110(5):339.

Mlakar J, Korva M, Tul N. Zika virus associated with microcephaly. *N Engl J Med*. 2016;374(10):951.

Monath TP. Review of the risks and benefits of yellow fever vaccination including some new analyses. *Expert Rev Vaccines*. 2012;11(4):427–448.

Mullegger RR. Dermatological manifestations of Lyme borreliosis. *Eur J Dermatol*. 2004;14(5):296.

Mung'Ala-Odera V, Snow RW, Newton CR. The burden of the neurocognitive impairment associated with Plasmodium falciparum malaria in sub-Saharan Africa. *Am J Trop Med Hyg*. 2004;71(suppl 2):64.

Nadelman RB, Luger SW, Frank E, Wisniewski M, Collins JJ, Wormser GP. Comparison of cefuroxime axetil and doxycycline in the treatment of early Lyme disease. *Ann Intern Med*. 1992;117(4):273.

Nadelman RB, Nowakowski J, Forseter G. The clinical spectrum of early Lyme borreliosis in patients with culture-confirmed erythema migrans. *Am J Med*. 1996;100(5):502.

Nelson CA, Saha S, Kugeler KJ. Incidence of clinician-diagnosed Lyme disease, United States, 2005-2010. *Emerg Infect Dis*. 2015;21(9):1625–1631.

Nocton JJ, Bloom BJ, Rutledge BJ. Detection of Borrelia burgdorferi DNA by polymerase chain reaction in cerebrospinal fluid in Lyme neuroborreliosis. *J Infect Dis*. 1996;174(3):623.

Nocton JJ, Dressler F, Rutledge BJ, Rys PN, Persing DH, Steere AC. Detection of Borrelia burgdorferi DNA by polymerase chain reaction in synovial fluid from patients with Lyme arthritis. *N Engl J Med*. 1994;330(4):229.

Nowakowski J, McKenna D, Nadelman RB. Failure of treatment with cephalexin for Lyme disease. *Arch Fam Med*. 2000;9(6):563.

Nowakowski J, Schwartz I, Liveris D. Laboratory diagnostic techniques for patients with early Lyme disease associated with erythema migrans: a comparison of different techniques. *Clin Infect Dis*. 2001;33(12):2023.

Oschmann P, Dorndorf W, Hornig C, Schäfer C, Wellensiek HJ, Pflughaupt KW. Stages and syndromes of neuroborreliosis. *J Neurol*. 1998;245(5):262.

Prusinski MA, Kokas JE, Hukey KT, Kogut SJ, Lee J, Backenson PB. Prevalence of Borrelia burgdorferi (Spirochaetales: Spirochaetaceae), Anaplasma phagocytophilum (Rickettsiales: Anaplasmataceae), and Babesia microti (Piroplasmida: Babesiidae) in Ixodes scapularis (Acari: Ixodidae) collected from recreational lands in the Hudson Valley Region, New York State. *J Med Entomol*. 2014;51(1):226.

Puius YA, Kalish RA. Lyme arthritis: Pathogenesis, clinical presentation, and management. *Infect Dis Clin North Am*. 2008;22(2):289.

Raoult D, Fournier PE, Fenollar F. Rickettsia africae, a tick-borne pathogen in travelers to sub-Saharan Africa. *N Engl J Med*. 2001;344(20):1504.

Rosenberg R, Lindsey NP, Fischer M. Vital signs: Trends in reported vectorborne disease cases - United States and territories, 2004-2016. *MMWR Morb Mortal Wkly Rep*. 2018;67(17):496.

Spielman A. The emergence of Lyme disease and human babesiosis in a changing environment. *Ann NY Acad Sci*. 1994;740:146.

Steere AC, Angelis SM. Therapy for Lyme arthritis: strategies for the treatment of antibiotic-refractory arthritis. *Arthritis Rheum*. 2006;54(10):3079.

Steere AC, Malawista SE, Snydman DR. Lyme arthritis: An epidemic of oligoarticular arthritis in children and adults in three Connecticut communities. *Arthritis Rheum*. 1977;20(1):7.

Steere AC, McHugh G, Damle N, Sikand VK. Prospective study of serologic tests for Lyme disease. *Clin Infect Dis*. 2008;47(2):188.

Steere AC, McHugh G, Suarez C, Hoitt J, Damle N, Sikand VK. Prospective study of coinfection in patients with erythema migrans. *Clin Infect Dis*. 2003;36(8):1078.

Steere AC, Schoen RT, Taylor E. The clinical evolution of Lyme arthritis. *Ann Intern Med*. 1987;107(5):725.

Steere AC, Sikand VK. The presenting manifestations of Lyme disease and the outcomes of treatment. *N Engl J Med*. 2003;348(24):2472.

Steere AC. Lyme disease. *N Engl J Med*. 2001;345(2):115.

Swanson SJ, Neitzel D, Reed KD, Belongia EA. Coinfections acquired from Ixodes ticks. *Clin Microbiol Rev*. 2006;19(4):708.

Urech K, Neumayr A, Blum J. Sleeping sickness in travelers—do they really sleep?. *PLoS Negl Trop Dis*. 2011;5(11):e1358.

Weaver SC, Lecuit M. Chikungunya virus and the global spread of a mosquito-borne disease. *N Engl J Med*. 2015;372(13):1231.

White NJ, Imwong M. Relapse. *Adv Parasitol*. 2012;80:113.

Wilson ME, Weld LH, Boggild A. Fever in returned travelers: results from the GeoSentinel Surveillance Network. *Clin Infect Dis.* 2007;44(12):1560.

Wormser GP, Dattwyler RJ, Shapiro ED. The clinical assessment, treatment, and prevention of Lyme disease, human granulocytic anaplasmosis, and babesiosis: clinical practice guidelines by the Infectious Diseases Society of America. *Clin Infect Dis.* 2006;43(9):1089.

Wormser GP, McKenna D, Carlin J. Brief communication: hematogenous dissemination in early Lyme disease. *Ann Intern Med.* 2005;142(9):751.

Zou S, Foster GA, Dodd RY, Petersen LR, Stramer SL. West Nile fever characteristics among viremic persons identified through blood donor screening. *J Infect Dis.* 2010;202(9):1354.

Sepsis

Micah Beachy ■ Kelly Cawcutt

Introduction

Sepsis is among the oldest medical conditions described, yet remains a leading cause of death. The Centers for Disease Control and Prevention estimate that 1.5 million people in the United States are affected each year, with a resulting 250,000 American deaths annually. For many, if not most, hospitals, sepsis is the main cause of mortality, and in a 2016 report contributed to $24 billion in annual costs (AHRQ-HC cost and utilization project; June 2016). From a global perspective, sepsis affects over 30 million people each year, with over 5 million deaths. For these reasons, it is imperative that sepsis be recognized early and treated as a medical emergency.

All providers will encounter patients with sepsis, regardless of their practice site or clinical focus; thus it is important for everyone to have an understanding of sepsis. How patients present with sepsis varies depending on age, and for the purposes of this review, pediatric patients will be excluded.

Epidemiology of Sepsis

The incidence of sepsis has increased over the last several decades. This is presumed to be secondary to increased rates of detection and diagnosis, aging populations, high numbers of patients who are immunocompromised, and use of more invasive and foreign medical devices (e.g., cardiovascular implantable electronic devices, ventricular assist devices, vascular catheters, prosthetic heart valves).

Seasonal variation of sepsis has also been described, with increased prevalence in the winter months, presumably due to influenza and other respiratory infections. Respiratory infections are the leading cause of sepsis throughout the year. Gram-positive organisms remain the primary pathogens, but Gram-negative organisms contribute a significant proportion of identified causes of sepsis. Fungi have continued to rise in incidence, possibly related to the increasing numbers of immunocompromised patients. Finally, a significant percentage of sepsis cases—between approximately 25% and 50%—have no pathogen identified and are therefore deemed to be culture-negative sepsis cases.

Pathophysiology and Definitions of Sepsis

Sepsis has long been considered the body's dysregulated host response to infection. During a 1992 consensus conference the phrase *systemic inflammatory response syndrome (SIRS)* was coined to refer to activation of the immune system, regardless of cause, hypothesizing that SIRS could be triggered by infection, trauma, or other inflammatory processes like pancreatitis. Thus early definitions of sepsis focused on the presence of two or more SIRS criteria in the setting of infection. Patients with sepsis plus organ dysfunction, evidence of hypoperfusion, or hypotension were defined as having severe sepsis, whereas septic shock was defined as persistent hypotension despite adequate fluid resuscitation. These sepsis syndrome definitions remained in place essentially unchanged until recently (2001 international sepsis definitions conference) (Table 16.1).

This all changed in 2016 with the publication of a task force's proposed revisions to the consensus definition. The task force was convened by two critical care societies to develop updated definitions to better reflect the advancements in the understanding of sepsis pathophysiology along with a desire to differentiate sepsis from uncomplicated infection. Noting that SIRS criteria did not necessarily indicate a dysregulated host response to infection and that many hospitalized patients have SIRS criteria who never develop infection, the task force determined that the inclusion of SIRS into the sepsis definition was unhelpful (i.e., SIRS + infection = sepsis). Instead, the task force elected to focus the new sepsis definition on patients already suspected of being infected. This infected population would be defined as sepsis if they had life-threatening organ dysfunction caused by a dysregulated host response to their infection. Additionally, the term *severe sepsis* was eliminated by the task force and septic shock was considered a subset of sepsis with profound circulatory or metabolic dysfunction associated with higher risk of mortality (JAMA sepsis 3). Table 16.2 compares old sepsis definitions with new ones. To reduce confusion throughout the remainder of this review, the term *sepsis 3* or *septic shock 3* will be utilized when referring to the new definitions. The new sepsis 3 definitions better reflect this pathophysiology along with pertinent clinical criteria for diagnosis.

TABLE 16.1 ■ **SIRS Criteria**

Two or More Of:
Temperature >38° C or <36° C
Heart rate >90/min
Respiratory rate >20/min or $PaCO_2$ <32 mmHg
White blood cell count >12,000/mm^3 or <4000/mm^3 or >10% immature band

TABLE 16.2 ■ **Comparison of Old and New Sepsis Definitions**

Old Sepsis 2 Definitions	New Sepsis 3 Definitions
SIRS • Two or more SIRS criteria	**SIRS** • Not included
Sepsis • SIRS *plus* • Suspected or confirmed infection	**Infection** • Suspected/confirmed infection without end-organ dysfunction
Severe Sepsis • Sepsis *plus* • End-organ dysfunction	**Sepsis 3** • Life-threatening organ dysfunction caused by dysregulated host response to infection
Septic Shock • Severe sepsis with persistent hypotension despite adequate fluid challenge *or* vasopressor support required	**Septic Shock 3** • Sepsis with circulatory and cellular/metabolic dysfunction associated with higher risk of mortality

The bottom line on definitions is that all definitions are still relevant. The Centers for Medicare and Medicaid Services (CMS) continues to utilize SIRS in their definition; thus administratively, the old definitions remain important. Hopefully, CMS will change to the new definitions in the future. Until that time, clinical practice and research will often utilize the newer definitions, given the increased simplicity and objectivity of the criteria.

With any infection, the host has a complex response, including proinflammatory and antiinflammatory cascades; activation of multiple immune cells, including macrophages and neutrophils; and normally remains regulated and does not harm a host. In sepsis 3, there is a dysregulated host response, which includes immune system dysregulation with sepsis-induced inflammation resulting in host injury via cellular damage and apoptosis leading to both organ failure and secondary immunosuppression. The immunosuppression of sepsis 3 is marked by lymphopenia that evolves within the first few days and predisposes patients to an increased risk of secondary infections.

Despite the emergence of sepsis 3, competing definitions remain, primarily in the form of the sepsis core measure. Due to the significant impact sepsis has had across the United States, CMS established the SEP-1 core measure in 2015, with its unique set of definitions for severe sepsis and septic shock. These definitions were developed to retrospectively monitor adherence to bundled sepsis treatment, hoping to highlight areas of opportunity for hospitals. The CMS severe sepsis definition is based on provider documentation of severe sepsis or the clinical criteria of SIRS, documentation of infection, and new organ dysfunction. The definition of septic shock is similar to severe sepsis, with the addition of either initial lactate ≥4.0 or persistent hypotension after fluid resuscitation (Table 16.3).

Screening and Diagnosis

To obtain optimal outcomes, sepsis should be recognized and treated promptly. Hence, a systematic screening process to identify patients at the earliest opportunity is key. Screening for sepsis should focus on evaluating signs and symptoms suggestive of underlying infection (e.g., dysuria, erythema, hypoxia). SIRS criteria may be part of this evaluation; however, it is important to remember that these criteria are also present in a variety of noninfectious disease conditions. Conversely, infection can be present without a patient manifesting SIRS criteria. This variable presence of SIRS during infection is the main reason it was removed as a criterion from sepsis 3 by the task force. Thus it is important to consider SIRS in the context of the overall clinical picture.

Once a clinician has concern for underlying infection, evaluation should commence to confirm or exclude the presence of infection with laboratory and/or diagnostic testing targeted at the source.

TABLE 16.3 ■ Severe Sepsis vs. Sepsis Shock

CMS: Severe Sepsis	CMS: Septic Shock

Clinical criteria (each within 6 hours of each other)
1. SIRS criteria (two or more)
2. Documentation of suspected/known infection
3. New organ dysfunction
	Clinical criteria (each within 6 hours of each other)
	1. SIRS criteria (two or more)
	2. Documentation of suspected/known infection
	3. New organ dysfunction
	4. Either:
	   a. Initial lactate ≥4.0
	   or
	   b. Persistent hypotension in the hour after 30 mL/kg of crystalloid fluids are complete

OR	OR
Provider documentation 1. Provider documents suspected, possible, or ruled-out severe sepsis	Provider documentation 1. Provider documents suspected, possible, or ruled-out septic shock

Determining the presumed source of infection is critical and often must be completed before obtaining laboratory or imaging results. A systematic approach to assessing for infection is recommended and includes a discussion with the patient about infection-related symptoms (e.g., fever, dysuria, diarrhea) and a head-to-toe examination, paying close attention to findings suggestive of underlying infection (e.g., erythema of a permanent pacemaker pocket, swollen tissue of a prosthetic joint, indwelling vascular catheters). A more detailed guide to a systematic infection assessment, including pertinent signs and symptoms that support empiric treatment, and useful laboratory and imaging screening results to support the concern for infection are included in Table 16.4. Blood cultures and other culture sites should be obtained before initiating antimicrobial therapy, unless doing so would significantly delay the start of antimicrobial therapy; otherwise, they should be obtained as soon as possible after the start of this therapy. Diagnostic testing has also evolved over recent years to include many rapid diagnostic methods for early identification of pathogens, such as antigen tests and polymerase chain reaction, including panels to identify pathogens causing meningitis, respiratory infections, bloodstream infections, and gastrointestinal infections, among others.

Despite adequate screening, however, the diagnosis of sepsis can be difficult in patients with multiple comorbidities and in those presenting in states of mixed shock.

With the advent of the electronic medical record and increasingly intelligent systems, automated screening tools and clinical decision-making support systems are evolving for sepsis with hopes of improving the rapidity, sensitivity, and specificity of sepsis detection and optimizing early management. Additionally, concurrent with technologic advances, there is increased assessment of biomarkers that may allow detection of sepsis before the onset of clinical symptoms.

Interventions for "Front-Line" Clinicians: Treatment Approaches and Trends

Sepsis is a medical emergency; thus time is of the essence. The complexities of sepsis management have been provided in various guidelines that are published both domestically and abroad and will not be delineated fully in this chapter. Key elements for primary care clinicians will be addressed, however, as delays in diagnosis and early resuscitation result in excess mortality. Early treatment of sepsis includes fluid resuscitation for those with an elevated lactate, evidence of end-organ dysfunction, or frank hypotension. Crystalloids (primarily normal saline and lactated Ringer) remain the recommended intravenous fluid of choice, with an initial target volume of 30 mL/kg for resuscitation per guideline recommendations, with additional fluid as needed if the patient is clinically determined to remain fluid responsive. The ideal amount of intravenous fluid must be individualized, and for those who remain hypotensive despite adequate fluid resuscitation, vasopressors should be initiated. Norepinephrine remains the vasopressor of choice for all patients presenting with septic shock.

Treatment with empiric antimicrobial agents based on the presumed source and potential pathogens of sepsis is critical. Guidelines recommend that antimicrobial agents be given within the first 60 minutes from the time of sepsis diagnosis. Once the site of infection, pathogen(s), and antimicrobial susceptibilities are known, antimicrobial therapy should be revised to specifically target the pathogen, with adequate tissue/fluid penetration of the infected site, to reduce the risk of potential adverse drug events secondary to antimicrobial therapy, such as acute kidney injury, *Clostridium difficile* infection, cytopenias, and emergence of multidrug-resistant pathogens. Equally, if a nonsepsis or noninfection-based diagnosis is confirmed, such as cardiogenic shock secondary to myocardial infarction, and no infection exists, antimicrobial agents should be discontinued promptly.

Antimicrobial administration is not the only management consideration in sepsis. Source control must be considered early and is the systematic approach to determine the site of infection and whether debridement, amputation, or other action is required. Additional examples of source control include removal of an infected central venous catheter, cholecystectomy for cholecystitis,

TABLE 16.4 ■ Systematic Infection Assessment

Source of Infection	Symptoms and Signs	Laboratory/Imaging	Other Information
Skin, soft tissue, or bone infection	• Examination is key. • Look for increasing redness, pain, tenderness, purulent drainage. • Examine all the skin if possible. • Look for surgical scars or swelling that may indicate septic arthritis or prosthetic joint infection	• WBC may or may not be elevated • PCT not useful • Imaging rarely useful unless severe infection	• Chronic ulcers should be examined and only considered a source of infection if there are clear signs of infection
Urinary tract infection (UTI)	• New onset • Lower UTI – dysuria, frequency, urgency, suprapubic pain, • Upper/pyelo – flank pain, CVA tenderness, nausea/vomiting	• Obtain urine microscopy • WBC <10 has high negative predictive value for infection • PCT not useful	• Do not treat patients without symptoms! • It is rare to have a UTI with single symptoms such as frequency or urgency alone.
Pneumonia	• Worsening • Cough, SOB, sputum production, chest pain, hypoxia	• Need to have infiltrate (exceedingly rare to have pneumonia "bloom") • PCT values <0.25 strong evidence against bacterial infection	• Evaluate for what kind of pneumonia (community acquired vs. health care associated vs. hospital acquired)
Intraabdominal infection	• Pain, nausea, vomiting. • Examination is key, especially serial examinations. • Look for increasing tenderness, guarding, rebound.	• WBC may or may not be elevated • PCT not as useful • Seriously consider CT if concern	• Patients with recent intraabdominal surgery are high risk
Intravascular catheter infection	• Intravascular catheter may look completely normal • Redness, tenderness, drainage at catheter site	• Obtain BCX from line and periphery • PCT typically elevated with bloodstream infection	• If tunnel tract infection, remove immediately
Meningitis	• Headache, neck stiffness, photophobia, mental status change, nausea/vomiting	• Lumbar puncture immediately • PCT elevated with bacterial infection	• If delay in diagnostic studies is anticipated, get BCX and start antibiotics

BCX, Blood culture; *CT,* computed tomography; *CVA,* costovertebral angle; *PCT,* procalcitonin; *SOB,* shortness of breath; *WBC,* white blood cell count (peripheral).

or tube thoracostomy for empyema. Not all sources of infection can be removed or drained, but clinicians must consider these options for all cases of sepsis.

The adoption of bundles by CMS has resulted in reporting of compliance on a national scale, with potential future punitive action for reimbursement if elements of a bundle are not met. Treatment recommendations for early sepsis have been historically bundled into 3- and 6-hour groupings in the Surviving Sepsis Campaign and adopted by CMS (Table 16.5). There is momentum toward a possible 1-hour bundle; therefore clinicians will need to be aware of future updates that may affect the "time-to-treatment" standard of care.

Novel treatment options are evolving, with clinical trials now assessing immunologic therapies and the combination of vitamin C, thiamine, and corticosteroids, although these therapies currently remain investigational. Many of the investigational therapies are targeted at the dysregulated host response to mitigate the risk of organ dysfunction; however, new antimicrobial agents have recently been approved, with more approvals anticipated in the future.

Outcomes

Sepsis results in increased in-hospital morbidity, mortality, and complications. Mortality generally remains >20% despite medical advances in the management of sepsis. Optimizing treatment via implementation of Surviving Sepsis Campaign bundles is associated with decreased mortality, and full compliance with the 3- and 6-hour bundles has resulted in a 40% reduction in in-hospital death.

Prediction of poor outcomes may be enhanced by the discovery of new laboratory findings and biomarkers in sepsis, which may provide insight into the prediction of organ failure, mortality, and immunosuppression, the latter of which may predispose to the risk for secondary infections or episodes of sepsis. For example, sepsis-induced lymphopenia is associated with worse 28-day and 1-year survival. Current literature suggests that the longer the persistence of lymphopenia, the worse the outcome.

With increasing rates of sepsis survival, there is an increasing patient population at risk for hospital readmissions and secondary infections. Sepsis is among the leading causes of hospital readmissions, resulting in increased patient morbidity, mortality, and excess costs for health care. Hospital readmissions after an initial hospitalization for sepsis are common, with approximately 25% being readmitted within 30 days and 48% within 180 days. Patients with medical comorbidities are at a higher risk of hospital readmission. The majority of readmissions are secondary to presumed recurrent or unresolved infections. Over time, there has been a small decrease in hospital readmission for sepsis; however, this comes at the cost of increased postsepsis emergency department visits. Due to the risk of hospital readmissions, close monitoring of patients who survive sepsis is of paramount importance.

Patients who survive sepsis often have long-term complications (mortality, secondary sepsis, hospital readmissions) that last for months to years later, and primary care clinicians should recognize them.

Quality of life may also be an issue after a bout of sepsis. Patients who were admitted to an intensive care unit (ICU) are at risk of post–intensive care syndrome (PICS). PICS is critical to understand for ambulatory care clinicians, as these patients, and often their immediate family

TABLE 16.5 ■ Surviving Sepsis Campaign Bundle

3-Hour Bundle	6-Hour Bundle
Lactate measurement	Repeat the lactate measurement
Obtain blood cultures before administration of antibiotics	Application of vasopressors for persistent hypotension
Give 30 mL/kg of intravenous crystalloid fluid for hypotension	Assessment of ongoing fluid responsiveness (e.g., measurement of central venous pressure, pulse pressure variation, passive leg raise)

members, may suffer from new or worsening cognitive, psychiatric, or physical function. A full discussion of PICS is beyond the scope of this chapter; however, clinicians must be aware of this syndrome to help provide screening and appropriate care to patients for optimal recovery. Some institutions have specific PICS clinics that patients can be referred to, and more information can be found through the Society of Critical Care Medicine's Thrive Initiative, the National Institute for Health and Care Excellence, the Acute Respiratory Distress Syndrome Support Center, and many other sources.

Prevention

Sepsis prevention is critical in decreasing the morbidity, mortality, and excess health care costs. It is noteworthy that in 2017, the World Health Assembly (WHA) included sepsis prevention in the adopted resolution entitled "Improving the Prevention, Diagnosis and Clinical Management of Sepsis." Strategies for prevention of sepsis include vaccinations, food safety screening and education, efficacious outbreak responses, and robust infection prevention programs to limit health care–associated infections. Among these, one of the most simple and powerful mechanisms for preventing sepsis remains hand hygiene, prompting the World Health Organization (WHO) campaign entitled "It's in Your Hands; Prevent Sepsis in Healthcare" in May 2018. Effective antimicrobial stewardship programs have also decreased sepsis, as recent antimicrobial therapy is a risk factor for the development of sepsis. Robust primary care to minimize the risk of infection among those with chronic conditions or high-risk exposures cannot be underestimated as a prevention modality for sepsis. Even preemptive care, such as counseling for smoking cessation, may result in decreased high-risk comorbidities such as cancer requiring immunosuppressive chemotherapy. This includes the concept of "pre-sepsis" management, when patients are treated for infections before the development of sepsis or admission to the hospital. Improvements in outpatient management of infections can augment sepsis by optimizing diagnosis and antimicrobial therapy to prevent evolution to sepsis.

Sepsis has become a public health concern; thus ongoing patient and community education on symptoms suggestive of sepsis, goals of seeking care early with onset of symptoms, and providing adequate resources for access to care must be publicly available. With this public health concern in mind, the CDC developed a national campaign to "Get Ahead of Sepsis" in September 2017, with the subsequent adoption of September as "Sepsis Awareness Month."

Conclusion and Key Points

Sepsis is a leading cause of death.
Clinicians must recognize that sepsis is a medical emergency and must be familiar with recommendations on early recognition and management to hopefully improve outcomes.
Postsepsis survivorship carries risks of physical, cognitive, and psychiatric complications and risks of recurrent sepsis and hospital readmissions.

Suggested Reading

Dantes RB, Epstein L. Combatting sepsis: a public health perspective. *Clin Infect Dis*. 2018;67(8):1300–1302.
De Backer D, Dorman T. Surviving sepsis guidelines: a continuous move toward better care of patients with sepsis. *JAMA*. 2017;317(8):807–808.
Han X, Edelson DP, Snyder A, et al. Implications of centers for medicare & medicaid services severe sepsis and septic shock early management bundle and initial lactate measurement on the management of sepsis. *Chest*. 2018;154(2):302–308.
Harvey MA, Davidson JE. Postintensive care syndrome: right care, right now, and later. *Crit Care Med*. 2016;44(2):381–385.

Mayr FB, Talisa VB, Balakumar V, et al. Proportion and cost of unplanned 30-day readmissions after sepsis compared with other medical conditions. *Jama*. 2017;3175:530–531.

Reinhart K, Daniels R, Kissoon N, Machado FR, Schachter RD, Finfer S. Recognizing sepsis as a global health priority—a WHO resolution. *New Engl J Med*. 2017;3775:414–417.

Rhodes A, Evans LE, Alhazzani W, et al. Surviving Sepsis Campaign: International guidelines for management of sepsis and septic shock: 2016. *Intensive Care Med*. 2017;433:304–377.

Rhodes A, Phillips G, Beale R, et al. The surviving sepsis campaign bundles and outcome: results from the International Multicentre Prevalence Study on Sepsis (the IMPreSS study). *Intensive Care Med*. 2015;419:1620–1628.

CHAPTER 17

Sexually Transmitted Infections

Arlene C. Seña ■ Srilatha Edupuganti

CHAPTER OUTLINE

Introduction

Sexually transmitted infections (STIs) contribute to the majority of reportable communicable diseases worldwide. More than a million STIs are acquired every day worldwide, with an estimated 357 million new infections annually with gonorrhea, chlamydia, syphilis, or trichomoniasis. Furthermore, there are emerging STIs such as *Mycoplasma genitalium* and viral STIs such as genital herpes that are highly prevalent on a global scale. The growing threat of antimicrobial resistance in *Neisseria gonorrhoeae* and *M. genitalium* underscores the need for enhanced public health strategies, novel diagnostics, and therapeutic agents for STIs.

In 2018, the Centers for Disease Control and Prevention (CDC) reported over 1.7 million cases of chlamydial infections, over 580,000 cases of gonococcal infections, and over 115,000 cases of syphilis in the United States. Adolescents and young adults 15 to 24 years of age account for half of the new STIs that occur in the United States each year. African Americans and men who have sex with men (MSM) in the United States are disproportionately affected by STIs, with the highest rates of bacterial STIs among all other racial/ethnic groups and compared with heterosexual persons, respectively.

A practical approach to STIs requires knowledge of the main clinical syndromes in men and women, including urethritis, vaginitis, cervicitis, pelvic inflammatory disease (PID), epididymitis, and genital ulcer disease (GUD)—and their associated pathogens (Table 17.1). Empiric therapy is generally recommended for STI syndromes to prevent sequelae (such as PID and infertility) and transmission to sexual partners. However, targeted therapy based on diagnostic testing is ideal for persons who are asymptomatic, are likely to return for treatment as needed, and/or are at lower risk for complications (e.g., nonpregnant women or persons not infected with human immunodeficiency virus [HIV]).

Adverse outcomes from STIs in pregnant women include premature rupture of membranes (PROM), preterm birth, neonatal ophthalmic infections, neonatal pneumonia, and fetal deaths. In addition to a heightened risk for complications (e.g., neurosyphilis) among HIV coinfected persons, STIs can increase the risk for HIV acquisition and transmission twofold to fivefold.

TABLE 17.1 ■ **Common Sexually Transmitted Syndromes, Infectious Agents, and Diagnostic Testing Options**

Clinical Syndrome	Major Infectious Agents	Diagnostic Testing Options
Urethritis (men)	*Neisseria gonorrhoeae*, *Chlamydia trachomatis*, *Mycoplasma genitalium*, *Trichomonas vaginalis*, herpes simplex virus type 2, adenovirus	*POC tests:* Urethral swab for Gram stain or methylene blue stain for NG and WBCs (nongonococcal urethritis) *NAATs:* Urine or urethral swab for NG/CT, MG, TV; lesion swab for HSV if present
Urethritis (women)	*Neisseria gonorrhoeae*, *Chlamydia trachomatis*, *Trichomonas vaginalis*	*POC tests:* Vaginal swab for TV by wet mount microscopy; vaginal swabs or urine for rapid TV test *Culture:* Vaginal swab for TV, urine for culture (as needed) *NAATs:* Cervical/vaginal swabs or urine for NG/CT, TV Urinalysis and microscopy as needed
Vaginitis	Bacterial vaginosis, *Trichomonas vaginalis, Candida albicans*	*POC tests:* Vaginal swabs for wet mount microscopy for BV, TV, and *Candida*; vaginal swabs for BV Gram stain or sialidase activity (BV); vaginal swabs for TV antigen or helicase dependent amplification tests *Culture:* Vaginal swab for TV *NAATs:* Vaginal swabs for TV
Cervicitis	*Neisseria gonorrhoeae*, *Chlamydia trachomatis*, *Mycoplasma genitalium*, *Trichomonas vaginalis*, herpes simplex virus type 2	*NAATs:* Cervical/vaginal swabs or urine for NG, CT, MG, TV; lesion swab from HSV if present
Pelvic inflammatory disease	*Neisseria gonorrhoeae*, *Chlamydia trachomatis*, anaerobic bacteria	*NAATs:* Cervical/vaginal swabs or urine for NG, CT
Epididymitis	*Neisseria gonorrhoeae*, *Chlamydia trachomatis*	*NAATs:* Urine or urethral swab for NG, CT
Proctitis	*Neisseria gonorrhoeae*, *Chlamydia trachomatis* (including L serovars), *Mycoplasma genitalium*, *Treponema pallidum*, herpes simplex virus types 1 or 2	*POC tests:* Rectal swab for Gram stain *NAATs:* Rectal swabs for NG, CT, HSV Dark-field microscopy and serology: TP
Pharyngitis	*Neisseria gonorrhoeae*, *Chlamydia trachomatis*, herpes simplex virus	*NAATs:* Oral swabs for NG, CT; lesion swab for HSV if present

Continued

TABLE 17.1 ■ Common Sexually Transmitted Syndromes, Infectious Agents, and Diagnostic
Testing Options—cont'd

Clinical Syndrome	Major Infectious Agents	Diagnostic Testing Options
Genital ulcers	Herpes simplex virus types 1 or 2, *Treponema pallidum* (syphilis), *Haemophilus ducreyi* (chancroid), *Chlamydia trachomatis* L serovars: (lymphogranuloma venereum)	*POC tests:* Type-specific serology for HSV *Culture:* Lesion swabs for HSV *NAATs:* Lesion swabs for HSV; lesion or rectal swabs, and lymph node specimens for CT (not FDA cleared, but commercially available) *Dark-field microscopy and serology:* TP *Serology:* CT/LGV
Non-ulcerative genital lesions	Human papillomavirus 6, 11 (genital warts), molluscum contagiosum	Visual inspection Biopsy for lesions that are atypical, have no response to therapy, immunocompromised patients

BV, Bacterial vaginosis; *CT, Chlamydia trachomatis*; *HSV*, herpes simplex virus; *LGV*, lymphogranuloma venereum; *MG, Mycoplasma genitalium*; *NAATs*, nucleic acid amplification tests; *NG, Neisseria gonorrhoeae*; *PCR*, polymerase chain reaction; *POC*, point-of-care tests; *TP, Treponema pallidum*; *TV, Trichomonas vaginalis*; *WBCs,* white blood cells.

The key components of STI management include routinely obtaining sexual history (regardless of age), screening of at-risk individuals, testing of symptomatic persons for definitive diagnosis, initiation of appropriate therapy, and evaluation and treatment of sexual partners. A nonjudgmental approach is important to obtaining a thorough sexual history; clinicians should encourage an open dialogue with patients, with questions regarding sexual practices (Table 17.2). Many individuals with suspected STIs present for initial care at primary care centers, urgent care centers, and emergency departments. Therefore physicians in training and noninfectious disease clinicians can play a vital role in increasing awareness of sexual health issues in their practice, early disease recognition and diagnosis, and optimizing STI management.

Sexually Transmitted Syndromes

URETHRITIS

Urethritis (inflammation of the urethra) in men is typically characterized by urethral discomfort and a penile discharge, which may be clear or mucoid, mucopurulent, or purulent in appearance. Traditionally, urethritis has been differentiated into gonococcal or nongonococcal urethritis (NGU). *N. gonorrhoeae* is most common among men 15 to 24 years of age. *Chlamydia trachomatis, M. genitalium,* and *Trichomonas vaginalis* (trichomoniasis) (see Table 17.2) contribute to approximately 30% to 40%, 25% to 30%, and 10%, respectively, of infections among men with NGU. Less common causes of urethritis include herpes virus simplex-1 (HSV-1), HSV-2, *N. meningitidis,* and adenovirus (especially among MSM).

Urethritis in women may occur with concomitant cervicitis and vaginitis due to gonorrhea, chlamydia, or trichomonas. Urethritis should be differentiated from acute cystitis with laboratory testing, which is associated with abrupt onset of dysuria accompanied by frequency, urgency, suprapubic tenderness, or low back pain.

TABLE 17.2 ■ Key Discussion Points and Questions in a Sexual History

Taking a Sexual History

I am going to ask you a few questions about your sexual health and sexual practices. I understand that these questions are very personal, but they are important for your overall health.

Just so you know, I ask all of my patients these questions, regardless of age, gender, or marital status. Like the rest of your visits, this information is kept in strict confidence. Do you have any questions before we get started?

Sexual Partners

Are you currently sexually active? If no, when were you last sexually active?

In the last 2 months, how many sexual partners have you had?

Are your sexual partners men, women, or both? (If the patient answers "both," repeat the earlier question for both genders)

Sexual Practice

Do you and your partner(s) use any protection against sexually transmitted diseases (STDs)?

If so, what kind of protection do you use?

How often do you use this protection?

Past History of STDs

Have you ever been diagnosed with an STD? When? How were you treated?

Has your current partner or any former partners ever been diagnosed or treated for an STD?

Have you ever been tested for HIV or other STDs? Would you like to be tested?

Additional Questions

Are you or your partner using contraception or practicing any form of birth control?

What other concerns or questions regarding your sexual health or sexual practices would you like to discuss?

Clinical Presentation

Men may report an acute onset of dysuria, penile itching, irritation, or discomfort 2 to 5 days after sexual exposure, followed by a purulent discharge. Although this presentation is more suggestive of gonococcal urethritis, the color of the discharge may be indistinguishable among the bacterial STIs. A history of symptom onset 1 to 3 weeks after an exposure, accompanied by a scant, mucoid discharge is more consistent with chlamydial urethritis. Patients with NGU may report an intermittent discharge or crusting at the meatus. Despite treatment for NGU, a proportion of men will have persistent symptoms. In these patients, it is important to distinguish reinfections due to repeated sexual exposures from treatment failures.

Women with urethritis may present with dysuria, frequency, and lower abdominal pain. Dysuria may be classified as internal or external (due to contact of urine with the inflamed perineum). The symptoms of classic urinary tract infection such as fever, chills, urgency, and hematuria are not a feature of urethritis.

Evaluation and Diagnosis

The male genitourinary examination should include an inspection of the urethral meatus for erythema or visible discharge; if none is evident, the urethra should be milked from the base of the penis to the meatus. If a Gram stain or methylene blue (MB) stain is available as a point-of-care (POC) test, a calcium alginate swab should be used to collect a sample of the penile discharge at the meatus or from within the urethra by inserting a swab 2 to 3 cm into the urethra and then rolling the specimen onto a glass slide.

The presence of urethritis should be confirmed by one or more of the following findings: (1) mucopurulent or purulent discharge (Fig. 17.1); (2) ≥2 white blood cells (WBCs) per oil

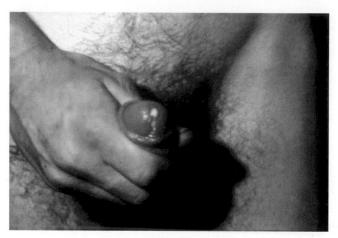

Fig. 17.1   Gonococcal urethritis.

immersion field from a urethral Gram stain or MB stain; and (3) a positive leukocyte esterase test on first-voided urine (the first 10 to 15 mL after voiding) or (4) the presence of ≥10 WBCs per high-power field in the spun sediment. Gonococcal urethritis is diagnosed by the finding of Gram-negative intracellular diplococci in the urethral exudate. NGU is defined by the absence of Gram-negative intracellular diplococci and presence of ≥2 WBCs per oil immersion field.

All men with urethritis should undergo testing for gonorrhea and chlamydia, which are typically combined in nucleic acid amplification tests (NAATs) using a first-void urine sample or a urethral swab (see Table 17.1) (see sections on gonorrhea and chlamydia). Recently, NAATs for detection of trichomonal infections and *M. genitalium* in men have received approval from the US Food and Drug Administration (FDA). Patients should also be screened for syphilis and offered tests for HIV. Among men with persistent or recurrent symptoms despite appropriate therapy, the presence of urethritis should be documented by the objective criteria noted earlier, with repeat STI testing depending on the likelihood of reinfection or treatment failure.

Women with symptoms of urethritis and risk for STIs based on the sexual history should undergo evaluation for vaginitis or cervicitis (see later). POC tests should include testing for trichomoniasis with vaginal swabs for wet mount microcopy or rapid testing (see Table 17.1). A urinalysis may reveal pyuria and a positive leukocyte esterase due to urethral inflammation, whereas a urinalysis in the setting of cystitis should have accompanying nitrites or blood present. Vaginal or cervical swabs should be obtained for gonorrhea, chlamydia, and *T. vaginalis* NAATs if POC tests are not available for the latter (see Table 17.1). In women, NAAT detection for gonorrhea, chlamydia, and trichomonas can be performed from urine, but have lower sensitivities compared with other specimens.

Treatment

Presumptive treatment for symptomatic patients with objective evidence of urethritis is recommended by the CDC to prevent complications and transmission of associated STIs. Targeted therapy based on NAAT results should be considered for individuals with minimal symptoms or those willing to abstain from sex until after diagnosis and treatment.

If gonorrhea is suspected based on the clinical presentation and/or POC tests, treat with ceftriaxone 250 mg as an intramuscular (IM) injection in the deltoid area plus azithromycin 1.0 g orally in a single dose (Table 17.3). Azithromycin is currently considered part of dual therapy for gonorrhea to minimize the development of antimicrobial resistance; however, azithromycin also has activity against *C. trachomatis* and *M. genitalium*. Patients treated with the recommended regimens need not return for a test of cure. However, if patients have persistent symptoms (given there is no

TABLE 17.3 ■ Sexually Transmitted Infection Syndromes and Empiric Therapies

Pathogens	Primary Therapy	Alternative Therapies and Treatment for Recurrences
Urethritis, nongonococcal	Azithromycin 1.0 g PO in single dose OR doxycycline 100 mg PO BID × 7 days	Levofloxacin 500 mg PO in single dose × 7 days OR ofloxacin 300 mg PO BID × 7 days *Persistent NGU:* Moxifloxacin 400 mg PO BID for 7 days PLUS metronidazole 2 g PO in a single dose
Cervicitis	Ceftriaxone 250 mg IM × 1 PLUS azithromycin 1.0 g PO in single dose	
Bacterial vaginosis	Metronidazole 500 mg PO BID × 7 days OR Metrogel 5 g intravaginally once daily for 5 days OR clindamycin cream 5gm intravaginally at bedtime for 7 days	Tinidazole 2 g PO daily for 2 days OR 1 g daily for 5 days OR secnidazole 2 g PO in a single dose OR clindamycin 300 mg PO BID for 7 days *Recurrent BV:* Metronidazole 2 g PO with fluconazole 150 mg PO in a single dose monthly Metrogel 0.75% twice weekly for 4 to 6 months
Pelvic inflammatory disease	*Inpatient therapy:* Cefotetan 2 g IV every 12 hours PLUS doxycycline 100 mg PO or IV every 12 hours OR cefoxitin 2 g IV every 6 hours PLUS doxycycline 100 mg PO or IV every 12 hours OR clindamycin 900 mg IV every 8 hours PLUS gentamicin 2 mg/kg loading dose IV followed by 1.5 mg/kg every 8 hours *Outpatient therapy:* Ceftriaxone 250 mg IM × 1 OR cefoxitin 2 g IM in a single dose and probenecid 1.0 g PO administered concurrently in a single dose PLUS doxycycline 100 mg PO BID × 14 days WITH or WITHOUT metronidazole 500 mg PO BID × 14 days	*Inpatient therapy:* Ampicillin/sulbactam 3 g IV every 6 hours PLUS doxycycline 100 mg orally or IV every 12 hours *Outpatient therapy:* Ceftriaxone 250 mg IM × 1 PLUS azithromycin 1 g PO every week × 2 weeks OR levofloxacin 500 mg PO once daily OR ofloxacin 400 mg twice daily OR moxifloxacin 400 mg orally once daily for 14 days, PLUS metronidazole 500 mg PO BID for 14 days
Epididymitis	Ceftriaxone 250 mg IM × 1 PLUS doxycycline 100 mg PO BID × 10 days	*Therapy for STIs and enteric pathogens:* Ceftriaxone 250 mg IM in a single dose PLUS levofloxacin 500 mg PO once a day for 10 days OR ofloxacin 300 mg PO twice a day for 10 days *Therapy for enteric pathogens:* Levofloxacin 500 mg PO once a day for 10 days OR ofloxacin 300 mg PO twice a day for 10 days
Proctitis	Ceftriaxone 250 mg IM × 1 PLUS doxycycline 100 mg PO BID × 7 days	*Therapy for LGV:* Doxycycline 100 mg PO BID × 3 weeks

BID, Twice a day; *BV,* bacterial vaginosis; *g,* gram; *IM,* intramuscular; *IV,* intravenous; *kg,* kilogram; *LGV,* lymphogranuloma venereum; *mg,* milligram; *NGU,* nongonococcal urethritis; *PO,* per os (oral); *STIs,* sexually transmitted infections.

reexposure), a culture for *N. gonorrhoeae* should be obtained and tested for antibiotic susceptibility. There have been concerns regarding increasing drug resistance among *N. gonorrhoeae* isolates worldwide to available antimicrobials used for treatment, including the fluoroquinolones, which should be avoided for therapy. In the United States, the proportion of gonococcal isolates with resistance to ceftriaxone remains low at <0.5%, but there has been an increase in azithromycin resistance to >4.0%.

For suspected NGU, the recommended therapy is azithromycin 1.0 g orally in a single dose, which provides empiric coverage for both chlamydial and *M. genitalium* infections. Doxycycline for 7 days may be more effective for chlamydial infections than azithromycin, but achieves only 30% cure rates for *M. genitalium*. Men with persistent urethritis should receive therapy with moxifloxacin 400 mg orally once daily for 7 days plus metronidazole 2 g orally in a single dose for presumptive azithromycin-resistant *M. genitalium* and trichomonal infections, respectively (see Table 17.3). Women with urethritis but without symptoms associated with cystitis (e.g., urinary frequency) should receive presumptive therapy for STIs, especially if there are signs or symptoms associated with concomitant vaginitis or cervicitis on evaluation. Patients who have persistent or chronic urethritis despite moxifloxacin therapy should be referred to a urologist or gynecologist for an additional evaluation. The differential diagnosis of bacterial cystitis, prostatitis, epididymitis, and Reiter syndrome should be considered in those individuals.

Management

Patients should be advised to abstain from sex or use condoms until they and their sexual partner(s) have been adequately treated, typically for 7 days after single-dose therapy. There is no need for follow-up unless there are recurrent or persistent symptoms.

Sexual partners of persons with urethritis within the preceding 60 days should be evaluated and treated appropriately as the initial patient. For heterosexual men and women with suspected or confirmed gonococcal infections, expedited partner therapy (EPT) can be offered with cefixime 400 mg and azithromycin 1 g orally in single doses. EPT is permissible in 44 states and the District of Columbia and allows the index patient to deliver therapy to the exposed partners. Written materials should accompany the provision of medications to educate partners about their exposure, the importance of therapy, and when to seek clinical evaluation for adverse reactions or complications. EPT may also be provided to sexual partners of index patients with chlamydial infection with azithromycin 1 g orally in a single dose.

VAGINITIS

An abnormal vaginal discharge may be due to vaginitis or vaginosis, cervicitis, or occasionally endometritis. The three most common causes of vaginal discharge are bacterial vaginosis (BV), vulvovaginal candidiasis (VVC), and trichomoniasis. An abnormal vaginal discharge may also result from cervicitis caused by *N. gonorrhoeae*, *C. trachomatis*, and *M. genitalium* (see Table 17.1). Although controversy remains on whether BV is sexually transmitted, trichomoniasis is one of the most common STIs. VVC is not sexually transmitted, but it is discussed briefly in this section, as it is frequently diagnosed in women with vaginitis.

BV results from a disruption of the normal vaginal flora, which consists primarily of *Lactobacillus* spp., with anaerobes, *Gardnerella vaginalis,* and *Mycoplasma hominis*. Risk factors associated with BV include a history of multiple sexual partners, douching, intrauterine device use, and prior pregnancy. Recurrent BV can occur in 25% to 30% of women due to persistent changes in the normal vaginal microbiome. BV has been known to cause upper genital tract disease, including PID, and has been associated with PROM, preterm labor, preterm birth, low birth weight, chorioamnionitis, and postcaesarean and postpartum endometritis.

T. vaginalis is a protozoan that infects the cervical and vaginal epithelial cells leading to vaginitis and cervicitis. It has also been isolated from the urethra, Bartholin glands, and Skene glands, which surround the vaginal opening and secrete mucus in women. In women, trichomoniasis is also associated with PID, infertility, and adverse pregnancy outcomes, including PROM, premature labor and low-birth-weight infants.

Clinical Presentation

Women with BV usually report an abnormal and malodorous ("fishy smelling") vaginal discharge that may be grayish or white in appearance without any vaginal irritation. Symptoms more suggestive of VVC include vulvar pruritus and vaginal discharge that may appear white, curdlike, or as a thin watery liquid. Women with acute vaginitis due to trichomoniasis may present with a yellow or green vaginal discharge accompanied with pruritus, dysuria, and dyspareunia (persistent or recurrent genital pain with sexual intercourse). A more chronic vaginal discharge due to trichomoniasis can present as scanty vaginal discharge with mild pruritis and dyspareunia.

Evaluation and Diagnosis

Women with symptoms of vaginitis should undergo a pelvic examination to visualize the vaginal mucosa and cervix and to determine the presence of vaginal and/or cervical discharge. The color and consistency of the vaginal discharge and whether it adheres to the vaginal walls should be noted. The vaginal wall and cervix should be inspected for punctate hemorrhages (called *colpitis macularis* or *"strawberry cervix"*) associated with *T. vaginalis*, although this is present in only a minority of women with trichomoniasis.

Vaginal fluid should be assessed for vaginal pH (using a pH strip of the vaginal secretions from the speculum) and presence of a fishy odor characteristic of BV. Vaginal specimens should be collected for POC tests (see Table 17.1) such as wet mount microscopy (WM), if available. A swab is used to collect material from the vaginal fornix and should be placed into 0.5 to 1.0 mL of normal saline. A drop of the saline preparation is placed on a slide and viewed with a microscope.

BV can be diagnosed based on the pelvic examination and WM using the Amsel criteria, which require three of the following: a homogeneous, thin, white discharge that smoothly coats the vaginal walls; "clue cells" (which refers to vaginal epithelial cells studded with adherent coccobacilli on microscopic examination; Fig. 17.2); a pH of vaginal fluid >4.5; and a positive "whiff test," or a fishy odor of vaginal discharge with the addition of 10% potassium hydroxide (KOH) on the vaginal swab or speculum. A vaginal pH >4.5 and a positive "whiff" test upon the addition of KOH may be present in both BV and trichomoniasis; concurrent infections are common in women with vaginitis.

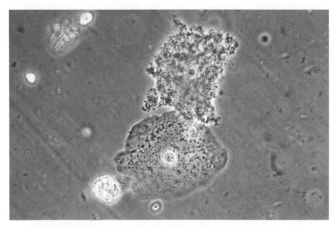

Fig. 17.2 Wet mount microscopy with clue cells.

   Trichomoniasis is diagnosed by identifying the organism on WM; motile trichomonads can be visualized on microscopy with a distinctive asynchronous motion (Fig. 17.3). However, this test is only 50% to 70% sensitive for detection from the vaginal discharge. The diagnosis of VVC can be made by the presence of vaginal erythema; a white, curdlike discharge on pelvic examination; and visualization of yeast and hyphae on WM after staining with 10% KOH.

   Other tests are available for the diagnosis of vaginitis. A Gram stain of the vaginal discharge is the "gold standard" for BV using the Nugent criteria, which is a scoring system of 0 to 10 points based on the most important bacterial morphotypes: lactobacilli, *G. vaginalis*, and *Mobilincus* species (Table 17.4). For *T. vaginalis*, culture can be performed from a vaginal swab specimen. Although culture for trichomoniasis was considered to be the "gold standard," use of this test has been limited since the development of highly sensitive NAATs for *T. vaginalis* using vaginal, cervical, or urine specimens.

   Newer POC tests for BV and trichomoniasis include rapid tests, such as vaginal fluid sialidase activity for BV and *T. vaginalis* antigen tests. Additionally, there are molecular-based assays that can provide results in 45 to 60 minutes. A nucleic acid hybridization test is available that can detect *G. vaginalis*, *Candida albicans*, and *T. vaginalis*, but has poor sensitivity for the latter. A real-time polymerase chain reaction (PCR) to detect the microorganisms responsible for BV, VVC, and trichomoniasis is also available.

Treatment

Metronidazole 500 mg orally twice daily for 7 days is the primary treatment for BV in nonpregnant and pregnant women (see Table 17.3). There is no evidence that the use of metronidazole in the first trimester of pregnancy leads to teratogenic or mutagenic complications. Topical metronidazole or clindamycin regimens are equally efficacious as the oral regimens but are not recommended for pregnant women.

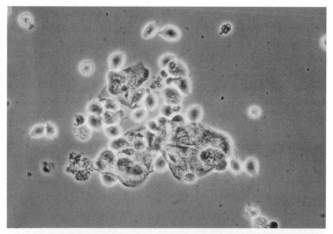

Fig. 17.3   Wet mount microscopy with trichomonads.

TABLE 17.4 ■ **Diagnosis of Bacterial Vaginosis Using Gram Stain and Nugent Score**

Nugent score, based on number of *Lactobacilli*, *Gardnerella*, and *Mobiluncus* spp.	
Score	Interpretation
0–3	Normal flora
4–6	Intermediate flora
7–10	Presence of bacterial vaginosis

Women with trichomoniasis, irrespective of HIV status, should be treated with metroni-dazole for 7 days, as it has demonstrated better cure rates than single-dose therapy (see Table 17.3). However, men with trichomoniasis should be treated empirically with single-dose ther-apy due to lack of data to support extended-dose regimens in this population. Women with VVC can be treated with fluconazole 150 mg orally in a single dose or be advised to use over-the-counter intravaginal products (e.g., clotrimazole or miconazole vaginal creams).

Recurrent BV and VVC are common and may be due to the development of biofilms or communities of resistant microorganisms in the vagina. Intermittent or longer courses of metro-nidazole and antifungal therapies have been shown to reduce recurrent BV and VVC, respectively (see Table 17.3) in some women. Reinfection with trichomoniasis is common, but resistance to metronidazole and tinidazole has been estimated in 5% to 10% and 1% of infections, respectively (see Table 17.3). Some patients may not respond to repeated courses of therapy, including higher doses of metronidazole for an extended course; those cases should be referred to a specialist or managed in consultation with the CDC.

Management

Women with trichomoniasis should abstain from sex or use condoms until they and their sexual partner(s) have been adequately treated. Sexual partners of persons with trichomoniasis within the preceding 60 days should be evaluated and treated. There are no data to support the routine treatment of sexual partners of women with BV or VVC.

Women with persistent or chronic vaginitis should be referred to a gynecologist for further evaluation. Women with recurrent or complicated VVC may need a vaginal culture to evaluate for resistant *Candida* species. For women with suspected metronidazole-resistant trichomoniasis, a consultation should be obtained with the CDC for determination of metronidazole susceptibility testing. Noninfectious causes of vaginal discharge include chemical or irritant vaginitis, trauma, pemphigus, collagen vascular diseases, and Behçet disease.

CERVICITIS

Cervicitis (inflammation of the cervix) may be caused by *N. gonorrhoeae, C. trachomatis, M. genita-lium, T. vaginalis,* and HSV-2 (see Table 17.1). However, most cases have no identifiable etiology. The presence of mucopurulent cervicitis has been used as a basis for presumptive chlamydial or gonococcal infection in settings where the prevalence of these infections is high and the patients are unlikely to return for follow-up. Mucopurulent cervicitis is defined by the presence of a muco-purulent discharge noted from the endocervix, together with friability or easily induced bleeding with the first endocervical swab.

Clinical Presentation

Women with cervicitis may present with an abnormal vaginal discharge, postcoital bleeding, or bleeding between menstrual periods. Women may also report dyspareunia or pain deep within the pelvis with sexual intercourse. The majority of women with chlamydial cervicitis are as-ymptomatic; overall, about 75% to 90% of cervicitis cases are asymptomatic and may persist for years.

Evaluation and Diagnosis

The evaluation should include a pelvic examination with inspection of the vaginal mucosa and cervical opening for erythema, punctate hemorrhages suggestive of trichomoniasis, or ulcerations suggestive of HSV infection. The cervix should be examined for the presence of a mucopurulent discharge and whether the mucosa bleeds easily upon introduction of a swab into the cervical opening (Fig. 17.4). The examination should also assess for cervical motion, as well as uterine or

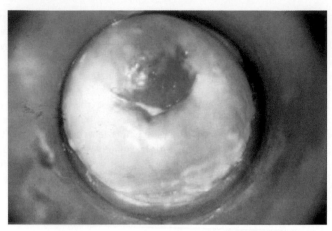

Fig. 17.4   Cervicitis with mucopurulent discharge.

adnexal tenderness suggestive of upper tract involvement. Vaginal swabs should be collected for WM or other POC testing, as already described for BV and *T. vaginalis* (see "Vaginitis" section). Vaginal or cervical swabs should be collected for *N. gonorrhoeae, C. trachomatis, T. vaginalis,* and *M. genitalium* NAATs, and HSV testing should be considered with culture or PCR if visible lesions are present (see Table 17.1). Testing for syphilis and HIV should be offered.

Treatment

Women with cervicitis should be provided presumptive treatment for chlamydia and/or gonorrhea if determined to be at high risk (e.g., <25 years of age, new sexual partner, multiple sexual partners) (see Table 17.3). Otherwise, treatment should be based on laboratory testing for the etiologic causes. Women with persistent cervicitis despite azithromycin should undergo testing for *M. genitalium*; if positive, treatment with moxifloxacin (Table 17.5) should be considered due to an increasing proportion of azithromycin-resistant *M. genitalium* infections.

Management

Patients should be advised to abstain from sex or use condoms until they and their sexual partner(s) have been adequately treated, which is typically 7 days after taking single-dose therapy or completion of their antibiotic regimen. Management of sexual partners should be based on the suspected or detected infection in the index patient if contact occurred within the preceding 60 days.

Women with chronic cervicitis despite treatment should be referred to a gynecologist. In the absence of an STI, cervicitis may be due to systemic illnesses such as autoimmune diseases, Stevens–Johnson syndrome, measles, neoplasia, and mechanical or chemical trauma.

PELVIC INFLAMMATORY DISEASE

PID refers to inflammation of the upper female genital tract and its related structures. Clinical syndromes include endometritis, salpingitis, adnexitis, tubo-ovarian abscess, pelvic peritonitis, or perihepatitis; however, there is a significant proportion of subclinical infections. Most cases of PID are secondary to *C. trachomatis* or *N. gonorrhoeae.* About 10% to 20% of women with acute gonorrhea can develop acute salpingitis or PID, with or without perihepatitis. The organisms that result in BV have been associated with endometritis and PID primarily after invasive gynecologic procedures. The major sequelae of acute PID are infertility, ectopic pregnancy, and chronic pelvic pain. The risk of developing tubal factor infertility is 7% after one episode of PID and increases

TABLE 17.5 ■ Sexually Transmitted Pathogens and Targeted Therapeutic Regimens

Pathogens	Primary Therapy	Alternative Therapies and Treatment for Recurrences
Candida albicans	Over-the-counter intravaginal agents Butoconazole OR terconazole intravaginal creams Fluconazole 150 mg PO in single dose	Recurrent vulvovaginal candidiasis Topical therapy for 7–14 days OR fluconazole every third day for total of three doses Oral fluconazole weekly for 6 months
Chlamydia trachomatis	Azithromycin 1.0 g PO in a single dose OR doxycycline 100 mg PO BID × 7 days	Levofloxacin 500 mg PO in a single dose × 7 days OR ofloxacin 300 mg PO BID × 7 days
Haemophilus ducreyi (chancroid)	Azithromycin 1.0 g PO in a single dose OR ceftriaxone 250 mg IM in a single dose OR ciprofloxacin 500 mg PO BID × 3 days OR erythromycin base 500 mg PO TID × 7 days	Fluctuant buboes: Incision and drainage
Herpes simplex virus (genital herpes)	First clinical episode: Acyclovir 400 mg PO TID × 7–10 days OR valacyclovir 1.0 g PO BID × 7–10 days OR famciclovir 250 mg PO TID × 7–10 days	Recurrent genital herpes: Acyclovir 400 mg PO TID × 5 days OR 800 mg PO BID × 5 days OR valacyclovir 500 mg PO BID × 3 days OR 1.0 g PO BID once daily for 5 days, OR famciclovir 125 mg PO BID × 5 days OR 1.0 mg BID × 1 day Suppressive therapy: Acyclovir 400 mg PO BID OR valacyclovir 500 mg PO once daily OR 1.0 g once a day OR famciclovir 250 mg PO BID
Human papilloma virus (genital warts)	Patient-applied: Imiquimod 3.75% at bedtime × 16 weeks OR 5% cream at bedtime three times weekly × 16 weeks OR podofilox 0.5% solution or gel BID × 3 days, followed by no therapy × 4 days for four cycles OR sinecatechins 15% ointment Provider-administered: Cryotherapy, surgical removal, OR trichloroacetic acid or bichloroacetic acid 80%–90% solution applied weekly	Provider-administered: Podophyllin resin 10%–25% preparation thoroughly washed off 1–4 hours after application
Lymphogranuloma venereum (LGV)	Doxycycline 100 mg PO BID for 21 days	Erythromycin base 500 mg PO QID for 21 days
Klebsiella granulomatosis (granuloma inguinale or donovanosis)	Azithromycin 1 g PO once per week or 500 mg daily for at least 3 weeks and until all lesions have completely healed	Doxycycline 100 mg PO BID for at least 3 weeks OR ciprofloxacin 750 mg PO BID for at least 3 weeks OR erythromycin base 500 mg PO QID for at least 3 weeks OR trimethoprim–sulfamethoxazole one double-strength (160 mg/800 mg) PO BID or at least 3 weeks and until all lesions have completely healed

Continued

TABLE 17.5 ■ Sexually Transmitted Pathogens and Targeted Therapeutic Regimens—cont'd

Pathogens	Primary Therapy	Alternative Therapies and Treatment for Recurrences
Mycoplasma genitalium	Azithromycin 1.0 g PO in a single dose	Moxifloxacin 400 mg BID for 7 days
Neisseria gonorrhoeae	Uncomplicated urogenital, pharyngeal, and rectal infections: Ceftriaxone 250 mg IM × 1, PLUS Azithromycin 1.0 g PO in single dose	Uncomplicated urogenital: Cefixime 400 mg PO in a single dose PLUS azithromycin 1.0 g PO in a single dose OR gentamicin 240 mg IM × 1 OR gemifloxacin 320 mg PO in a single dose PLUS azithromycin 2.0 g PO in a single dose
Treponema pallidum (syphilis)	Primary, secondary, early latent syphilis: Benzathine penicillin 2.4 mu IM in a single dose	Primary, secondary, early latent syphilis: Doxycycline 100 mg PO BID × 14 days
Trichomonas vaginalis	Metronidazole 2.0 g PO in a single dose OR tinidazole 2.0 g PO in a single dose HIV-infected women: Metronidazole 500 mg PO BID × 7 days	Metronidazole 500 mg PO BID × 7 days Persistent trichomoniasis: Metronidazole or tinidazole at 2 g PO for 7 days

BID, Twice a day; *g,* gram; *IM,* intramuscular; *IV,* intravenous; *mg,* milligram; *mu,* million units; *PO,* per os (oral); *QID,* four times a day; *TID,* three times a day.

to 28% after three or more episodes. Furthermore, women with PID have a sevenfold to tenfold increased risk of ectopic pregnancy and a fivefold increased risk of chronic pelvic pain.

Clinical Presentation

Women with symptomatic PID may present with lower abdominal pain; dyspareunia; vaginal discharge; menstrual irregularities; or systemic symptoms of fever, chills, and malaise. Women with gonococcal PID may present with abdominal pain of less than 3 days' duration, compared with women with chlamydial PID, who tend to present with abdominal pain for more than 1 week. The clinical findings may consist of lower abdominal tenderness, cervical motion tenderness, adnexal tenderness, or mucopurulent cervical discharge.

Evaluation and Diagnosis

The diagnosis of PID may be made on the basis of signs and symptoms alone, but the burden of subclinical disease warrants a more thorough evaluation that includes abdominal and pelvic examination, as well as testing for the causative pathogens. A presumptive diagnosis can be based on the presence of one or more of the following minimum clinical criteria: (1) cervical motion tenderness, (2) uterine tenderness, and/or (3) adnexal tenderness. Additional criteria that can be used to support a diagnosis of PID include oral temperature >101° F (>38.3° C); abnormal cervical mucopurulent discharge or cervical friability; presence of abundant numbers of WBCs on saline microscopy of vaginal fluid; elevated erythrocyte sedimentation rate; elevated C-reactive protein; and laboratory documentation of cervical infection with *N. gonorrhoeae* or *C. trachomatis*. In severe or complicated cases of PID, procedures such as endometrial biopsies, transvaginal sonography, or laparoscopy may be needed to confirm the diagnoses.

The evaluation for PID should therefore include an abdominal examination to assess for tenderness, especially in the right upper quadrant; this may be indicative of Fitz–Hugh–Curtis syndrome or perihepatitis as a complication of PID when accompanied with fever. A pelvic examination should include careful inspection of the cervix for friability or presence of a mucopurulent discharge consistent with cervicitis. Pain upon palpation of the cervix during the speculum examination or with movement during the bimanual examination are indicators of cervical motion tenderness. The ovaries and fallopian tubes should be palpated during the bimanual examination for tenderness or masses. Vaginal swabs should be collected for WM or other POC testing, as already described for BV and *T. vaginalis* (see "Vaginitis" section). Vaginal or cervical swabs should be collected for gonorrhea, chlamydia, trichomoniasis, and *M. genitalium* NAATs (see Table 17.1). Urine pregnancy testing to rule out ectopic pregnancy and syphilis and HIV testing should be offered to women with evidence of PID.

Treatment

Presumptive treatment for PID should be initiated based on the minimal clinical criteria, because a delay in therapy may lead to untoward long-term sequelae. Antimicrobial therapy should include coverage against *N. gonorrhoeae*, *C. trachomatis*, and anaerobic bacteria.

Ceftriaxone 250 mg IM in single dose plus doxycycline 100 mg by mouth (PO) twice a day (BID) for 14 days is the recommended outpatient regimen for women with mild-to-moderately severe acute PID. Due to the potential contribution of anaerobes to PID and the lack of anaerobic coverage with third-generation cephalosporins, patients should also receive metronidazole 500 mg PO BID for 14 days. Cefoxitin or other parenteral third-generation cephalosporins can be used instead of ceftriaxone in the treatment regimen. Alternative therapies for penicillin- or cephalosporin-allergic patients can include a fluoroquinolone plus metronidazole for 14 days (see Table 17.3) if the community prevalence and individual risk for gonorrhea are low. Patients with severe illness (e.g., with nausea, vomiting, or high fever), inability to take oral medications, pregnancy, suspected tubo-ovarian abscess, or a possible surgical emergency (e.g., appendicitis cannot be excluded) may require hospitalization. Inpatient treatment regimens are provided in Table 17.3.

Management

The approach to management of PID includes patient education, follow-up, and treatment of sexual partners. Patients treated with an outpatient regimen for PID should have a follow-up visit within 72 hours to assess for improvement in fever, abdominal tenderness, cervical motion tenderness, and adnexal tenderness. Patients who fail an outpatient treatment regimen should be hospitalized.

Patients with PID should abstain from intercourse until all symptoms have resolved. Sexual partners of patients with PID who had contact with the patient 60 days before the onset of symptoms should be evaluated and treated empirically with regimens effective against *N. gonorrhoeae* and *C. trachomatis*. All women with a diagnosis of chlamydial or gonococcal PID should be retested 3 months after treatment, regardless of whether their sexual partners were treated. All cases of PID are considered an STI unless proven otherwise.

Women with atypical acute symptoms or complications from PID such as infertility and chronic pelvic pain should be referred to a specialist. The differential diagnosis of PID includes ectopic pregnancy and other gynecologic conditions (ovarian cyst rupture, bleeding, or torsion), acute appendicitis, urinary tract infection, renal or ureteral stones, mesenteric lymphadenitis, and inflammatory bowel disease.

EPIDIDYMITIS

Inflammation of the upper male genital tract may lead to epididymitis, orchitis, epididymo-orchitis, and prostatitis. In men younger than 35 years of age, epididymitis is usually a complication of asymptomatic gonococcal or chlamydial urethritis. About 70% of cases of epididymitis among young sexually active men are caused by chlamydia. Enteric pathogens such as *Escherichia coli* are likely pathogens in MSM who practice insertive anal sex, in men older than 35 years of age, in men who have undergone recent urinary tract instrumentation or surgery, and in men with anatomic abnormalities of the genitourinary tract.

Clinical Presentation

Epididymitis usually presents as acute, unilateral scrotal and inguinal pain. Unilateral epididymitis may progress to bilateral epididymo-orchitis. Physical examination may reveal an erythematous scrotum with a tender, swollen epididymis. Concurrent urethritis may also be present. Testicular torsion, a surgical emergency, must be considered in evaluating a patient with testicular pain. Testicular torsion is more common among adolescents and may be associated with sudden, severe pain.

Evaluation and Diagnosis

The scrotum should be inspected for any enlargement; both testicles and epididymis should be palpated for any tenderness, enlargement, or abnormalities. Inguinal areas should be evaluated for lymphadenopathy. It is also important to inspect for evidence of urethritis (see "Urethritis" section).

Urethral swabs or a first-void urine specimen should be collected for gonorrhea and chlamydia NAATs testing. Serology for syphilis and HIV testing should also be obtained. A urinalysis and urine culture should be considered, as epididymitis can be due to genitourinary pathogens rather than pathogens commonly associated with STIs, especially in older men.

Treatment

Empiric therapy with ceftriaxone 250 mg IM in a single dose plus doxycycline 100 mg PO BID for 10 days is recommended while awaiting culture results (see Table 17.3). Alternative therapies, including fluoroquinolones, should be considered in men with epididymitis that may be secondary to enteric pathogens. In addition, scrotal elevation, analgesics, and ice packs will help lead to resolution.

Management

Patients should abstain from sex or use condoms until they and their sexual partner(s) have been adequately treated and symptoms have resolved. Sexual partners of patients with epididymitis presumed secondary to STIs, who had contact with the patient 60 days before the onset of symptoms, should be evaluated and treated empirically with regimens effective against *N. gonorrhoeae* and *C. trachomatis*.

Men with epididymitis should be asked to return for evaluation if symptoms fail to improve within 3 days, in which case evaluation for tumor, abscess, infarction, or mycobacterial or fungal disease should be pursued.

Patients with suspected testicular torsion, tumor, or abscess should be referred to a surgeon. Men with chronic epididymitis (persistent unilateral or bilateral testicular, epididymal, or scrotal pain) should be referred to a urologist to determine other etiologies, including tuberculosis among persons with risk factors.

PROCTITIS

Proctitis (inflammation of the rectum) is usually seen among male or female patients who practice anal intercourse and may be due to *N. gonorrhoeae* and other STIs (see Table 17.1). Proctocolitis (inflammation of the rectum and colon) may also be due to enteric pathogens such as *Salmonella*, *Shigella*, *Campylobacter*, *Giardia*, and *Entamoeba histolytica* that can be transmitted through oral–anal sexual exposures.

Clinical Presentation

Symptoms of proctitis include tenesmus (continual or recurrent inclination to evacuate the bowels), anorectal pain, mucopurulent or bloody anal discharge, and constipation. Proctocolitis is associated with diarrhea and cramps in addition to the symptoms of proctitis.

Evaluation and Diagnosis

The anal area should be inspected for lesions or visible discharge. Anorectal swabs should be collected for gonorrhea and chlamydia testing (see Table 17.1). If the *C. trachomatis* NAAT is positive on a rectal swab, PCR to distinguish lymphogranuloma venereum (LGV) should be performed, if available. Testing for syphilis, HSV, and HIV should also be performed. There are no currently available tests for *M. genitalium* from rectal swabs. Evaluation of patients who present with symptoms of acute proctitis includes stool culture for enteric pathogens. Anoscopy may reveal rectal exudates or rectal bleeding.

Treatment

In a person with acute proctitis and a history of recent unprotected anal intercourse, presumptive therapy for gonorrhea and chlamydia is indicated (see Table 17.3). If LGV is suspected (based on exclusion of herpes or syphilis), doxycycline should be extended to 100 mg PO BID for 3 weeks.

Management

Patients treated for acute proctitis should be instructed to abstain from sexual intercourse until they and their partner(s) have been adequately treated. Partners who have had sexual contact with persons treated for STI pathogens within the past 60 days before the onset of symptoms should be offered evaluation and treatment. Persons with persistent symptoms despite therapy should be referred to a gastrointestinal specialist. The differential diagnosis includes malignancy, trauma, and inflammatory bowel diseases such as ulcerative colitis.

GENITAL ULCER DISEASE

Genital, anal, or perianal ulcers, defined as breaches in the skin or mucosa of the affected areas, may be single or multiple and may be associated with inguinal or femoral lymphadenopathy. Causative agents include HSV-1 and -2, *Treponema pallidum* (syphilis), *Haemophilus ducreyi* (chancroid), L-serovars of *Chlamydia trachomatis* (LGV), and *Klebsiella granulomatis* (granuloma inguinale or donovanosis) (see Table 17.1). HSV is by far the most common cause of GUD in the United States. HSV-1 accounts for 5% to 30% of the first-episode cases of genital herpes, but the vast majority in the United States are caused by HSV-2.

Primary syphilis should be considered in most situations in light of the increase in early syphilis cases, especially among MSM. In the presence of syphilitic genital ulcers, there is a fivefold increase in susceptibility to HIV. Primary syphilis may overlap with signs of secondary syphilis, especially among HIV-coinfected persons, which include dermatologic (maculopapular rash involving the palms and soles) (Fig. 17.5), central nervous system (CNS) (aseptic meningitis, cranial neuropathy), ocular (iritis, uveitis, or keratitis), hepatic (hepatitis), and renal (immune complex glomerulonephritis) manifestations. The other pathogens associated with GUD are primarily seen outside the United States, although LGV-associated proctitis has increased in North America.

Clinical Presentation

The presentation of GUD can vary depending on the etiologic agent (Table 17.6). Patients with genital herpes typically present with a history of grouped vesicles or pustules that lead to shallow ulcers. Symptoms of low-grade fever, tender bilateral lymphadenopathy, and severe pain or

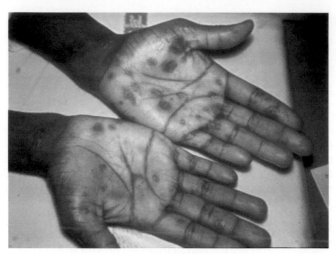

Fig. 17.5   Rash due to secondary syphilis.

paresthesias are associated with a primary first episode of genital herpes (i.e., there is no pre-existing antibody to HSV-1 or HSV-2). Occasionally, diffuse cutaneous disease, pneumonitis, hepatitis, or CNS infection may be present. Recurrent genital herpes is usually less severe and not preceded by prodromal symptoms. In comparison, a patient presenting with primary syphilis may report a painless solitary ulcer (chancre) accompanied with inguinal adenopathy. Patients with chancroid present with painful single or multiple genital ulcers with significant inguinal lymphadenopathy (called a *bubo*), usually with a history of travel and sexual exposure abroad. GUD can be complicated by systemic involvement or the disseminated stage of infection with HSV or syphilis.

Physical examination may reveal a deep solitary ulcer with a well-demarcated border and non-purulent base (primary syphilis) or multiple shallow ulcers with an erythematous base (genital herpes). A chancre can develop on the oral or anorectal mucosa as well as in the genital mucosa. Other physical examination findings that are important to the differential include whether the ulcers are painful and accompanied with inguinal lymphadenopathy (see Table 17.6). Inguinal lymphadenopathy is present in approximately 50% of patients with GUD.

Evaluation and Diagnosis

The clinical presentation of lesions, associated pain, inguinal lymphadenopathy, and history of travel can assist with narrowing the differential for GUD (see Table 17.6). At a minimum, diagnostic testing should be conducted for syphilis and genital herpes (see Table 17.1). Dark-field microscopy for direct detection of spirochetes, if available, and serologic testing for syphilis and should be performed even when lesions appear atypical. A specimen can be obtained by gently abrading an ulcer with gauze and applying the serous exudate on a slide with a cover slip to avoid drying. PCR for *T. pallidum* is not used routinely for syphilis testing due to lack of an FDA-cleared assay.

Nontreponemal tests detect anticardiolipin antibodies and include the rapid plasma reagin (RPR), toluidine red unheated serum test (TRUST), and Venereal Disease Research Laboratory (VDRL). However, the sensitivity of the nontreponemal tests varies from 70% in primary syphilis (due to a "window period" of detection in the first 2 weeks of infection) to 100% in secondary syphilis. Confirmation of the nontreponemal tests is necessary with the specific treponemal antibody tests, which detect immunoglobulin M (IgM) and immunoglobulin G (IgG) to *T. pallidum*. Treponemal tests include the *T. pallidum* particle agglutination assay (TP-PA), new automated enzyme immunoassays (EIAs), immunoblots and chemiluminescence assays, and the fluorescent

TABLE 17.6 ■ Differential Diagnosis for Genital Ulcer Disease

Feature	Genital Herpes	Primary Syphilis	Chancroid	Lymphogranuloma Venereum	Granuloma Inguinale
Etiologic agent	Human simplex virus 1 and 2	Treponema pallidum	Haemophilus ducreyi	Chlamydia trachomatis L1, L2, and L3 serovars	Klebsiella granulomatosis
Distribution of cases	Worldwide	Worldwide	Africa, Caribbean, rare in United States	Mainly in tropical and subtropical areas; increasing in United States (proctitis)	India, New Guinea, Caribbean, Australia, Africa, rare in United States
Incubation period	2–7 days	2–4 weeks	3–7 days	10–14 days	1–4 weeks
Number of lesions	Multiple	Single	Usually 1–3	Single	Single or multiple
Genital lesion appearance	Superficial, grouped vesicles, or ulcerations	Defined ulcer	Deep, defined, or irregular ulcer	Papule, pustule, vesicle, or ulcer (transient)	Defined or irregular ulcer, hypertrophic or verrucous
Base	Red, smooth	Red, smooth, shiny	Yellow-gray, rough	Variable	Red, beefy, rough, usually friable
Induration	None	Firm	Soft	None	Firm
Pain	Common[a]	None	Common	Variable	Rare
Inguinal lymphadenopathy	Bilateral, tender[a]	Unilateral or bilateral; nontender; no suppuration	Unilateral or bilateral; tender; may suppurate	Unilateral or bilateral; tender, may suppurate	None; inguinal swelling
Constitutional symptoms	Common	Rare	Rare	Frequent	Rare

[a]Occurs more commonly in primary episodes of genital herpes than in recurrences.

treponemal antibody absorption test (FTA-ABS), which are 80% to 100% sensitive, depending on the stage of disease.

Genital herpes can be clinically diagnosed by the presence of typical lesions; however, HSV culture or NAATs can confirm the diagnosis when uncertain. Culture is more sensitive during the vesicle stage (100%) than the ulcer stage (33%). Vesicles should be unroofed and the base should be swabbed for culture or NAATs. Several antigen detection kits are available, but they do not distinguish between HSV-1 and HSV-2. The sensitivity of type-specific serology for HSV-2 ranges from 70% to 90% and the specificity ranges from 95% to 99%.

Unfortunately, testing for LGV, chancroid, and granuloma inguinale is very limited. NAATs for *C. trachomatis* are not FDA-cleared for GUD. Chlamydia serologies with complement fixation or microimmunofluorescence titers can be considered for the diagnosis of LGV in the appropriate clinical context. Patients with GUD should undergo testing for other STIs and HIV due to the likelihood of coinfections.

Treatment

Probable or confirmed primary syphilis should be treated with 2.4 mu benzathine penicillin IM given as a single dose or doxycycline 100 mg orally BID for 14 days for penicillin-allergic patients (see Table 17.5). Patients may develop a Jarisch–Herxheimer reaction 2 to 8 hours after antimicrobial therapy for syphilis. This is an acute febrile reaction characterized by headache, myalgias, tender lymphadenopathy, and pharyngitis; it may be treated with acetaminophen, but preventive measures are not known.

Patients with primary or recurrent genital herpes should be treated with antiviral therapies and provided education and counseling (see Table 17.5). Recurrent episodes of genital herpes may be treated episodically or with continuous suppressive therapy. Patient-initiated treatment should begin at the first sign of the prodrome or within 1 day after the onset of genital lesions for recurrent disease. Treatment with daily suppressive therapy reduces the frequency of recurrences (especially among patients with 4 to 12 episodes per year) and decreases the duration of viral shedding and improves the quality of life. After 1 year, the need for continued therapy should be reassessed, as the frequency of recurrences decreases with time.

Treatment for chancroid, LGV, and granuloma inguinale are also provided in Table 17.5 and will need additional consideration for management of fluctuant buboes that can occur with the former.

Management

Patients should be asked to return for follow-up and re-examination of the genital ulcers 3 to 7 days after initiation of therapy if the diagnosis is uncertain. Persons with HSV do not need to return for re-evaluation unless symptoms persist or worsen. Persons diagnosed with primary syphilis, however, need clinical and serologic follow-up to ensure response to therapy. An appropriate serologic treatment response is at least a fourfold decline in nontreponemal antibody titers (for example, from 1:32 to 1:8) within 6 to 12 months after treatment. Seroreversion to nonreactive nontreponemal titers also indicates serologic cure. However, approximately 12% of patients will exhibit less than a fourfold decline in nontreponemal titers and may be serologic "nonresponders." A high proportion of patients also have "lack of seroreversion" with persistent nontreponemal antibody titers despite therapy. A sustained fourfold increase in nontreponemal antibody titers from baseline values is indicative of treatment failure or reinfection. In cases of treatment failure, the following should be done: recheck HIV status, consider cerebrospinal fluid evaluation for persons with neurologic signs/symptoms, and retreat with three weekly IM doses of benzathine penicillin. In cases of reinfection, a repeat course of benzathine penicillin IM should be administered. HIV-infected patients with syphilis may have a higher risk of treatment failure and a slower decline in nontreponemal antibody titers than non-HIV-infected patients. Therefore closer clinical and serologic follow-up at 3, 6, 9, 12, and 24 months is recommended for this population.

Patients with syphilis and their sexual partners must be managed in conjunction with the health department. Sexual partners of patients with primary syphilis within the past 90 days should receive 2.4 million units of benzathine penicillin, regardless of their serologic results; those with sexual contact >90 days should be treated presumptively if serologic test results are not immediately available and follow-up is uncertain.

Sexual partners of patients with genital herpes who are symptomatic should be evaluated and treated. Asymptomatic sexual partners should be evaluated, counseled, and encouraged to examine themselves for genital lesions. Persons who have had sexual contact with a patient with suspected chancroid, LGV, or granuloma inguinale within the 60 days before onset of the patient's symptoms should be examined and offered therapy.

Patients with persistent genital, anal, or perianal ulcers should be referred to a gynecologist, urologist, or gastrointestinal specialist. Possible reasons for persistence of symptoms include malignancy, trauma, fixed drug eruption, Behçet disease, and Reiter syndrome. Primary HIV infection should also be considered in the differential diagnosis of mucocutaneous ulcers and a mononucleosis-like syndrome.

Other Sexually Transmitted Infections

HUMAN PAPILLOMAVIRUS INFECTION

HPV infection is the most common viral sexually transmitted disease worldwide. From 2013 to 2014, the prevalence of genital HPV infection in the United States was estimated to be 42.5% among adults 18 to 59 years of age. HPV infections are transmitted primarily through sexual contact. Several transmission studies noted that 75% to 95% of male partners of women with HPV-genital lesions also had genital HPV infection. Vertical transmission can cause laryngeal papillomatosis in infants and children. Approximately 100 types of HPV have been identified. Over 40 types infect the anogenital area and can be divided into low risk (e.g., 6, 11, 42, 43, 44) and high risk (e.g., 16, 18, 31, 33, 35, 39, 45, 52, 55, 56, 58) based on their association with anogenital cancer. Low-risk types 6 and 11 cause genital warts and respiratory papillomatosis. The high-risk, oncogenic types, especially 16 and 18, have been associated with malignant transformation; squamous intraepithelial neoplasia; and squamous cell carcinoma of the vulva, vagina, cervix, penis, anus, and oropharynx. A substantial burden of cancers and anogenital warts are due to HPV infection worldwide.

Clinical Presentation

Most patients with genital warts are asymptomatic, but some report itching, burning, pain, and bleeding. Condyloma acuminata describes multiple nodular or large, exophytic, pedunculated, cauliflower-like lesions usually noted on the penis, vulva, vagina, cervix, perineum, and anal region. Flat condylomas are usually subclinical and not visible to the naked eye. They are most commonly noted on the cervix, but may also be present on the vulva and the penis. They may also present as white plaquelike lesions.

Other clinical manifestations include benign plantar and external genital warts, precancerous conditions (cervical intraepithelial neoplasia, squamous intraepithelial neoplasia), and cancers (cervical, anal, vaginal, vulvar, penile, oropharynx).

Diagnosis

Diagnosis of HPV infection is made by clinical examination, by pathology (Pap smear), or by HPV deoxyribonucleic acid (DNA) detection. The clinical diagnosis is based on the appearance of the lesions on visual examination, which may be enhanced by bright light and a magnifying glass. Routine use of the "acetowhite" test (brief soaking of skin with 3% to 10% acetic acid), which causes HPV lesions to appear white, is not recommended, as this test in not specific for HPV. When the diagnosis is uncertain, the patient should be referred to a gynecologist or urologist. Biopsy of the lesions is recommended when the lesions are ulcerated, fixed to the underlying tissue, indurated, or greater than 1 cm in size. Biopsy is also recommended if the lesions do not respond to or worsen with therapy. Cervical flat warts are not visible to the naked eye and require cytologic or colposcopic examination.

All women with external genital warts or with a history of contact with external genital warts should have cervical cytologic screening. Cervical cancer screening should be performed at age 21 using Pap smears every 3 years. For women >30 years, screening could include FDA-approved oncogenic or high-risk HPV tests that detect viral nucleic acids. During age 30 to 65, women could be tested with either a Pap test every 3 years or Pap test plus HPV test every 5 years.

Treatment

The goal of treatment of external genital warts is to eliminate the physical symptoms and the relief of emotional distress associated with the presence of lesions. Treatment of external genital warts does not cure the infection, may not decrease infectivity, and may not alter the course of infection. Untreated genital warts may resolve on their own.

The treatment modality of genital warts should be based on patient preference, provider experience, and available resources (see Table 17.5). In general, the treatment of external genital warts is divided into patient applied or provider applied; all modalities are equally efficacious. Patient-applied therapies include imiquimod, podofilox (podophyllotoxin), and sinecatechins, which should not be continued for longer than 16 weeks. Imiquimod is a topically active immune enhancer that stimulates production of interferon and other cytokines. Sinecatechins is a green tea extract; its mechanism of action against HPV is not fully known. Podophyllotoxin is a plant-derived product, with derivatives that have antiviral activity. Podofilox is contraindicated in pregnancy; data regarding the safety of imiquimod and sinecatechins in pregnancy are limited. Cryotherapy is an effective provider-applied therapy, but health care providers must be trained on its proper use because overtreatment and undertreatment can result in complications or low efficacy.

Management

Patients with genital warts and their sexual partners should be counseled and evaluated for other STIs. Examination of sexual partners is not necessary, as they are most likely subclinically infected with HPV. As for all sexually active females, female sexual partners of patients with genital warts should be encouraged to receive Pap smears for cervical cancer screening.

Most anogenital warts respond within 3 months of therapy. If the lesions fail to respond to a treatment regimen, an alternative modality should be pursued. Immunosuppressed patients may not respond as well as immunocompetent patients and may experience more recurrences.

The treatment of warts on mucosal surfaces such as cervical, intravaginal, and rectal areas should be managed in consultation with a gynecologist. Atypical or persistent lesions despite therapy should also be referred for further evaluation. The differential diagnosis of papular genital warts includes condyloma lata of secondary syphilis, molluscum contagiosum, normal pearly papules of the glans penis, seborrheic keratosis, Crohn disease, lichen planus, and melanocytic nevi. The differential diagnosis of flat warts includes erythema from psoriasis, seborrheic dermatitis, circinate balanitis of Reiter syndrome, Bowen disease, squamous intraepithelial neoplasia, or carcinoma.

Prevention

Three HPV vaccines are licensed in the United States, but only the 9-valent vaccine is being distributed, which prevents oncogenic HPV types (16, 18, 31, 33, 45, 52, and 58) and two HPV types that cause most genital warts (6 and 11). The 9vHPV vaccine is licensed for females and males ages 9 through 45 years. All HPV vaccines have been recommended for females and males ages 11 to 12 years with catch-up vaccination until age 26.

Suggested Reading

Brunham RC, Gottlieb SL, Paavonen J. Pelvic inflammatory disease. *N Engl J Med.* 2015;372(21):2039–2048.
Centers for Disease Control and Prevention. Sexually transmitted diseases treatment guidelines, 2015. *MMWR Morb Mortal Week Rep.* 2015;64:1–137.
Ghanem KG. Management of adult syphilis: key questions to inform the 2015 Centers for Disease Control and Prevention Sexually Transmitted Diseases Treatment Guidelines. *Clin Infect Dis.* 2015;61:S818–S836.
Gnann Jr JW, Whitley RJ. Genital herpes. *N Engl J Med.* 2016;375(7):666–674.
Kidd S, Workowski KA. Management of gonorrhea in adolescents and adults in the United States. *Clin Infect Dis.* 2015;61(suppl 8):S785–S801.
Park IU, Introcaso C, Dunne EF. Human papillomavirus and genital warts: a review of the evidence for the 2015 Centers for Disease Control and Prevention Sexually Transmitted Diseases Treatment Guidelines. *Clin Infect Dis.* 2015;61(suppl 8):S849–S855.
Wiesenfeld HC, Manhart LE. *Mycoplasma genitalium* in women: current knowledge and research priorities for this recently emerged pathogen. *J Infect Dis.* 2017;216(suppl 2):S389–S395.

CHAPTER 18

HIV Infection

Jessica S. Tischendorf ■ James M. Sosman

Introduction

Human immunodeficiency virus (HIV) infection in the United States has evolved over the past three decades from an untreatable illness that predictably led to death to a chronic disease that can be medically managed, with life expectancy for many patients similar to that for the general population. Most patients who take combination antiretroviral therapy (ART) experience immune reconstitution and resume normal lives.

Natural History of HIV Infection

PATHOGENESIS

HIV infection is characterized by an initial, occasionally symptomatic acute phase followed by an asymptomatic period of variable length, culminating in clinically evident immunodeficiency unless treatment is initiated. In HIV infection, persistent immune activation is manifested by increased turnover of T cells, monocytes, and natural killer; high levels of CD4 and CD8 T-cell apoptosis; and polyclonal B-cell activation with hypergammaglobulinemia. Immune activation is strongly predictive of HIV disease progression.

Continuous CD4 T-cell loss and replenishment lead to immunodeficiency because the regenerative capacity of CD4 cells dwindles despite apparent excess of homeostatic cytokines in the peripheral blood and lymphoid tissue. Exhaustion of the T-cell reserve may be due to direct killing by the virus, virus-induced apoptosis, immunologic senescence, and destruction of lymphoid tissue from fibrosis induced by inflammatory cytokines.

Transmission of HIV and progression of disease can be accelerated by bacterial and viral coinfections, which may augment immune activation through upregulation of HIV replication.

When the CD4 lymphocyte count falls below 200 cells/μL of blood, the patient has progressed to the acquired immunodeficiency syndrome (AIDS), characterized by profound deficiency in cell-mediated immunity and resultant increased susceptibility to opportunistic infections (OIs) and certain forms of cancer.

HIV VIRAL TRANSMISSION

The majority of new HIV infections are acquired through sexual intercourse. In resource-limited areas, vaginal sex is the most common means of acquisition. In the United States, male-to-male sexual intercourse is the most common route. Perinatal transmission and exposure to infected blood, such as through intravenous drug use, account for the remaining infections. The risk of transmission correlates with HIV viral load (measured as the number of virus ribonucleic acid [RNA] copies per milliliter [mL] of blood), and risk of sexual transmission increases in the presence of other sexually transmitted infections.

ACUTE AND EARLY HIV INFECTION

After the HIV virus enters the body through a mucosal surface or the bloodstream, it infects CD4 T lymphocytes (Table 18.1). There is a period of rapid viral replication leading to an abundance

---

TABLE 18.1 ■ Stages of HIV Infection

Viral Transmission

Acute HIV Infection
Also known as *primary HIV infection,* infection occurring within the first several weeks after acquisition. During this phase, HIV RNA and/or p24 antigen are detectable and HIV antibodies are not yet present. Acute retroviral syndrome refers to the clinical manifestations many patients develop during acute HIV infection.

Early HIV Infection
The 6-month period after acquisition.

Chronic HIV Infection
Subclassified as asymptomatic disease, early symptomatic disease, AIDS, or advanced HIV infection.
- Acquired immunodeficiency syndrome (AIDS): CD4 T-cell count (CD4 count) <200 cells/μL or the presence of an AIDS-defining illness.
- Advanced HIV infection: CD4 T-cell count <50 cells/μL

of virus in the peripheral blood. During primary infection, the level of HIV may reach several million viral copies per milliliter of blood. Clinicians must have a high index of suspicion for acute HIV infection, given implications of the high viremia for the patient and public health due to increased risk of transmission.

This high viremia is accompanied by a marked drop in circulating CD4+ T cells. Acute viremia is associated with the activation of CD8+ T cells, which kills HIV-infected cells, and subsequently with antibody production, or seroconversion. The CD8+ T-cell response is thought to be important in controlling virus levels, which peak and then decline, as the CD4+ T-cell counts partially rebound. A good CD8+ T-cell response does not eliminate the virus but has been linked to slower disease progression and a better prognosis.

By about 6 months after the primary infection, plasma viremia reaches a steady state, known as the viral set point. The set point, which is variable among patients, can be predictive of the rate of clinical progression to AIDS in the absence of ART.

CHRONIC HIV INFECTION

During the chronic phase of HIV infection, the consequences of generalized immune activation coupled with the gradual loss of the ability to generate new T cells appear to account for the gradual reduction in CD4+ T cells. Many patients with chronic HIV infection are asymptomatic. Often, it is not until a substantial decline in the CD4 count occurs that patients manifest symptoms. Some patients with HIV infection experience symptoms even before significant CD4 declines, including vaginal candidiasis, recurrent herpes simplex, reactivation of herpes zoster, oral hairy leukoplakia, seborrheic dermatitis, folliculitis, cervical and anal dysplasia, chronic diarrhea, and thrombocytopenia (idiopathic thrombocytopenic purpura).

AIDS

CD4+ T-cell depletion and chronic inflammation drive HIV pathogenesis and progression to AIDS. In patients not on ART, CD4 count progressively declines over time. The largest percentage in CD4 cell decline is seen in early infection, with a more gradual decline once out of the early stage of infection. The symptoms of immune deficiency characteristic of AIDS typically do not appear for years after a person is infected. AIDS is defined as a CD4 cell count below 200 cells/μL or the occurrence of any AIDS-defining condition, as outlined later in this chapter. Certain OIs, namely disseminated *Mycobacterium avium* complex (MAC) and cytomegalovirus (CMV) disease, are more likely to occur with advanced HIV infection, when the CD4 cell count is below 50 cells/μL. Once the infection has progressed to advanced HIV disease, life expectancy is usually less than 12 to 18 months unless ART is initiated.

ELITE CONTROLLERS

Elite controllers are a rare group (1%) of HIV-positive individuals who maintain undetectable viral loads and a high CD4 cell count in the absence of ART. They appear to be long-term nonprogressors for clinical HIV disease and do not progress to AIDS-defining illness. This condition is not fully understood and may be associated with certain human leukocyte antigen (HLA) haplotypes. These patients still exhibit immune activation but at a much lower level. Thus they may still be at risk for noninfectious complications of HIV compared with non–HIV-infected patients. It is not known if elite control is an indefinite state. These individuals may eventually require treatment to avoid the development of HIV complications or AIDS.

TABLE 18.2 ■ Signs and Symptoms of Acute HIV Infection

Feature	%
Fever	75
Fatigue	68
Myalgia	49
Skin rash	48
Headache	45
Pharyngitis	40
Cervical adenopathy	39
Arthralgia	30
Night sweats	28
Diarrhea	27

HIV-2 INFECTION

HIV-1 is responsible for the vast majority (95%) of HIV infections worldwide. HIV-2 is rarely reported in the United States and is largely confined to persons from West Africa. Compared with HIV-1 infection, the clinical course of HIV-2 infection is generally less aggressive. HIV-2 infection is characterized by a longer asymptomatic stage, lower plasma HIV-2 RNA levels, and lower mortality; however, progression to AIDS does occur. HIV-2 causes a significant number of infections in West Africa and in areas with strong socioeconomic ties to West Africa (e.g., France, Spain, Portugal, and former Portuguese colonies such as Brazil, Angola, Mozambique, and parts of India).

Acute and Early HIV Infection: Clinical Manifestations and Diagnosis

CLINICAL MANIFESTATIONS OF THE ACUTE RETROVIRAL SYNDROME

The acute retroviral syndrome refers to the manifestations many develop during acute infection. These symptoms can range from asymptomatic infection, to a "mononucleosis"-like syndrome, to a severe febrile illness. Symptoms typically manifest within 28 days of infection and most commonly include fever, fatigue, myalgia, rash, headache, pharyngitis, and adenopathy (Table 18.2). Symptoms persist for a median 14 days. Occasionally, acute infection can cause a significant decline in CD4 counts, which may lead to oropharyngeal candidiasis or other OIs.

LABORATORY DIAGNOSIS OF ACUTE AND EARLY HIV INFECTION

HIV can be diagnosed through blood and saliva tests, most of which can detect HIV between 2 and 12 weeks after infection (Fig. 18.1). The fourth-generation p24 antigen–HIV antibody test is the most accurate in use (>99.7% sensitivity and >99.3% specificity) and is recommended as the initial screening test for HIV infection, unless acute infection is suspected. The p24 antigen is a viral core protein that appears in the blood as the viral RNA level rises after HIV infection. In patients suspected of having acute HIV infection, both HIV RNA and HIV antibody testing is recommended. If HIV antibody testing is negative and p24 antigen is positive, individuals should have follow-up testing to document HIV antibody seroconversion.
- *HIV RNA (viral load)*: detectable approximately 10 days after HIV infection
- *Fourth-generation p24 antigen–HIV antibody test*: detectable 15 to 20 days after HIV infection Detection of p24 antigen occurs approximately 1 week sooner than the HIV

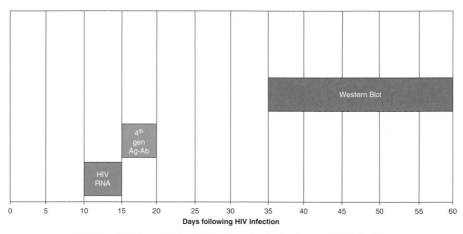

Fig. 18.1 Time to positivity of laboratory studies to diagnose HIV infection.

antibody, providing an advantage over third-generation testing. See Fig. 18.2 for interpretation of the fourth-generation antigen–antibody test.

■ *HIV antibody testing by Western blot*: Detectable between 3 and 6 weeks after infection.

HIV Screening

Health care professionals should offer HIV testing to anyone who requests it, and everyone should be tested at least once (Table 18.3). All pregnant women should also be offered testing, usually twice during the pregnancy. Individuals at high risk for HIV infection should be offered testing at least once a year. Risk-based testing alone has not been effective, as providers seldom adequately assess risk. Due to deficiencies in assessing risk and failure to optimize screening, approximately 10% to 25% of persons with undiagnosed HIV are unaware of any risk factors or are uncomfortable disclosing them, and almost half of patients are identified late in the course of disease.

Initial Evaluation of the HIV-Infected Adult

The goals of the initial evaluation of the HIV-infected adult are to (1) confirm diagnosis, (2) assess stage of HIV infection, (3) determine risk for and presence of any concurrent infectious diseases, (4) identify any comorbid conditions that may influence HIV treatment, and (5) select an appropriate antiretroviral regimen. These goals are achieved through a comprehensive history and physical examination and evaluation of laboratory studies and imaging data. Educating the patient about their HIV infection and establishing a therapeutic alliance is of utmost importance at the initial visit.

CONFIRMING HIV INFECTION

For patients with a prior diagnosis of HIV infection, every effort should be made to review documentation of prior HIV antibody and HIV viral load testing. If this documentation is not available, confirming diagnosis with HIV antibody testing is prudent. Rarely, misdiagnosis or factitious HIV infection has occurred.

For those with a suspected infection, confirm with the appropriate diagnostic test (see Fig. 18.2). For patients with suspected acute HIV infection, HIV viral load is the most sensitive and specific means of identifying early infection. Even our best serologic test, the fourth-generation combined antigen–antibody test, may take up to 20 days to turn positive. For those undergoing

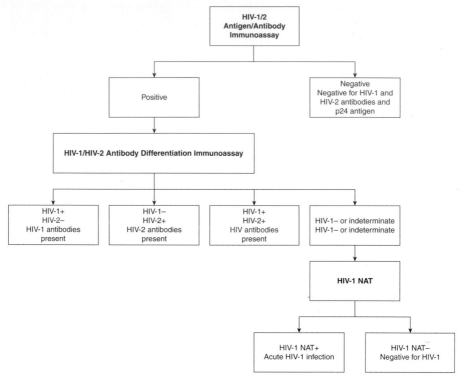

Fig. 18.2 Interpretation of fourth-generation p24 antigen–HIV antibody screening test with confirmatory HIV-1/HIV-2 antibody differentiation assay.

TABLE 18.3 ■ **HIV Screening Recommendations**

Organization	Screening Recommendation
Centers for Disease Control and Prevention (CDC)	Screen everyone between age 13 and 64 at least once using an opt-out approach. Screen high-risk patients annually.
US Preventive Services Task Force (USPSTF)	Screen all adolescents and adults age 15–65, younger adolescents and older adults at higher risk, and pregnant women.
American Academy of HIV Medicine	Screen all adults regardless of risk.

routine screening or those in whom acute infection is not clinically suspected, the fourth-generation HIV antigen–antibody testing is appropriate.

COMPREHENSIVE MEDICAL HISTORY

A comprehensive medical history should focus on HIV-specific issues, the presence of other infectious diseases, medical comorbidities that may affect prognosis or treatment, and risk factors for HIV transmission or acquisition of other infections. For those patients with an established HIV diagnosis, a detailed history of prior treatment regimens is essential.

TABLE 18.4 ■ AIDS-Defining Conditions

Candidiasis, esophageal or respiratory
Invasive cervical cancer
Coccidioidomycosis
Cryptococcosis
Cryptosporidiosis
Cytomegalovirus disease
Encephalopathy, HIV-related
Herpes simplex virus disease
Histoplasmosis
Isosporiasis
Kaposi sarcoma
Lymphoma, multiple forms
Tuberculosis
Nontuberculous mycobacterium infections, pulmonary or extrapulmonary
Pneumocystis jirevicii pneumonia
Pneumonia, recurrent
Progressive multifocal leukoencephalopathy
Salmonella septicemia, recurrent
Toxoplasmosis, brain
Wasting syndrome of HIV

Adapted from AIDSinfo.

HIV-Specific History

HIV-specific issues to discuss at the initial evaluation include:
- Method and date of suspected acquisition
- Duration of infection, if known
- Behaviors that increase the risk of transmission, such as unprotected sexual intercourse or injection drug use
- Any prior use of pre-exposure prophylaxis (PrEP) or postexposure prophylaxis (PEP)

HIV-specific issues to discuss for patients with a prior HIV diagnosis additionally include prior treatment regimens, prior history of OIs, HIV-related malignancies or other comorbid conditions, and prior CD4 count and viral load results.

Past Medical History

A thorough past medical history should include assessment of prior OIs or AIDS-defining conditions (Table 18.4), common coinfections, and underlying comorbidities that may affect the course and treatment of HIV infection.

Common coinfections include hepatitis B and C and other sexually transmitted infections, including gonorrhea, chlamydia, syphilis, anogenital warts, and herpes simplex virus. A history of tuberculosis or risk for exposure to tuberculosis should be sought, given the greater risk of activation of latent infection among HIV-infected patients. Prior anocervical dysplasia should also be assessed.

All patients should be assessed for cardiometabolic risk factors and disease because their presence may alter HIV treatment. Evelute for smoking, hypertension, diabetes mellitus, dyslipidemia, renal insufficiency, bone disease, peripheral neuropathy, and coronary artery disease. The presence of non–AIDS-defining malignancy, prior cancer screening, and family history of malignancy should be determined. An assessment of a patient's psychiatric and substance use history is essential to promoting treatment adherence and retention in care.

A current medication and allergy history is necessary to safely prescribe ART. Prior immunization history should be obtained, and immunity to hepatitis A and B should be documented even if previously vaccinated.

Social History

Social history allows the provider to determine the risk of HIV transmission and acquisition of other infectious diseases and to identify barriers to retention in care.
- Employment history and insurance status
- Housing security, safety, and stability
- Thorough travel history to assess potential infectious exposures
- Substance use, past and current
- Tobacco history
- Sexual history, including all exposure sites, use of contraception, and status of partners, if known
- Social support

Family History

A family history of cardiometabolic disease and malignancy should be ascertained.

Review of Systems

A thorough review of systems can identify symptoms concerning for OI or other HIV-related illness. Particular attention should be paid to visual symptoms, respiratory symptoms such as chronic cough or shortness of breath, gastrointestinal symptoms such as dysphagia or odynophagia, skin changes, neurologic changes such as headache, cognitive changes, and weakness or paresthesias.

COMPREHENSIVE PHYSICAL EXAMINATION

A complete examination should be performed at the initial encounter, with particular attention paid to:
- General appearance, weight, lipodystrophy, or wasting
- Skin, including bruising, rashes, or lesions
- Lymph nodes
- Eye, including retinal examination and visual acuity
- Oropharynx, including dentition
- Genitourinary
- Anorectal
- Neurologic, including presence of neuropathy or weakness
- Cognitive status

INITIAL LABORATORY TESTS

Laboratory testing should evaluate HIV-specific parameters, organ function, and presence of coinfections (Table 18.5).
Other testing may be indicated based on the clinical scenario, including:
- Glucose-6-phosphate dehydrogenase deficiency (G6PD) screening among those of African, Asian, or Mediterranean descent.
- Anti-CMV antibody for those with a low risk of acquiring CMV. Men who have sex with men (MSM) and injection drug users are presumed positive, and screening is not recommended.
- Anti–varicella zoster virus (VZV) immunoglobulin G (IgG) in patients without a history of chickenpox or prior vaccination.

TABLE 18.5 ■ Initial Laboratory Evaluation of New HIV Infection

HIV-Specific Tests	Tests for Coinfection	Other Routine Tests
Laboratory confirmation of HIV infection CD4 count with percentage HIV RNA level (viral load) HIV genotypic drug-resistance testing HLA-B*5701 (if abacavir treatment is considered) Coreceptor tropism testing (if maraviroc treatment is considered)	Hepatitis A antibody Hepatitis B surface antigen, surface antibody, and core antibody Hepatitis C antibody Tuberculin skin testing or interferon-gamma release assay Antitoxoplasma IgG Syphilis screening *Neisseria gonorrhea* at all sites of exposure *Chlamydia trachomatis* at all sites of exposure *Trichomonas vaginalis*, for women Cervical cancer screening, for women	Complete blood cell count with differential Basic metabolic and renal panel Liver function tests Urinalysis Fasting lipid panel Fasting glucose or hemoglobin A1c Pregnancy test, for women

- MAC screening with acid-fast bacillus (AFB) blood culture, to be considered in patients with ≤50 cells/µL before initiation of MAC prophylaxis.
- Anal cancer screening, which should be considered in MSM, women with history of receptive anal intercourse or abnormal cervical Pap, and all persons with HIV infection and genital warts.

PREVENTION OF OPPORTUNISTIC INFECTIONS IN HIV-INFECTED PATIENTS

HIV-related OIs are infections that occur more frequently or are more severe because of HIV-mediated immunosuppression. Historically, OIs were often the first manifestation of underlying AIDS. Today, OIs may also herald a diagnosis of AIDS in patients previously unaware of their infection, those not engaged in care, or those without durable viral suppression.

Before the advent of highly active ART, OIs portended a very poor prognosis. During this era, antimicrobial prophylaxis and vaccination were introduced to prevent OIs. Today, viral suppression with ART is the most effective means of preventing OIs, though some occur regardless of CD4 count.

Antimicrobial agents can be administered to decrease the risk of developing an OI (Table 18.6). This is most effective for individuals with CD4 count <200 cells/µL, in conjunction with starting ART, to decrease the risk of developing certain OIs, including *Pneumocystis jirovecii* pneumonia (PJP) and toxoplasmosis. Antimicrobial prophylaxis can generally be discontinued in patients on ART with maximal viral suppression and CD4 count recovery to >200 cells/µL for ≥3 months. Antimicrobials are not generally recommended to prevent active infection with other pathogens such as *Bartonella* spp., *Coccidioides* spp., *Cryptococcus* spp., *Cystoisospora*, or CMV.

Antiretroviral Therapy in HIV Infection

GOALS OF TREATMENT

Prompt treatment of HIV infection offers benefit not just to the patient but to public health as well. Treatment must be aimed at achieving the following goals:

- Maximal, sustained suppression of HIV RNA viral load below the limit of detection (currently <20 RNA copies/mL, or "undetectable")
- Reconstitute and preserve immune system function

- Decrease risk of HIV-related comorbidities
- Prolong survival
- Improve quality of life
- Prevent transmission of HIV

TABLE 18.6 ■ Opportunistic Infections and Associated Prevention Strategies

Opportunistic Infection	Indication	Preferred Regimen
Antimicrobial Prevention		
Pneumocystis jirovecii pneumonia (PJP)	CD4 count <200 cells/μL or CD4 <14%	Trimethoprim/sulfamethoxazole 1 single strength or 1 double-strength tab PO daily
Toxoplasma gondii encephalitis	Toxoplasma IgG–positive patients with CD4 count <100 cells/μL	Trimethoprim/sulfamethoxazole 1 double-strength tab PO daily
Disseminated Mycobacterium avium complex (MAC) disease	Primary prophylaxis is not recommended for patients who immediately initiate ART. Recommended for those with CD4 count <50 cells/μL, not on fully suppressive ART, after disseminated MAC has been ruled out	Azithromycin 1200 mg PO once weekly or Azithromycin 600 mg PO twice weekly or Clarithromycin 500 mg PO BID
Histoplasma capsulatum	CD4 count ≤150 cells/μL and: • Occupational exposure or • Live in hyperendemic region	Itraconazole 200 mg PO daily
Preemptive Antimicrobial Therapy		
Coccidioidomycosis	CD4 count <250 cells/μL and Newly positive serologic test in patient who lives in endemic area	Fluconazole 400 mg PO daily
Cryptococcus	Preventive therapy is generally not recommended. In certain settings, patients with CD4 count <100 cells/μL who screen positive for cryptococcal antigen can receive preemptive therapy to prevent symptomatic infection	Fluconazole 400 mg PO daily
Mycobacterium tuberculosis, latent infection (LTBI)*	Positive screening for LTBI with no evidence of active TB, no prior treatment for LTBI or active TB, or Close contact with a patient with infectious TB without evidence of active TB, regardless of screening test	Isoniazid 300 mg + pyridoxine 25–50 mg PO daily for 9 months or Isoniazid 900 mg PO twice weekly (by DOT) + pyridoxine 25–50 mg PO daily for 9 months or Isoniazid 15 mg/kg plus rifapentine† (≥50 kg: 900 mg) PO weekly (by DOT) for 3 months or Rifampin† 10 mg/kg (maximum dose 600 mg) PO daily for 4 months
Syphilis	Patient exposed to partner with primary, secondary, or early latent syphilis within the past 90 days or Patient exposed to sex partner >90 days before syphilis diagnosis in the partner, if test results are not available and follow-up is not certain	Benzathine penicillin G 2.4 million units IM for 1 dose

TABLE 18.6 ■ Opportunistic Infections and Associated Prevention Strategies—cont'd

Opportunistic Infection	Indication	Preferred Regimen
Vaccine-Preventable Infections		
Hepatitis A	Patient susceptible to HAV, including those with chronic liver disease, injection drug users, or men who have sex with men	Hepatitis A vaccine, 2 doses 6 months apart *or* If at risk for HAV and HBV, combined HAV and HBV vaccine 3- or 4-dose series
Hepatitis B	Patient without chronic HBV infection without evidence of immunity to HBV Recommended when CD4 count CD4 count <350 cells/μL	HBV vaccine, either 3- or 4-dose regimen depending on vaccine *or* Conjugated HBV 2-dose series *or* If at risk for HAV and HBV, combined HAV and HBV vaccine 3- or 4-dose series
Human papillomavirus (HPV)	Females and males aged 13–26 years	HPV recombinant vaccine 9-valent at 0, 1–2, and 6 months
Varicella zoster virus (VZV)	Patients with CD4 count ≥200 cells/μL, not previously vaccinated, no history of varicella or herpes zoster, or who are seronegative for VZV	Primary varicella vaccination, 2 doses administered 3 months apart
Influenza	All HIV-infected patients	Inactivated influenza vaccine annually Live-attenuated influenza vaccine is contraindicated in HIV-infected patients
Streptococcus pneumoniae	For any patient regardless of CD4 count	One dose of PCV13 followed by one dose of PPSV23 at least 2 months later *and* Second dose of PPSV 23 5 years after first dose of PPSV23 *and* If most recent PPSV23 administered before age 65, administer additional dose at age 65 or older at least 5 years after last PPSV23 dose
Neisseria meningitides	All HIV-infected patients age 2 months or older	Two doses of MenACWY vaccine at least 2 months apart; revaccinate every 5 years Adolescents and young adults may receive MenB, two-dose series, decided on an individual basis

*There are several effective latent TB treatment regimens appropriate for patients with HIV. Clinicians should prescribe the more convenient shorter regimens, when possible, as patients are more likely to complete shorter treatment regimens.
†For those taking antiretroviral medications with clinically significant drug interactions with once-weekly rifapentine or daily rifampin, 9 months of daily isoniazid is a preferred treatment.
ART, Antiretroviral therapy; *BID,* twice a day; *DOT,* directly observed therapy; *IgG,* immunoglobulin G; *IM,* intramuscular; *HAV,* hepatitis A virus; *HBV,* hepatitis B virus; *PO,* per os (oral); *TB,* tuberculosis.

WHO TO TREAT

All patients with HIV infection, regardless of stage, should be considered for treatment. Before initiating treatment, a thorough psychosocial assessment should be performed. If there are active mental health, substance use, or social factors that would significantly affect the patient's ability to initiate and maintain ART, treatment can be delayed until adherence is more assured. In the setting of some OIs, namely cryptococcal disease and tuberculous meningitis, a short delay (2 weeks) before initiation of ART may lessen the occurrence of the immune reconstitution inflammatory syndrome (IRIS). With other OIs, early initiation of ART confers a survival advantage.

DRUG SELECTION

Genotypic drug resistance testing should be performed after the initial diagnosis of HIV infection to guide ART selection. Infection with a virus that harbors at least one drug resistance mutation is estimated to occur in up to 20% of newly infected patients. Empiric ART can be initiated before results of drug resistance testing are known. The following regimens are recommended for the empiric treatment of acute and early HIV infection while awaiting results of drug resistance testing.

- Bictegravir (BIC)/tenofovir alafenamide (TAF)/emtricitabine (FTC)
- Dolutegravir (DTG) with (TAF or tenofovir disoproxil fumarate [TDF]) plus (FTC or lamivudine [3TC])
- Boosted darunavir (DRV) with (TAF or TDF) plus (FTC or 3TC)

Darunavir is attractive for acute infection, as protease inhibitors (PIs) have a high genetic barrier to resistance and transmission of PI-resistant virus is rare. Dolutegravir, an integrase strand transfer inhibitor (INSTI), is also reasonable, but given concern for neural tube defects, should be avoided in women of childbearing age with the potential to become pregnant or those in their first trimester of pregnancy. Bictegravir, a newer INSTI, is also an alternative; however, data on use in acute HIV infection are lacking.

The decision between tenofovir DF and tenofovir AF should be made based on patient comorbidities. Tenofovir DF has been associated with nephrotoxicity and bone demineralization to a greater degree than tenofovir AF. Tenofovir AF may negatively affect lipids to a greater degree than tenofovir DF.

MODIFICATION OF ART REGIMEN

When the patient's drug resistance profile is known, treatment can be modified and, if possible, transitioned to a coformulated combination medicine recommended for the treatment of chronic HIV infection. Once treatment is initiated, it should continue indefinitely with the goal of maximal viral suppression.

Selecting Antiretroviral Regimens for the Treatment-Naïve HIV-Infected Patient

There are six major classes of antiretroviral medications, each with a different target. However, we predominantly use medication from four of these classes (Table 18.7). All recommended initial regimens consist of an INSTI anchor drug with a two–nucleoside reverse transcriptase inhibitor (NRTI) backbone.

Another two classes of ART work by blocking HIV entry into the CD4 cell. Three drugs with separate mechanisms make up these classes: enfuvirtide, maraviroc, and ibalizumab. These drugs are used infrequently and mostly for individuals with multiclass drug-resistant virus.

When to Start Antiretroviral Therapy

ART is recommended in all patients with HIV infection, regardless of CD4 cell count. On an individual basis, delayed ART may be appropriate based on assessment of psychosocial factors or the presence of certain OIs, namely central nervous system (CNS) tuberculosis or CNS cryptococcosis.

TABLE 18.7 ■ Four Major Classes of Antiretrovirals

Class	Nucleoside Reverse Transcriptase Inhibitors (NRTIs)	Non-Nucleoside Reverse Transcriptase Inhibitors (NNRTIs)	Integrase Strand Transfer Inhibitors (INSTIs)	Protease Inhibitors (PIs)
Mechanism	Prevents transcription of HIV RNA into double-stranded DNA. NRTIs mimic human nucleotides, which terminate elongation of HIV DNA strand during transcription.	Prevents transcription of HIV RNA into double-stranded DNA. Binds to reverse transcriptase, inducing a conformational change blocking HIV reverse transcription.	Blocks integration of HIV DNA into host DNA.	Impedes viral protein maturation by inhibiting HIV protease.
Selected Drugs	Abacavir Lamivudine Emtricitabine Tenofovir AF Tenofovir DF Zidovudine	Doravirine Efavirenz Etravirine Rilpivirine	Dolutegravir Elvitegravir* Raltegravir Bictegravir	Atazanavir* Darunavir* Lopinavir†

*Coformulated with the pharmacologic booster cobicistat.
†Coformulated with the pharmacologic booster ritonavir.

What to Start

All preferred initial regimens for treatment-naïve patients without drug-resistant HIV consist of an INSTI in combination with two NRTIs. Although the following are generally recommended for treatment initiation, patient-specific factors should be considered. Detailed US Department of Health and Human Services (DHHS) recommendations for ART can be found at the AIDSinfo website (aidsinfo.nih.gov).

Recommended initial regimens:

- Bictegravir–tenofovir AF–emtricitabine (Biktarvy)
- Dolutegravir–abacavir–lamivudine (Triumeq)
- Dolutegravir (Tivicay) plus tenofovir AF–emtricitabine (Descovy)
- Dolutegravir (Tivicay) plus tenofovir DF–emtricitabine (Truvada)
- Raltegravir (Isentress) plus tenofovir AF–emtricitabine (Descovy)
- Raltegravir (Isentress) plus tenofovir DF–emtricitabine (Truvada)
- Dolutegravir–lamivudine (Dovato)

The latest data on neural tube defects (NTDs) in infants born to women who received dolutegravir around the time of conception have shown that the prevalence of NTDs is lower than initially reported (the rate has been reduced from 0.9% to 0.3%). However, this rate is still higher than the rate reported for infants born to individuals who received ART that did not contain DTG (0.1%). Providers should discuss the benefits of using DTG and the risk of NTDs with the person of childbearing potential to allow the person to make informed decisions about care.

In patients with chronic kidney disease (estimated glomerular filtration rate [eGFR] <60 mL/min) tenofovir DF should be avoided, if eGFR <30 mL/min, tenofovir AF should also be avoided. Tenofovir DF should not be prescribed for patients with existing osteoporosis. Abacavir is contraindicated in patients with the HLA*B5701 haplotype due to increased risk of abacavir hypersensitivity reaction, a syndrome of multiorgan dysfunction that leads to significant morbidity and, rarely, mortality if not promptly recognized.

Among the INSTIs, bictegravir and dolutegravir are preferred, as they have a higher barrier to resistance than raltegravir. Bictegravir is only available in a once-daily, fixed-dose combination pill with tenofovir AF and emtricitabine (Biktarvy). Dolutegravir is dosed once daily, whereas raltegravir can be dose once or twice daily.

Additional data now support the use of the two-drug regimen dolutegravir plus lamivudine for initial treatment of people with HIV. However, this combination should not be used for individuals with HIV RNA > 500,000 copies/mL or HBV coinfection.

Patient Monitoring During HIV Antiretroviral Therapy

Patients need close monitoring after initiation of ART. At each visit, medication adherence and tolerability should be assessed, along with an appropriate evaluation for opportunistic or sexually transmitted infections.

VISIT FREQUENCY

After initiating ART, patients should return to the clinic in 2 to 4 weeks to assess adherence and tolerability of the new regimen and to address questions that may arise during the early stages of treatment. If there are issues with adherence or medication intolerance, frequent follow-ups should be scheduled. Once patients are adhering to a well-tolerated antiretroviral regimen, visits can be separated out to every 3 to 6 months.

Adherence to ART and adverse medication effects should be assessed at each visit. A thorough review of systems and examination are particularly important early in treatment to assess for signs of IRIS in patients with high viral loads and low CD4 counts. Follow-up visits should also provide ongoing patient education on reducing transmission and preventing acquisition of other infectious diseases.

LABORATORY MONITORING OF HIV INFECTION

HIV viral load and CD4 count measurements are routinely used to monitor the efficacy of ART and the risk of OIs (Table 18.8). Patients should have an HIV viral load checked at 4 to 8 weeks after initiation of ART. If viral load remains detectable at that time, repeat viral load testing every 4 to 8 weeks is indicated until virologic suppression is achieved. Once suppressed, the viral load should be measured every 3 to 6 months and with any modification to the ART regimen.

Within the first 2 years on ART, CD4 counts are measured every 3 to 6 months. They are also indicated this frequently for patients with CD4 count <300 cells/μL or those with detectable viremia on ART. After 2 years of ART, patients without detectable viremia and with CD4 counts >300 cells/μL can be followed with annual CD4 counts. For patients with stable CD4 counts >500 cells/μL, routine monitoring of the CD4 count is not necessary.

HIV genotypic resistance testing is recommended at baseline, when patients do not achieve virologic suppression at 24 weeks, or when patients have detectable viremia after a period of suppression on two consecutive measurements. In patients with virologic suppression, resistance testing is not indicated when switching ART regimens. Genotypic resistance assays are preferred and detect the presence of specific drug resistance mutations in the regions of the HIV genome encoding protease, reverse transcriptase, and integrase. Each report summarizes which drugs may have reduced activity based upon the viral sequence. The International Antiviral Society-USA provides an updated list of mutations associated with HIV drug resistance to all Food and Drug Administration (FDA)-approved drugs (www.iasusa.org). The Stanford drug resistance database (hivdb.stanford.edu) provides access to a genotypic resistance algorithm. Most commercially available resistance assays cannot be performed if the viral load is less than 500 to 1000 RNA copies/mL.

DRUG SAFETY MONITORING

Antiretrovirals are generally well tolerated, though many carry a risk of adverse metabolic effects. Within 4 to 8 weeks after initiation or modification of ART, basic chemistries and renal function,

TABLE 18.8 ■ Laboratory Monitoring in HIV Infection

Baseline	Four to Eight Weeks After Treatment Initiation	Every Three to Six Months	Annually
HIV viral load	HIV viral load, then every 4–8 weeks until virologic suppression	HIV viral load, once virologic suppression is achieved	
CD4 count		CD4 count, during first 2 years of therapy of if <300 cells/μL	CD4 count, after 2 years of therapy and >300 cells/μL
Genotype testing*			
Basic chemistry, renal function, liver function tests	Basic chemistry, renal function, liver function tests	Basic chemistry, renal function, liver function tests	
CBC with differential	CBC with differential	CBC with differential	
Urinalysis			Urinalysis
Fasting lipid profile		Fasting lipid profile, if abnormal (6 months)	Fasting lipid profile, if normal
Fasting blood glucose or hemoglobin A1c		Fasting blood glucose or hemoglobin A1c, if abnormal	Fasting blood glucose or hemoglobin A1c, if normal
Pregnancy test, if female of reproductive potential†			

*Repeat genotype testing if virologic suppression is not achieved by 24 weeks or patients develop detectable viremia after a period of suppression on two consecutive measurements of HIV viral load.
†Pregnancy test should be repeated with change of antiretroviral therapy.
CBC, Complete blood count.

alanine aminotransferase (ALT), aspartate aminotransferase (AST), total bilirubin, and complete blood count with differential should be measured. These parameters should then be assessed every 3 to 6 months along with routine monitoring of HIV viral load. Urinalysis, specifically urine glucose and protein, should be obtained after changes in ART and then at least annually to monitor for nephrotoxicity.

Antiretrovirals can affect lipids and glucose tolerance. A fasting lipid profile should be performed at treatment initiation and after modification, every 6 months if abnormal or every 12 months if normal. Fasting blood glucose or hemoglobin A1c should be assessed with treatment initiation and modification, every 3 to 6 months if abnormal or annually if normal at the last measurement.

For women of reproductive age, pregnancy tests should be checked with initiation or change in ART.

DRUG INTERACTIONS

Drug interactions between antiretrovirals and other medications are common. Interactions can affect absorption, metabolism, or elimination of antiretrovirals and other drugs patients are taking. For example, acid-reducing agents impair the absorption of rilpivirine and atazanavir, and polyvalent cations can reduce the absorption of INSTIs. Many antiretrovirals (PIs, NNRTIs, maraviroc, elvitegravir) use the cytochrome P450 enzyme pathway for metabolism. Pharmacologic boosters (ritonavir and cobicistat) inhibit the CYP3A4 enzyme, which can lead to higher exposure to drugs metabolized through this pathway.

Before initiating or modifying ART or concomitant drugs, a thorough assessment for drug interactions must be undertaken. Consultation with a pharmacist knowledgeable in ART is recommended.

Role of Primary Care in HIV

With widespread adoption of ART, life expectancy is increasing, and HIV infection has become a chronic disease. The rates of non-AIDS comorbid conditions are rising, including cardiovascular disease and non–AIDS-defining malignancies. Primary care clinicians play a key role in the identification and management of these conditions.

CARDIOVASCULAR DISEASE RISK

Individuals living with HIV are at a 1.5- to 2-fold greater risk of developing cardiovascular disease than the general population. Dyslipidemia, obesity, smoking, and metabolic side effects of ART contribute to this risk, as do the HIV-specific factors of chronic immune activation and inflammation.

Although the benefit of ART outweighs the risk of cardiovascular disease, certain ART medications and drug classes have a greater effect on cardiac and metabolic health. For example, there is conflicting evidence that PIs and abacavir increase cardiovascular risk.

HYPERTENSION

Hypertension is a common comorbidity in patients living with HIV infection and independently raises the risk for acute myocardial infarction. It is not known whether HIV infection or ART increases the risk of hypertension. There are no specific guidelines for managing hypertension in patients living with HIV, although clinicians should be mindful of medication interactions, particularly between certain antiretrovirals (PIs, cobicistat) and dihydropyridine calcium channel blockers.

HYPERLIPIDEMIA

Lipid disorders are independently associated with HIV infection and ART. The mechanism of the excess risk attributable to HIV infection is thought to be the result of HIV-associated chronic inflammation, elevated low-density lipoprotein (LDL) cholesterol and serum triglycerides, and decreased high-density lipoprotein (HDL) cholesterol. After initiating ART, lipid levels may partially normalize, with the exception of HDL, which remains low. Each class of ART has a differing effect on lipid parameters, with the PIs causing the largest change in lipids and INSTIs being the most lipid neutral. The decision to change ART for a more favorable lipid effect must not compromise virologic suppression.

The Primary Care Guidelines for the Management of Persons Infected with HIV recommend the following for management of lipid disorders in patients infected with HIV:

- Fasting lipid panel should be monitored at entry into care, before starting ART, within 3 months of starting ART, and at least annually thereafter.
- Patients with abnormal lipids should be treated according to current American College of Cardiology/American Heart Association (ACC/AHA) guidelines.
- If statin therapy is indicated, a lower dose should be initiated and subsequently titrated based on efficacy and tolerability.

- Drug interactions must be checked before initiation of a statin. PIs, NNRTIs, and cobicistat can increase serum levels of simvastatin and lovastatin, increasing the likelihood of adverse drug reactions. These agents are contraindicated in the presence of a pharmacologic booster (ritonavir or cobicistat).
- Pravastatin, low-dose atorvastatin, and rosuvastatin have less interaction with ART.
- Clinicians should emphasize a heart-healthy diet, physical activity, managing blood glucose, and weight control.
- In patients with hypertriglyceridemia despite dietary modifications, fibrates can be used to lower triglyceride levels.

DIABETES

Patients living with HIV have a higher risk of diabetes. In addition to traditional risk factors for diabetes, HIV infection and ART appear to independently contribute to insulin resistance. Patients with HIV infection should be screened for diabetes at entry into care, within 3 months of starting ART, and annually thereafter. Patients with HIV infection and diabetes mellitus should be managed according to currently available guidelines by the American Diabetes Association, with special attention to potential drug interactions and their expected effect on blood glucose levels.

CHRONIC KIDNEY DISEASE

Patients living with HIV are at higher risk of chronic kidney disease (CKD). Risk factors include lower CD4 counts and higher HIV viral loads, black race, older age, female sex, history of injection drug use, coinfection with hepatitis C, diabetes, and hypertension. Renal impairment can be from HIV-associated nephropathy or from ART. In patients with HIV-associated nephropathy, ART should be initiated at diagnosis. Tenofovir DF, a commonly used agent, has been associated with renal insufficiency and Fanconi syndrome.

Renal function should be monitored at entry into care, with changes in medication, and at least twice annually in clinically stable patients. Both serum creatinine and eGFR should be measured. Urinalysis with quantitative assessment of albumin and protein should be measured at entry into care, with change in therapy, and at least annually in stable patients. In patients taking tenofovir DF or tenofovir AF, monitoring should be performed more frequently. Among patients on INSTIs and cobicistat, the tubular secretion of creatinine is inhibited, leading to an elevation in serum creatinine and decline in eGFR, but without a true decline in renal function. Patients with eGFR of less than 60 mL/min/1.73 m^2 should be referred to a nephrologist if there is no improvement after limiting nephrotoxins. Patients with HIV infection and pre–end-stage renal disease (ESRD) should be given statin therapy, and those with CKD should be considered for low-dose aspirin for primary prevention of cardiovascular disease.

METABOLIC BONE DISEASE: OSTEOPENIA AND OSTEOPOROSIS

Patients with HIV infection are at higher risk of osteopenia and osteoporosis due to HIV-specific effects and ART effects on bone metabolism. Tenofovir DF is associated with the greatest risk for ART-induced osteoporosis. Among patients with HIV infection, men 50 years or older, postmenopausal women, patients with a history of fragility fracture, those on chronic corticosteroids, and those at high risk of falls should be screened for osteoporosis with bone densitometry. Earlier assessment is based on individual risk factors. Repeat screening is based on the presence of bone loss: in those with advanced osteopenia, every 2 to 3 years; in those with mild osteopenia, every 5 years. If normal at initial screening, bone densitometry can be repeated after 5 years. Bisphosphonate therapy with alendronate and zoledronic acid have shown efficacy in maintaining and improving bone density in patients with HIV infection. Calcium supplementation can inhibit the absorption of INSTIs.

CHRONIC LUNG DISEASE

Patients living with HIV have a higher rate of chronic obstructive pulmonary disease. No HIV-specific guidelines for the management of chronic obstructive pulmonary disease exist. The use of inhaled steroids may increase the risk of certain infections, including oral candidiasis, and can interact with PIs and pharmacologic boosters. Rarely, these interactions can lead to significantly elevated levels of corticosteroid.

SMOKING

Patients with HIV infection are twice as likely to smoke as those without HIV infection. Smokers have poorer response to ART, progress to AIDS at a higher rate, and have an increased risk of mortality. Patients with HIV infection should be screened and counseled regarding smoking and assisted with cessation when they are ready.

CANCER SCREENING

Persons with HIV are at increased risk of malignancy. AIDS-defining malignancies include Kaposi sarcoma, non-Hodgkin lymphoma, and cervical cancer; these are among the most common malignancies in patients with HIV infection. Lung, anal, liver, and oropharyngeal cancers occur at a high rate. There does not appear to be excess risk for breast, prostate, or colon cancers, and screening recommendations are not influenced by HIV status. In addition to routinely recommended age-appropriate cancer screening, patients living with HIV infection are more aggressively screened for cervical cancer and are considered for anal cancer screening.

Cervical cancer screening should be performed for patients with HIV infection with the following considerations:

- Among sexually active women, perform at entry into care and 12 months later.
- Begin screening within 1 year of onset of sexual activity or at age 21, whichever is sooner.
- Continue cervical cancer screening throughout the lifespan—do not end at age 65.
- Annual Pap is recommended for women younger than 30, unless three serial screens are normal, and then Pap can be done every 3 years. Human papillomavirus (HPV) cotesting is not recommended in this age group.
- In women 30 years or older, Pap and HPV cotesting is recommended and, if negative, can be done every 3 years.

Anal cancer incidence is higher among patients with HIV infection, particularly among MSM. Although optimal screening has not yet been defined, the Primary Care Guidelines for Persons Infected with HIV recommends anal Pap for MSM, women with receptive anal intercourse history or abnormal cervical Pap results, and all those with genital warts. HPV cotesting is not currently recommended. Abnormal anal cytology, including atypical squamous cells of undetermined significance (ASCUS), should be followed by high-resolution anoscopy with biopsy, if indicated. If anal cancer screening is going to be initiated, adequate services for follow-up of abnormal tests must be available and accessible.

Suggested Reading

Aberg JA, Gallant JE, Ghanem KG, Emmanuel P, Zingman BS, Horberg MA. Primary care guidelines for the management of persons infected with HIV: 2013 updated by the HIV Medicine Association of the Infectious Diseases Society of America. *Clin Infect Dis*. 2014;58(1):e1–e34.

AETC National Curriculum HIV. *AETC National Coordinating Resource Center*. Available at http://aidsetc. org/nhc.

Feinberg J, Keeshin S. Management of newly diagnosed HIV infection. *Ann Intern Med*. 2017;167(1):ITC1–ITC16.

Panel on Antiretroviral Guidelines for Adults and Adolescents. *Guidelines for the Use of Antiretroviral Agents in Adults and Adolescents with HIV. Department of Health and Human Services*. Available at http://aidsinfo.n ih.gov/contentfiles/lvguidelines/AdultandAdolescentGL.pdf.

Panel on Opportunistic Infections in HIV-Infected Adults and Adolescents. *Guidelines for the Prevention and Treatment of Opportunistic Infections in HIV-Infected Adults and Adolescents: Recommendations from the Centers for Disease Control and Prevention, the National Institutes of Health, and the HIV Medicine Association of the Infectious Diseases Society of America*. Available at http://aidsinfo.nih.gov/contentfiles/lvguidelines/adult_oi .pdf

CHAPTER 19

Bacteremia

Aditya Shah ■ Daniel C. DeSimone

CHAPTER OUTLINE

What Is Bacteremia?

In Which Patients Should We Suspect Bacteremia?

What Is the Likelihood of Bacteremia in Different Clinical Settings?

How Do We Establish a Diagnosis of Bacteremia?

How Do We Interpret Blood Culture Results: True Positive, True Negative, False Positive, False Negative?

What Should Be Done When There Is Uncertainty About the Clinical Significance of a Positive Blood Culture?

What Are the Components of a Complete and Thorough History That Are Particularly Relevant to Bacteremia?

What Are the Components of a Complete and Thorough Physical Examination That Are Particularly Relevant to Bacteremia?

What Additional Testing Should Be Considered to Further Evaluate Positive Blood Cultures: Inflammatory Markers, Imaging Studies, Echocardiogram, etc?

When Should an Endovascular Source Be Suspected?

A General Approach to Managing Bacteremia: Antimicrobial Treatment, Source Control, Monitoring for Response, Safety Laboratory Monitoring, Duration of Treatment, etc

When Should Referral Be Made to Infectious Diseases?

What Is Bacteremia?

Human blood is supposed to be a sterile environment. Bacteremia is defined as the presence and detection of bacteria in blood. The body has several defense mechanisms against this, mainly barrier and immunologic defenses. There are several ways in which bacteria can enter the bloodstream. Bacteria can compromise the internal mucosal barrier of the body when the integrity of the gastrointestinal tract is compromised due to inflammation, chemotherapy, obstruction, or surgery. In addition to this, bacteremia can also be low grade and transient in settings such as chewing, brushing, or flossing. Bacteria can also enter the bloodstream when external barriers of the body are compromised, such as skin wounds or diabetic foot ulcerations. In addition, bacteremia may be a complication of a local infection such as pneumonia, osteomyelitis, cellulitis, or meningitis. Due to expansion of health care facilities, increased access to health care, and advanced diagnostic and therapeutic techniques, there are an increasing number of patients with health care exposures resulting in patients with long-term central venous catheters for hemodialysis, cardiac devices including pacemakers, prosthetic heart valves, and prosthetic joints. The presence of any of these devices increases the risk of bacteremia.

Bacteremia can overwhelm the body's immune response resulting in significant adverse outcomes for the patient. Once bacteria gain access to the bloodstream, they may cause foci of infection in organs causing, for example, infective endocarditis, pyelonephritis, abscess formation, or

TABLE 19.1 ■ Signs and Symptoms of SIRS

Temperature	<36° C or >38° C
Heart rate	>90 beats/min
White blood cell count	<4 or >12 µg/L
Respiratory rate	>20 breaths/min

osteomyelitis. Patients with bacteremia may present with sepsis, severe sepsis, or septic shock. Sepsis is a syndrome where the body's immune system reacts to the circulating bacteria and chemicals released in response, resulting in an elevated body temperature, elevated heart rate, and increased respiratory rate with a probable or confirmed infection. In severe sepsis, there is development of organ failure such as mental status changes, decreased urine output, difficulty breathing, or abdominal pain. Septic shock occurs when there are signs and symptoms of severe sepsis with hypotension that does not respond to intravenous (IV) fluid resuscitation and requires vasopressor support.

Sepsis and septic shock can result in significant mortality and morbidity, along with significant financial implications on the health care system. Prompt recognition, diagnosis, and treatment with antibiotics of bacteremia are paramount to limit morbidity and mortality.

In Which Patients Should We Suspect Bacteremia?

A clinician should suspect bacteremia when a patient presents with certain signs and symptoms. These signs and symptoms are due to the intense immune response from circulating bacteria in the bloodstream. Patients can present with a temperature less than 36° C or greater than 38° C, rigors, elevated heart rate of more than 90 beats/min, white blood cell count of less than 4 µg/L or more than 12 µg/L, and elevated respiratory rate of more than 20 breaths/min. These signs and symptoms collectively are recognized as systemic inflammatory response syndrome (SIRS) (Table 19.1).

If prompt identification and treatment are not made, this can progress to hemodynamic instability with a dangerous fall in a patient's blood pressure leading to shock. Scoring systems have been proposed to prompt physicians to have a low threshold to suspect infection and bacteremia, like the Sequential (Sepsis-related) Organ Failure Assessment (SOFA) score, which includes:

Respiratory rate ≥22 breaths/min
Altered mentation
Systolic blood pressure ≤100 mmHg

In summary, every patient who meets these clinical parameters with a suspected source of infection should prompt the physician to suspect an underlying bacteremia as the cause of a patient's clinical decompensation. In a minority of patients, there will be no fever but rather hypothermia, as mentioned above, or euthermia.

What Is the Likelihood of Bacteremia in Different Clinical Settings?

1. The likelihood of bacteremia can vary and is based on three important factors: host factors, virulence of the organism, and site of infection. Table 19.2 lists host factors.
2. Virulent organisms causing infections at alternative sites that include but are not limited to long-term catheters, artificial or damaged joints, and artificial or abnormal heart valves comprise the following:

TABLE 19.2 ■ Host Factors

Immunocompromising conditions, including HIV/AIDS, systemic lupus erythematosus, and vasculitis
Immunocompromising medications, including steroids, monoclonal antibodies, and chemotherapy drugs
Diabetes mellitus
Kidney disease, with or without hemodialysis dependence
Chronic indwelling catheters or prosthetic devices
Solid organ transplantation
Hematologic transplantation
Malignancy

TABLE 19.3 ■ Pathogen Distribution of Bacteremic Gram-Negative Urinary Tract Infection, 1998–2007

	Gender		Site of Infection Acquisition			
Pathogen	Female	Male	CA	HCA	Nosocomial	Total N (%)
Escherichia coli	291	115	252	128	26	406 (74.9)
Klebsiella pneumoniae	29	23	25	25	2	52 (9.6)
Proteus mirabilis	14	11	11	13	1	25 (4.6)
Pseudomonas aeruginosa	7	11	4	11	3	18 (3.3)
Klebsiella oxytoca	2	9	6	3	2	11 (2.0)
Citrobacter freundii	1	5	2	3	1	6 (1.1)
Enterobacter aerogenes	2	3	4	0	1	5 (0.9)
Enterobacter cloacae	1	3	0	4	0	4 (0.7)
Serratia marcescens	0	3	2	1	0	3 (0.6)
Acinetobacter spp.	2	1	1	2	0	3 (0.6)
Morganella morganii	0	2	0	0	2	2 (0.4)
Achromobacter spp.	0	2	0	2	0	2 (0.4)
Other	4	1	4	1	0	5 (0.9)

CA, Community-acquired; HCA, health care associated.
From Al-Hasan MN, Eckel-Passow JE, Baddour LM. Bacteremia complicating Gram-negative urinary tract
  infections: A population-based study. *J Infect.* 2010;60(4):278–285. https://doi.org/10.1016/j.jinf.2010.01.007.

- Methicillin-resistant *Staphylococcus aureus* (MRSA)
- Methicillin-sensitive *S. aureus* (MSSA)
- *Pseudomonas aeruginosa*
- *Enterococcus faecalis*
- Beta-hemolytic streptococcus

3. Source of infection

Large-scale retrospective reviews of patients with community-acquired pneumonia estimate an overall rate of bacteremia between 12% and 16%. It is important to note that the presence of clinical signs and objective data significantly increases the chance that the patient has bacteremia.

In patients who present with a urinary tract infection, studies estimate an overall rate of bacteremia between 10% and 15%. The most common organisms causing bacteremia are summarized in Table 19.3.

The most common pathogens isolated from cultures in patients with cellulitis are group A beta-hemolytic streptococcus *(Streptococcus pyogenes)* and non–group A beta-hemolytic streptococci (groups B, C, F, and G). *S. aureus* is a rare cause of bacteremia due to cellulitis. *Streptococcus* species–related cellulitis usually presents with diffuse and sudden-onset redness without purulence.

In meningitis, pneumococcal and meningococcal meningitis are the most common causes, with the likelihood of bacteremia at approximately 20%. However, an important caveat to these percentages of bacteremia, regardless of what the studies estimate, is that all studies do mention that if the patient has signs of clinical instability, as documented in the SIRS and SOFA criteria, the chance of bacteremia increases significantly.

How Do We Establish a Diagnosis of Bacteremia?

Blood cultures should be collected from peripheral venous blood at two separate sites. If central venous catheters are present, blood should be draw through a catheter at the same time as peripheral venous blood cultures to determine whether the central catheter is a potential source of infection. Adequate sterile precautions (alcohol-based product to clean skin) ought to be taken while drawing blood cultures. Due to improved diagnostic techniques and laboratory procedures, skin colonizers like *Staphylococcus epidermidis* and *Cutibacterium acnes* often result in positive blood cultures. The presence of these organisms in blood cultures is most often due to contamination from incorrect sterile techniques. However, the growth of pathogenic bacteria such as *Escherichia coli*, *Pseudomonas aeruginosa*, *Klebsiella* species, and *S. aureus* are seldom considered to be contaminants.

How Do We Interpret Blood Culture Results: True Positive, True Negative, False Positive, False Negative?

When interpreting blood culture results, correlating them with the clinical presentation of the patient is critical. Due to advanced microbiologic techniques in most standardized laboratories in the country, a true positive blood culture occurs when two sets of blood cultures are collected with adequate sterile technique from two separate sites growing the same organism. Alternatively, if only one of the two sets of blood cultures grows an organism, then its pathogenicity needs to be taken into account. Growth of usual skin flora like *S. epidermidis* or *C. acnes* in only one set of blood cultures should raise suspicion for a false positive. If the organism is not usual skin flora such as *S. aureus* and only grows in one set of blood cultures, you must consider this to be a true positive. Negative blood cultures are achieved when both sets are negative after 5 days of incubation. Most cultivatable organisms will grow within 5 days using current media and culturing technique. Organisms that are fastidious (require additional growth factors in media, storage at different temperatures) or noncultivatable organisms include *Coxiella burnetii* (Q fever), *Bartonella*, and *Brucella*. Brucella can grow in "routine" BC media, though growth can be delayed. The use of targeted serologic and polymerase chain reaction (PCR) testing of blood has been helpful in identifying these organisms that will not grow on standard blood cultures.

What Should Be Done When There Is Uncertainty About the Clinical Significance of a Positive Blood Culture?

Blood cultures are typically obtained in a set consisting of one aerobic and one anaerobic bottle from two separate peripheral sites. Uncertainty about the clinical significance of a positive blood culture often arises due to the number of positive blood culture sets, as well as the bacteria, especially when the isolate is part of the normal human skin flora such as coagulase-negative staphylococci, *Corynebacterium* species, and *C. acnes*. Additional blood cultures would be indicated if there is high suspicion of bacteremia, especially if there is concern that the infecting organism is part of the skin flora, such as pacemakers, prosthetic heart valves, or prosthetic vascular grafts. Pathogens such as *S. aureus*, *P. aeruginosa*, Enterobacteriaceae such as *E. coli* and *Klebsiella* species, and *Candida* species are clinically important, and a single positive blood culture with any of these organisms should prompt additional evaluation and initiation of antibiotic therapy.

When uncertainty remains when a less clinically relevant organism is identified in blood cultures, it would be reasonable to repeat blood cultures before initiating antibiotic therapy; antibiotics may be held if the patient remains clinically stable, afebrile, and without evidence of sepsis. If the repeat blood cultures remain negative, it would most likely be consistent with a blood culture contaminant. However, if blood cultures grow the same organism, it would most likely be a true pathogen and require additional evaluation to identify the infectious source, such as endocarditis, osteomyelitis, or intraabdominal abscess. In some patients, there may be a role for surveillance, with repeat blood cultures obtained about 1 to 2 weeks later to see if the same organism is isolated. This is especially helpful in patients with indwelling catheters or foreign bodies such as a prosthetic joint, pacemaker, or vascular graft. If antibiotics were given, surveillance blood cultures should be obtained about 1 to 2 weeks after antibiotics are completed, and if cultures are positive, additional evaluation is warranted at that time to identify the source of infection.

What Are the Components of a Complete and Thorough History That Are Particularly Relevant to Bacteremia?

The key components of a history that are relevant to bacteremia are those that elucidate any potential exposures that would explain the pathogen identified. A thorough infectious diseases history would include the following:
- Recreational drugs (including injection)
- Hobbies
- Farm animal exposure
- Sexual exposure
- Pets
- Childhood infections history
- Known tick, other insect, or animal bites
- Travel to the southwestern United States
- International travel history
- Tuberculosis (TB) exposure
- Water source
- Raw meat/fish consumption
- Raw salads
- Nonpasteurized dairy products (milk, cheese)
- Occupation
- Outdoor activities
- Recent contact with ill persons

What Are the Components of a Complete and Thorough Physical Examination That Are Particularly Relevant to Bacteremia?

The goal of the physical examination in bacteremia is to look for signs of a source of infection or portal of entry. A head-to-toe examination is required in all patients with bacteremia. Examination of the entire body is necessary to look for any evidence of rash, cellulitis, masses or lymphadenopathy, and open or draining wounds. Another goal of the examination is to identify the infectious syndrome. For example, a patient with bacteremia complicated by meningitis will often be toxic appearing and have confusion with altered mental status, severe headache, photo-phobia, phonophobia, nuchal rigidity, and positive Kernig and Brudzinski signs. Another example includes beta-hemolytic streptococcal bacteremia in a patient with recurrent lower extremity cel-lulitis (Fig. 19.1). Examination may show evidence of lymphedema and tinea pedis, which can be complicated by cellulitis that can be recurrent. Non–group A, beta-hemolytic streptococci can often colonize sites of tinea pedis and likely are operative in the pathogenesis of cellulitis.

Examination of the mouth to look for dental infection and auscultation of the lungs and heart are critical in the diagnosis of pneumonia and endocarditis, respectively. Palpation of the abdomen may result in pain and be concerning for an occult intraabdominal abscess. Assess all joints for erythema, swelling, tenderness, and range of motion.

Combining the history with pertinent physical examination findings and blood culture results will help determine the source of infection and assist in defining an appropriate course of antibi-otic therapy.

What Additional Testing Should Be Considered to Further Evaluate Positive Blood Cultures: Inflammatory Markers, Imaging Studies, Echocardiogram, etc?

Additional testing to support blood culture results may include inflammatory markers, specifi-cally erythrocyte sedimentation rate (ESR), C-reactive protein (CRP), and pro-calcitonin. These inflammatory markers, although nonspecific, are helpful in the diagnosis of certain infections such as prosthetic joint infections and vascular graft infections. Also, they may be helpful in the treatment and resolution of infection. However, these tests take time to return a result. Imaging studies include ultrasound, computed tomography (CT), magnetic resonance imaging (MRI), and echocardiography and can be extremely important in establishing a primary nidus of infection and the extent of infection.

When Should an Endovascular Source Be Suspected?

Persistent bacteremia (>72 hours) is the hallmark of an endovascular source of infection. Endovascular infections include infective endocarditis (native and prosthetic valve); cardiac im-plantable electronic devices (CIED) such as a pacemaker, an implantable converter/defibrillator (ICD), or cardiac resynchronization therapy (CRT); and vascular graft infections. All of these in-fectious syndromes involve direct access to the bloodstream, and when infected, there is a constant presence of bacteria in the bloodstream. Other infections such as pyelonephritis, osteomyelitis, septic arthritis, and pneumonitis may be complicated by bacteremia but often lack persistent bacteremia in the bloodstream. However, it is possible that a nonendovascular source of infection could seed the heart valves causing infective endocarditis, CIED infections, and vascular graft infections. These patients will often have signs or symptoms of infective endocarditis, such as con-duction abnormalities of the heart including heart block, septic pulmonary emboli, cardioembolic stroke, and vascular phenomena such as splinter hemorrhages and Janeway lesions (Fig. 19.2).

A General Approach to Managing Bacteremia: Antimicrobial Treatment, Source Control, Monitoring for Response, Safety Laboratory Monitoring, Duration of Treatment, etc

The first step is to obtain an accurate and thorough history and physical examination, followed by a review of vital signs, laboratory studies, and available imaging. The initial information provided from the microbiology laboratory will be a Gram stain of the positive blood cultures, which will

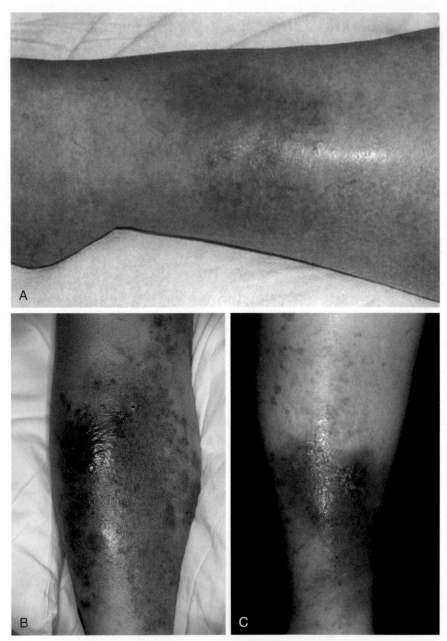

Fig. 19.1 Cellulitis. (A, from Klieger D, Shiland MDB. Shiland Medical Assistant: Integumentary, Sensory Systems, Patient Care and Communication—Module A. Elsevier. Figure 1-6. B, from Bolognia JL, Schaffer JV, Duncan KO, Ko CJ. Bolognia Dermatology Essentials. 7th ed. Elsevier. Fig. 61.5. C, from Dinulos J. Habif's Clinical Dermatology: A Color Guide to Diagnosis and Therapy. 7th ed. Elsevier: 50.)

give the first clue of what the pathogen may be. Empiric antibiotic therapy (given before availability of Gram stain of a positive blood culture) will need to cover a wide spectrum of bacteria, including drug-resistant organisms, specifically MRSA and *P. aeruginosa*. Typical empiric regimens include IV vancomycin plus cefepime, piperacillin/tazobactam, and meropenem. If there

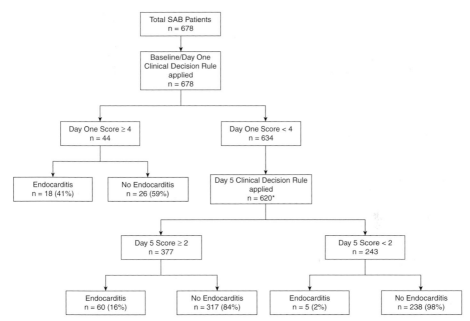

Fig. 19.2 Algorithm for *S. aureus* bacteremia when evaluating an endovascular source. (From https://www.semanticscholar.org/paper/Predicting-Risk-of-Endocarditis-Using-a-Clinical-to-Palraj-Baddour/b92e7c71426ba3e69a87ecd9c0006e312425d5fc.)

is a concern for anaerobic infection, such as aspiration pneumonia, esophageal rupture, intraabdominal abscess, or bowel perforation, the addition of metronidazole may be needed (this is not needed if piperacillin/tazobactam or meropenem was used). Factors in the patient's history, such as recent broad-spectrum antibiotic use, known colonization with vancomycin-resistant enterococcus (VRE), or other multidrug-resistant organisms, may affect the empiric regimen.

The next step is to identify the source of infection. Often, the use of CT, MRI, or echocardiography is needed. Depending on the findings, surgical or interventional radiology may be needed for source control, such as drainage of an abscess. The patient should be monitored closely for the next 48 to 72 hours. At the same time, blood cultures will be further identified, and antimicrobial susceptibility testing should be performed—antibiotics can be deescalated when this information becomes available. If the patient is not improving during this period, it may be necessary to repeat blood cultures, obtain additional imaging and laboratory tests, and adjust antibiotics to cover additional organisms and/or consider other infectious etiologies, such as viral or fungal infection, depending on patient risk factors.

Laboratory tests should be closely monitored initially until the patient is clinically improved. Patients with bacteremia are commonly treated with 2 weeks of IV antibiotics and in some cases oral antibiotics. If we are dealing with a complicated bacteremia—infectious syndromes such as infective endocarditis, vertebral osteomyelitis, vascular graft infections, or extensive intraabdominal abscesses—this may require 4 to 6 weeks of antibiotic therapy. Typically, laboratory monitoring will be performed on a weekly basis with a complete blood count (CBC) with differential, creatinine, and aspartate aminotransferase (AST). Depending on the antibiotics used and patient factors, closer monitoring and additional laboratory tests may be necessary.

Furthermore, most patients with a complicated bacteremia will often require outpatient infectious diseases follow-up with repeat imaging to evaluate the response to antibiotic therapy and resolution of infection. Some patients may require additional antibiotic therapy and possibly life-long antibiotic suppressive therapy.

When Should Referral Be Made to Infectious Diseases?

Most patients with bacteremia would benefit from an infectious diseases consultation to determine appropriate antibiotic therapy, including de-escalation of antibiotics from empiric therapy to targeted therapy to limit unnecessary antibiotic exposure, development of antibiotic resistance, and duration and route of antibiotics.

Patients with a straightforward cause of bacteremia, such as a urinary tract infection, could be treated by the health care provider without infectious diseases referral/consultation. This assumes that the pathogen is identified, antibiotic susceptibility testing is available, and the patient is responding to treatment. Conversely, if the patient is worsening clinically despite appropriate antibiotic therapy, infectious diseases referral would be most appropriate.

There are certain infectious diseases syndromes that always warrant an infectious diseases referral, such as infective endocarditis; pacemaker/ICD infections; vascular graft infections; prosthetic joint infections; and infections in significantly immunosuppressed patients with solid organ transplant, stem cell transplant, human immunodeficiency virus/acquired immune deficiency syndrome (HIV/AIDS), and active immunosuppressive therapy, among others. Certain pathogens such as *S. aureus*; *Streptococcus pneumoniae*; *P. aeruginosa*; and multidrug-resistant organisms should have an infectious diseases referral for additional evaluation and treatment—especially considering that there is established evidence of improved outcomes with infectious diseases consultation in patients with *S. aureus* bacteremia.

Suggested Reading

Al-Hasan MN, Eckel-Passow JE, Baddour LM. Bacteremia complicating gram-negative urinary tract infections: a population-based study. *J Infect*. 2010;60(4):278–285.

Falguera M, Trujillano J, Caro S, et al. CAP: a prediction rule for estimating the risk of bacteremia in patients with community-acquired pneumonia. *Clin Infect Dis*. 2009;49(3):409–416.

Kaplan SL, Schutze GE, Leake JA, et al. Meningitis: multicenter surveillance of invasive meningococcal infections in children. *Pediatrics*. 2006;118(4):e979.

Peralta G, Padrón E, Roiz MP, et al. Cellulitis: risk factors for bacteremia in patients with limb cellulitis. *Eur J Clin Microbiol*. 2006;25(10):619–662.

Page numbers followed by "*f*" indicate figures and "*t*" indicate tables.

Fever of unknown origin (FUO)
  causes, 80–82, 81t
  classic, 79
  diagnostic evaluation, 84t–85t
  diagnostic strategy, 86–89
  drugs associated with, 82t
  episodic, 83t
  etiology, 86t
  historical clues, 82–83
  laboratory testing and imaging, 86–89
  physical examination clues, 83–85
  routine laboratory tests, 87t–88t
  testing, 87t
  treatment, 89
  understanding fever, 80–85
Fishy smelling vaginal discharge, 235. *See also*
    Vaginitis
Flucytosine, 77
Fosfomycin, 72
Fungal arthritis, 177–178
Fungal meningitis, 197
Fungi, 43–45, 44t
Furuncles, 166

G

Gastritis, 133
Genital ulcer disease, 243–246, 245t
Genital warts, 248
Glycopeptides, 67
Gonococcal arthritis, 175
Gonococcal urethritis, 232f
Group A β-hemolytic streptococci (GABHS), 160
Guillain-Barré syndrome, 215

H

Hand-foot-mouth disease, 109–111
  erythematous bullous lesions, 110f
  small vesicles and papules, 110f
Health care–associated pneumonia (HAP), 128–131
Helicobacter pylori, 133
Helminths, 47
Hepatitis B and C, 178–179
Herpes simplex virus (HSV), 130, 193
Herpes zoster (shingles), 111–112, 111f–112f
Histoplasmosis, 197
Human granulocytic anaplasmosis, 209–210
Human immunodeficiency virus (HIV) infection
  acute and early HIV infection, 250–251
    clinical manifestations, 252
    laboratory diagnosis, 252–253, 253f
  AIDS, 251
  antiretroviral therapy regimen, 249
    classes of, 261t
    drug interactions, 263–264
    goals of treatment, 257–259

Human immunodeficiency virus (HIV) infection
    (Continued)
      modification, 260
      patient monitoring during, 262–264
      recommendation, 260–261
      treatment, 260
      visit frequency, 262
  chronic, 251
  comprehensive medical history, 254–256
  comprehensive physical examination, 256
  confirmation of, 253–254
  drug safety monitoring, 262–263
  drug selection, 260
  elite controllers, 251
  family history, 256
  fourth-generation p24 antigen-HIV antibody
      screening test, 254f
  HIV-2 infection, 252
  initial evaluation, 253–257
  initial laboratory tests, 256–257, 257t
  in United States, 249
  laboratory monitoring, 262, 263t
  natural history of, 250–252
  past medical history, 255–256
  pathogenesis, 250
  prevention of opportunistic infections, 257,
      258t–259t
  primary care role
    cancer screening, 266
    cardiovascular disease risk, 264
    chronic kidney disease, 265
    chronic lung disease, 266
    diabetes, 265
    hyperlipidemia, 264–265
    hypertension, 264
    metabolic bone disease, 265–266
    smoking, 266
  review of systems, 256
  screening, 253
    recommendations, 254t
  signs and symptoms, 252t
  social history, 256
  specific issues, 255
  stages of, 250–251, 250t
  treatment, 259–260
  viral transmission, 250
Human monocytic ehrlichiosis (HME), 211–212
Human papillomavirus (HPV) infection, 247–248
Hyperlipidemia, 264–265
Hypertension, 264

I

Impetigo, 162f, 166
Infectious arthritis
  acute bacterial arthritis, 172–177